Principles of Biomedical Ethics

Principles of Biomedical Ethics

FIFTH EDITION

TOM L. BEAUCHAMP, PH.D.
Kennedy Institute of Ethics and
Department of Philosophy
Georgetown University
Washington, D.C.

JAMES F. CHILDRESS, PH.D.
Department of Religious Studies
University of Virginia
Charlottesville, Virginia

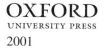
UNIVERSITY PRESS
2001

OXFORD
UNIVERSITY PRESS

Oxford   New York
Athens   Auckland   Bangkok   Bogotá   Buenos Aires   Calcutta
Cape Town   Chennai   Dar es Salaam   Delhi   Florence   Hong Kong   Istanbul
Karachi   Kuala Lumpur   Madrid   Melbourne   Mexico City   Mumbai
Nairobi   Paris   São Paulo   Shanghai   Singapore   Taipei   Tokyo   Toronto   Warsaw

and associated companies in
Berlin   Ibadan

Library of Congress Cataloging-in-Publication Data
Beauchamp, Tom L.
Principles of biomedical ethics /
Tom L. Beauchamp, James F. Childress.—5th ed.
p. cm.   Includes bibliographical references and index.
ISBN 0-19-514331-0—ISBN 0-19-514332-9 (pbk.)
1. Medical ethics.   I. Childress, James F.   II. Title.
R724.B36 2001   174'2.—dc21   00-062394

9 8 7 6 5 4 3 2 1

Printed in the United States of America
on acid-free paper

To
Georgia, Ruth, and Don

I can no other answer make but thanks,
And thanks, and ever thanks.

Twelfth Night

Preface

We have thoroughly revised this edition of *Principles of Biomedical Ethics,* taking account of suggestions by friends and critics, developments in moral, social, and political philosophy and in biomedical ethics, and new issues in research, medicine, and health care.

We have modified the book's structure in order to accommodate the needs of diverse readers. Chapter 1 now introduces our framework through a discussion of moral norms, with particular attention to prima facie principles and rules and to specifying and balancing them for moral deliberation and decision-making. Chapter 2 focuses on moral character, especially moral virtues and ideals, which are too often neglected or downplayed in biomedical ethics. The next four chapters (Chapters 3 through 6) present four basic groups of principles—respect for autonomy, nonmaleficence, beneficence, and justice. Chapter 7 examines the moral rules of veracity, privacy, confidentiality, and fidelity in the context of relationships between health care professionals and patients and between researchers and participants in research. We have retained our examination of methods and theories in biomedical ethics, now including a detailed explication and defense of our preferred method and theory. These topics appear in the final two chapters (8 and 9). We believe that this revised edition will be more accessible to readers who do not come to the subject with substantial background in moral theory. Those grounded in or more interested in moral theory may choose to examine the last two chapters immediately after the first two chapters.

With each edition, our debts of gratitude grow. We remain indebted to colleagues and students who provided suggestions, insights, cases, and so forth for previous editions, though we cannot identify all of them by name here. In addition to the valuable discussions of our framework in various books and articles, numerous students, colleagues, health professionals, and teachers who use the book have contributed immeasurably to this fifth edition. In particular, we want to thank John Arras, Marcia Day Childress, the late Dan Clouser, John Fletcher, Bernie Gert, Jonathan Moreno, and Sven Sherman-Peterson for direct questions, challenges, and critiques, as well as supportive conversation. Moheba Hanif has provided remarkable assistance, as has the staff of the Kennedy Institute's library and information retrieval system. Jim also expresses his deep appreciation to Ezekiel Emanuel, Frank Miller, and other colleagues in the Department of Clinical Bioethics at the National Institutes of Health, where he was a visiting scholar in 1999–2000; the department provided a most stimulating and enjoyable context for much of his work on this edition.

We also want to take this opportunity to express our deep gratitude for our wonderful relationship with Jeffrey House, our editor at Oxford University Press, who has worked with us on different editions of this book for over a quarter of a century.

We dedicate this edition, just as we have dedicated each of the previous four editions, to Georgia, Ruth, and Don. Georgia, Jim's wife, died in 1994, just after the fourth edition appeared. Our dedication honors her memory and pays tribute to Ruth Faden and Donald Seldin.

Washington, D.C.   T. L. B.
Charlottesville, Va.   J. F. C.

Contents

PART III

Principles of Biomedical Ethics

1

Moral Norms

Medical ethics enjoyed a remarkable degree of continuity from the days of Hippocrates until the middle of the twentieth century. Developments in the biological and health sciences then led to critical reflection on conventional conceptions of the moral obligations of health professionals and society in preventing disease and injury and meeting the needs of the sick and injured. Although major writings in ancient, medieval, and modern health care contain a rich storehouse of reflection on the relationship between the professional and the patient, these writings are inadequate for contemporary biomedical ethics. This historical record often neglects problems of truthfulness, privacy, justice, communal responsibility, and the like.

To avoid a similar narrowness, we begin with philosophical reflection on morality and ethics that is remote from the history of professional ethics. Such reflection affords some distance from assumptions still evident in the biomedical sciences and health care.

Ethics and Morality

Ethics

The term *ethics* needs attention before we turn to the term *morality*. *Ethics* is a generic term for various ways of understanding and examining the moral life. Some approaches to ethics are normative, others nonnormative.

Normative ethics. General normative ethics is a form of inquiry that attempts to answer the question, "Which general moral norms for the guidance and evaluation of conduct should we accept and why?" Ethical theories attempt to identify and justify these norms. We examine such theories together with an ideal set of criteria for assessing them in Chapter 8.

Many practical questions would remain unanswered even if a fully satisfactory general ethical theory were available. *Practical ethics* (often called *applied ethics*) is the attempt to implement general norms and theories for particular problems and contexts. The term *practical* refers to the use of theory, argument, and analysis to examine moral problems, practices, and policies in professions, institutions, and public policy. Often no straightforward movement from theory or principles to particular judgments is available in these contexts. Theory and principles are only starting points and general guides for the development of norms of appropriate conduct. They are supplemented by paradigm cases of right action, empirical data, organizational experience, and the like. (Chapter 9 pays detailed attention to the methods involved in practical ethics.)

Nonnormative ethics. There are two broad types of nonnormative ethics. First, *descriptive ethics* is the factual investigation of moral conduct and beliefs. It uses scientific techniques to study how people reason and act. For example, anthropologists, sociologists, psychologists, and historians determine which moral norms and attitudes are expressed in professional practice; in professional codes, institutional mission statements, and rules; and in public policies. They study such matters as surrogate decision-making, treatment of the dying, and the nature of consent obtained from patients.

Second, *metaethics* involves analysis of the language, concepts, and methods of reasoning in ethics. For example, it addresses the meanings of ethical terms such as *right, obligation, virtue, justification, morality,* and *responsibility.* It also treats moral epistemology (the theory of moral knowledge) and the logic and patterns of moral reasoning and justification, as well as investigating whether morality is objective or subjective, relative or nonrelative, and rational or emotional.

Descriptive ethics and metaethics are grouped together as *nonnormative* because their objective is to establish what factually or conceptually *is* the case, not what ethically *ought to be* the case. Often in this book we cite descriptive ethics—for example, when discussing current professional codes of ethics. However, our underlying interest is usually in whether the prescriptions of such codes are justifiable, which is a normative issue.[1]

Morality and the Common Morality

In its most familiar sense, *morality* refers to norms about right and wrong human conduct that are so widely shared that they form a stable (although usually incomplete) social consensus. Morality, as a social institution, encompasses many standards of conduct, including moral principles, rules, rights, and virtues. We all learn about basic moral standards and responsibilities as we grow up. They predate us and are transmitted across generations. We also learn to distinguish the general morality that holds for all persons from norms that bind only members of special groups, such as physicians, nurses, or public health officials. This section examines general morality, while a later section examines professional morality.

Since virtually everyone grows up with a basic understanding of the institution of morality, its norms are readily understood. All persons who are serious about living a moral life already grasp the core dimensions of morality. They know not to lie, not to steal property, to keep promises, to respect the rights of others, not to kill or cause harm to innocent persons, and the like. All persons serious about morality are comfortable with these rules and do not doubt their relevance and importance. They know that to violate these norms without having a morally good and sufficient reason is immoral and should lead to feelings of remorse. Because we are already convinced about such matters, the literature of ethics does not debate them. Such debate would be a waste of time.

We will refer to the set of norms that all morally serious persons share as *the common morality*. The common morality contains moral norms that bind all persons in all places; no norms are more basic in the moral life. In recent years, the favored category to represent this universal core of morality in public discourse has been human rights,[2] but moral obligation and moral virtue are no less vital parts of the common morality.

Morality consists of more than the *common morality,* and we should never confuse or conflate the two. For example, morality includes *moral ideals* that individuals and groups voluntarily accept, *communal norms* that bind only members of specific moral communities, extraordinary *virtues*, and the like. The common morality, by contrast, comprises all and only those norms that all morally serious persons accept as authoritative. Here two distinctions are crucial: The first is between "morality" in the universal sense and "morality" in a community-specific sense; and the second is between *nonnormative* (that is, empirical) claims about what is universal in moral belief and *normative* claims about what should be universal in moral belief. These distinctions are indispensable for understanding this book's assumptions and arguments.

Universal morality and community-specific morality. The universal norms of the common morality comprise a small set of all actual and possible moral norms. "Morality" in this universal sense refers exclusively to the norms in the common morality. By contrast, "morality" in the community-specific sense includes the moral norms that spring from particular cultural, religious, and institutional sources. For example, different social standards of allocating resources for health care and different religious and communal standards of giving to charitable causes are parts of morality in this sense.

Sometimes, persons who suppose that they speak with an authoritative moral voice operate under the false belief that they have the force of the common morality (that is, universal morality) behind them. The particular moral viewpoints that such persons represent may be acceptable and even praiseworthy, but they also may not bind other persons or communities. For example, persons who believe intensely that scarce medical resources, such as transplantable organs, should be distributed by lottery rather than by medical need may have very good moral reasons for their views, but they cannot claim the force of the common morality for those views. At the same time, the common morality's norms do require interpretation if we are to have workable practical ethics. Such interpretation is often subject to vigorous dispute in order to resolve particular problems, such as how to allocate organs.

Normative and nonnormative claims. The appeals we have made to the common morality might be understood as normative, nonnormative, or both. If the appeals are *normative*, the claim is that the common morality actually has normative force: It establishes obligatory moral standards for everyone. To fail to abide by these standards is to engage in improper conduct. The present authors do, indeed, understand the common morality in this way: This morality is morally authoritative for the conduct of all persons and it provides the basis for the normative theses and rudimentary moral theory that we develop in this book.

Appeals to the common morality might also be *nonnormative*, or empirical, in which case they describe what all people believe. This thesis is more difficult to defend and requires caution and qualification. It would be absurd to suppose that all persons do, in fact, accept the norms of the common morality. Many amoral, immoral, or selectively moral persons do not care about or identify with these or any other moral demands. Nonetheless, we believe that all persons in all cultures who are *serious about moral conduct* do accept the demands of the common morality.

Some readers will think that we are tripping over our own distinction and begging the question by conflating the difference between *empirical claims* about what *is* universal in moral belief and *normative claims* about what *should be* universal in moral belief. Our formulation may seem to simply pack *our conception* of morality into the notion of morally serious persons, while failing to take seriously the empirical claims of multiculturalists. This criticism misunderstands our position. We accept the thesis that morality in the community-specific sense reflects significant cultural differences; but we think it is an institutional fact about morality, not merely our view of it, that it contains fundamental precepts. These fundamental precepts alone make it possible for persons to make cross-temporal and cross-cultural judgments and to assert firmly that not all practices in all cultural groups are morally acceptable. Enslavement, racial and gender discrimination, and many other unacceptable practices have appeared throughout history, but the fact of their existence does not make them morally acceptable, even if a particular society regards them as morally acceptable.

Are the norms absolute? It is no objection to the norms in the common morality (or any other part of morality) that, in some circumstances, they can be justifiably overridden by other moral norms with which they conflict. All moral norms can be justifiably overridden in some circumstances. For example, we might not tell the truth in order to prevent someone from killing another person; and we might have to disclose confidential information about one person in order to protect the rights of another person. Principles, duties, and rights are not absolute or unconditional merely because they are universal. We discuss this feature of moral norms in the sections below on "specification," "balancing," and "prima facie norms" (and then return to these topics in Chapter 9).

Morality and theories of ethics. Morality, as delineated above, is a social institution that exists prior to moral reflections of the sort found in philosophical and theological ethics. When we say that the norms in this book are grounded in the common morality, we mean that they are not grounded in a particular philosophical or theological theory or doctrine. We will make numerous recommendations in this book that are controversial and involve appeals to theory, but these recommendations should not be confused with the common morality that forms our starting point. To say that we build on the common morality is not to say that we can validly claim its authority for everything we build.

Professional Morality

Just as the common morality is accepted by all morally serious persons, so most professions contain, at least implicitly, a professional morality with standards of conduct that are generally acknowledged by those in the profession who are serious about their moral responsibilities. In medicine, professional morality specifies general moral norms for the institutions, practices, and traditions of medicine. Special roles and relationships in medicine require rules that other professions may not need. For example, as we maintain in Chapters 3 and 7, rules of informed consent and medical confidentiality are rooted in the more general moral requirements of respecting the autonomy of persons and protecting them from harm. However, these rules of consent and confidentiality may not be serviceable or appropriate outside of medicine.

The professions often informally transmit moral guidelines. However, formal instruction and attempts to codify professional morality have increased in recent years through codes of medical and nursing ethics, codes of research ethics, and reports by public commissions. Before we assess these developments, the nature of professions needs brief discussion.

According to Talcott Parsons, a profession is "a cluster of occupational roles, that is, roles in which the incumbents perform certain functions valued in the society in general, and, by these activities, typically earn a living at a full-time job."[3] Under this definition, circus performers, exterminators, and garbage collectors are professionals; prostitutes probably are not (because their function is not "valued in the society in general"), despite prostitution's reputation as "the world's oldest profession." Today, it is not surprising to hear all these activities characterized as professions, inasmuch as the word *profession* has come, in common use, to mean almost any occupation in which a person earns a living. The once honorific sense of *profession* is now reflected in the term *learned profession*, which assumes an extensive education in the arts or sciences.

We thus need a more restricted meaning for the term *profession* in order to appreciate the context of professional ethics. Professionals in the relevant sense are usually identified by their specialized training and by their commitment to provide important services to clients or consumers. Professions maintain self-regulating organizations that control entry into occupational roles by formally certifying that candidates have acquired the necessary knowledge and skills. In learned professions, such as medicine, nursing, and public health, the professional's background knowledge derives from closely supervised training, and the professional provides a service to others.

Health care professions typically specify and enforce obligations for their members, thereby seeking to ensure that persons who enter into relationships with these professionals will find them competent and trustworthy. The obligations that professions attempt to enforce are role obligations, that is, obligations determined by an accepted role. Problems of professional ethics usually arise from conflicts over professional standards or conflicts between professional commitments and commitments of persons outside the profession. The rules of professional morality are vague, so that different interpretations emerge of the duties stated in these rules. To avoid moral confrontation and legal struggles, some professions codify their standards in order to reduce this vagueness.

Codes often specify rules of etiquette as well as professionals' moral responsibilities. For example, one historically significant version of the code of the American Medical Association instructed physicians not to criticize a fellow physician previously in charge of a case. This code also urged all physicians to offer professional courtesy.[4] Such professional codes tend to foster and reinforce member-identification with the prevailing values of the profession. They are beneficial if they effectively incorporate defensible moral norms. Unfortunately, some professional codes oversimplify moral requirements, make them indefensibly rigid, or claim more completeness and authority than they are entitled to claim. As a consequence, professionals may mistakenly suppose that they satisfy all relevant moral requirements if they obediently follow the rules of the code, just as many people believe that they discharge their moral obligations when they meet all relevant legal requirements.

A pertinent question concerns whether the codes specific to areas of science, medicine, and health care are comprehensive, coherent, and plausible. Medical codes sometimes mention general principles, such as "Do no harm," and rules, such as those of medical confidentiality. Only a few codes have much to say about the implications of other principles and rules, such as veracity, respect for autonomy, and justice, which have been the subjects of intense contemporary discussion in biomedical ethics. From ancient medicine to the present, physicians have generated codes without subjecting them to the scrutiny or acceptance of patients and the public, which the codes are intended to serve. Also, these codes have rarely appealed to more general ethical standards or to a source of moral authority beyond the traditions and judgments of physicians. In some cases, the special rules in codes for professionals seem to conflict with more general moral norms. The pursuit of professional norms in these circumstances may do more to protect the profession's interests than to introduce a broad and impartial moral viewpoint.

Psychiatrist Jay Katz once poignantly expressed his own reservations about such codes of medical ethics. Initially inspired by his outrage over the fate of Holocaust victims, Katz became convinced that only a persistent improvement in professional ethics and an educational effort that reached beyond traditional codes could provide meaningful guidance in research involving human subjects:

As I became increasingly involved in the world of law, I learned much that was new to me from my colleagues and students about such complex issues as the right to self-determination and privacy and the extent of the authority of governmental, professional, and other institutions to intrude into private life. . . . These issues . . . had rarely been discussed in my medical education. Instead it had been all too uncritically assumed that they could be resolved by fidelity to such undefined principles as *primum non nocere* ["First, do no harm"] or to visionary codes of ethics.[5]

Public Supervision of Professional Conduct

Additional moral direction for health professionals and scientists sometimes comes through the public policy process, which includes regulations and guidelines promulgated by government agencies. The term *public policy* in this text refers to a set of normative, enforceable guidelines accepted by an official public body, such as an agency of government or a legislature, to govern a particular area of conduct. The policies of corporations, hospitals, trade groups, and professional societies sometimes have a deep impact on public policy, but these policies are private rather than public (although these bodies are frequently regulated by public policies). A closer connection exists between law and public policy: All laws constitute public policies, but not all public policies are, in the conventional sense, laws. In contrast to laws, public policies need not be explicitly formulated or codified. For example, an official who decides not to fund a government program (that has no prior history of funding) may be formulating a public policy. Decisions not to act, as well as decisions to act, can constitute public policies.

Public policies, such as those that fund health care for the indigent or protect subjects of biomedical research, usually incorporate moral considerations. Indeed, moral analysis is part of good policy formation, not merely a method for evaluating existing policy. Efforts to protect the rights of patients and research subjects provide instructive examples. For instance, over the past 25 years the U.S. government has created several national commissions and advisory committees to formulate guidelines for research involving human subjects, as well as other areas of biomedical ethics. Morally informed policies have guided decision-making about life-sustaining treatment as well. For example, in 1991 the U.S. Congress passed the Patient Self-Determination Act (PSDA), which was the first federal legislation to ensure that health care institutions inform patients about institutional policies to accept or refuse medical treatment and about their rights under state law, including a right to formulate advance directives.[6]

The relevance of bioethics for public policy has now gained recognition in most developed countries. The French National Consultative Committee on Ethics in the Biological Sciences, the Japanese Ad Hoc Committee on Brain Death and Organ Transplantation, the Mexican National Bioethics Commission, and the Russian National Committee on Bioethics are examples of influential national bioethics committees. The studies, reports, and legislation developed by these bodies raise questions explored later in this book about the proper relation between government and professional groups in formulating and enforcing standards of practice.

These questions also emerge from the prominent role of the courts in developing case law that sets standards for science, medicine, and health care. Legal decisions often provide significant resources for ethical reflection on moral responsibilities and public policy. For example, the line of court decisions in the U.S. since the Karen Ann Quinlan case in the mid-1970s has constituted a nascent tradition of moral reflection that has been influenced by literature in ethics on topics such as whether artificial nutrition and hydration should be viewed as a medical treatment that is subject to the same standards of decision-making as other forms of treatment.

Policy formation and criticism involve more complex forms of judgment than ethical principles and rules can handle on their own.[7] Public policy is often formulated in contexts that are marked by profound social disagreements, uncertainties, and different interpretations of history. No body of abstract moral principles and rules can determine policy in such circumstances, because it cannot contain enough specific information or provide direct and discerning guidance. The specification and implementation of moral principles and rules must take account of problems of feasibility, efficiency, cultural pluralism, political procedures, uncertainty about risk, noncompliance by patients, and the like. Principles and rules provide the moral background for policy evaluation, but a policy must also be shaped by empirical data and by information available in fields such as medicine, nursing, economics, law, and psychology.

When using moral principles or rules to formulate or criticize public policies, we cannot move with assurance from a judgment that an *act* is morally right (or wrong) to a judgment that a corresponding *law* or *policy* is morally right (or wrong). The judgment that an act is morally wrong does not necessarily lead to the judgment that the government should prohibit it or refuse to allocate funds to support it. For example, one can argue, without inconsistency, that sterilization or abortion is morally wrong but that the law should not prohibit it or deny public funds to those who otherwise could not afford it. Similarly, the judgment that an act is morally acceptable does not imply that the law should permit it. For example, the thesis that voluntary, active euthanasia is morally justified if patients face uncontrollable pain and suffering is consistent with the thesis that the government should legally prohibit active euthanasia because it would not be possible to control abuses if it were legalized.

At this point, we are not defending any particular moral judgments. We are only maintaining that the connections between moral norms and judgments about policy or law are complicated and that a judgment about the morality of acts does not entail a corresponding judgment about law and policy. Factors such as the symbolic value of law, the costs of a program and its enforcement, and the demands of competing programs must often be considered.

Moral Dilemmas

Reasoning through dilemmas to conclusions and choices is a familiar feature of the human condition. Consider a particular case (Case 1 in the Appendix). Some years ago, the judges on the California Supreme Court had to reach a decision about a possible violation of medical confidentiality. A man killed a woman after confiding to a therapist his intention to commit the act. The therapist had attempted unsuccessfully to have the man committed but, in accordance with his duty of medical confidentiality to the patient, did not communicate the threat to the woman when the commitment attempt failed.

The majority opinion of the Court held that "When a therapist determines, or pursuant to the standards of his profession should determine, that his patient presents a serious danger of violence to another, he incurs an obligation to use reasonable care to protect the intended victim against such danger." This obligation extends to notifying the police and directly warning the intended victim. The justices in the majority opinion argued that therapists generally ought to observe the rule of medical confidentiality, but that this rule must yield in this case to the "public interest in safety from violent assault." Although they recognized that rules of professional ethics have substantial public value, they held that matters of greater importance, such as protecting others against violent assault, can override these rules.

In a minority opinion, a justice disagreed and argued that doctors violate patients' rights if they fail to observe standard rules of confidentiality. If it were common practice to break these rules, he reasoned, the fiduciary nature of the relationship between physicians and patients would erode. The mentally ill would refrain from seeking aid or divulging critical information because of the loss of trust that is essential for effective treatment. As a result, violent assaults would increase.

This case presents a straightforward moral dilemma (as well as a legal dilemma), because both judges cite good and relevant reasons to support their conflicting judgments. Moral dilemmas are circumstances in which moral obligations demand or appear to demand that a person adopt each of two (or more) alternative actions, yet the person cannot perform all the required alternatives. These dilemmas occur in at least two forms.[8] (1) Some evidence or argument indicates that an act is morally right, and some evidence or argument indicates that it is morally wrong, but the evidence or strength of argument on both sides is inconclusive. Abortion, for example, is sometimes said to be a terrible dilemma for women who see the evidence in this way. (2) An agent believes that, on moral grounds, he or she is obligated to perform two (or more) mutually exclusive actions. In a moral dilemma of this form, one or more moral norms obligate an agent to do x and one or more moral norms obligate the agent to do y, but the agent cannot do both in the same circumstance. The reasons behind alternatives x and y are good and weighty, and neither set of reasons is obviously overriding. If one acts on either set of reasons, one's actions will be morally acceptable in some respects but morally unacceptable in others. Some have viewed the intentional cessation of lifesaving therapies in the case of patients in a persistent vegetative state, such as Karen Ann Quinlan and Nancy Cruzan, as dilemmatic in this second way.

Conflicting moral principles and rules may create dramatic dilemmas, as popular literature, novels, and films often illustrate. For example, an impoverished person who steals to save a family from starvation or a person who lies to protect a confidential family document confronts such a dilemma. The only way to comply with one obligation in such situations is to contravene another obligation. No matter which course is elected, some obligation must be set aside or compromised. It is misleading to say that we are, in these dilemmatic circumstances, obligated to perform both actions. We should discharge the obligation that in the circumstances overrides what we would have been firmly obligated to perform were it not for the conflict. However, in some circumstances, the dilemma may be unresolvable in the sense that the agent cannot determine which obligation is overriding.

Conflicts between moral requirements and self-interest sometimes produce a *practical* dilemma rather than a *moral* dilemma. If moral reasons compete with nonmoral reasons, questions about priority can still arise even though moral dilemmas, strictly speaking, are not present. Numerous examples appear in the work of anthropologist William R. Bascom, who collected hundreds of "African dilemma tales" transmitted for decades or centuries in African tribal societies. One traditional dilemma posed by the Hausa tribe of Nigeria is called *cure for impotence*:

A friend gave a man a magical armlet that cured his impotence. Later he [the man with the armlet] saw his mother, who had been lost in a slave raid, in a gang of prisoners. He begged his friend to use his magic to release her. The friend agreed on one condition— that the armlet be returned. What shall his choice be?[9]

Hard choice? Perhaps, but not a hard *moral* choice. The obligation to the mother is moral in character, whereas retaining the armlet is a matter of self-interest. (We are assuming that no moral obligation exists to a sexual partner; in some circumstances, such an obligation could produce a moral dilemma.)

Some moral philosophers and theologians have argued that many *practical* dilemmas exist, but that no unresolvable *moral* dilemmas exist. They do not deny that agents experience moral perplexity, moral conflict, and moral disagreement in difficult cases, but they insist that if there were moral dilemmas, two moral *obligations* would conflict, so that agents could not fulfill one obligation without forgoing another. The belief that one *cannot* do what one *ought* to do seems to these writers a confusion about the nature of moral obligation and a failure to see that the purpose of a moral theory is to provide a principled procedure for resolving deep moral problems. Some major figures in the history of ethics have defended this conclusion, both because they accept one supreme moral value as overriding all other conflicting values (moral and nonmoral) and because they regard it as incoherent to allow contradictory obligations in a properly structured moral theory. The only *ought*, they maintain, is the *ought* generated by the supreme value.[10] We will examine theories of this sort (e.g., utilitarian and Kantian theories) in Chapter 8.

In contrast to the account of moral obligation found in these theories, we maintain throughout this book that various moral principles can and do conflict in the moral life. Explicit acknowledgment of the resulting moral dilemmas helps avert unwarranted expectations of moral principles and theories. On some occasions, moral dilemmas are so deep that specifying and balancing principles will not determine an overriding *ought*. Although we generally have ways of reasoning about what we should do, we may not be able to reach a clear resolution in many cases. In these cases, the dilemma only becomes more difficult and remains unresolved even after the most careful reflection.

An agent who can determine which act is the best act to perform under the circumstances still might violate a moral obligation in doing so. Even the morally best action under circumstances of a dilemma can leave a trace of a moral violation.[11]

A Framework of Moral Principles

The common morality contains a set of moral norms that includes principles that are basic for biomedical ethics. These principles form the structure of the chapters in Part II of this book (Chapters 3–6). Most classical ethical theories include these principles in some form,[12] and traditional medical codes presuppose at least some of them.

Basic Principles

A set of principles in a moral account should function as an analytical framework that expresses the general values underlying rules in the common morality. These principles can then function as guidelines for professional ethics. In Chapters 3–6, we defend four clusters of moral principles that serve this function. The four clusters are (1) *respect for autonomy* (a norm of respecting the decision-making capacities of autonomous persons), (2) *nonmaleficence* (a norm of avoiding the causation of harm), (3) *beneficence* (a group of norms for providing benefits and balancing benefits against risks and costs), and (4) *justice* (a group of norms for distributing benefits, risks, and costs fairly).

Nonmaleficence and beneficence have played a central historical role in medical ethics, whereas respect for autonomy and justice were neglected in traditional medical ethics but came into prominence because of recent developments. To illustrate this traditional neglect, consider the work of British physician Thomas Percival. In 1803, he published *Medical Ethics*, which was the first well-formed account of medical ethics in the long history of the subject. This book served as the prototype for the American Medical Association's (AMA) first code of ethics in 1847. Easily the dominant influence in both British and American medical ethics of the period, Percival argued (using somewhat different language) that nonmaleficence and beneficence fix the physician's primary obligations and triumph over the patient's preferences and decision-making rights in circumstances of serious conflict.[13] Percival failed to appreciate the power of principles of respect for autonomy and distributive justice, but, in fairness to him, we must acknowledge that these considerations are now ubiquitous in discussions of biomedical ethics in a way they were not when he wrote at the turn of the nineteenth century.

That four clusters of moral "principles" are central to biomedical ethics is a conclusion the authors of this work have reached by examining *considered moral judgments* and the way *moral beliefs cohere*—two notions we explain in Chapter 9. The selection of these four principles, rather than some other cluster of principles, does not receive an argued defense in Chapters 1 and 2. However, we will, in Chapters 3 through 6, defend the vital role of each principle in biomedical ethics.

Rules

Our framework encompasses several types of moral norms, including principles, rules, rights, virtues, and moral ideals. Rules, rights, and virtues are very important in the framework, though we believe that principles provide the most general and comprehensive norms. We also operate with only a loose distinction between rules and principles. Both are general norms that guide actions. The difference is that rules are more specific in content and more restricted in scope than principles. Principles are general norms that leave considerable room for judgment in many cases. They thus do not function as precise action guides that inform us in each circumstance how to act in the way that more detailed rules and judgments do.

We defend several types of rules that specify principles (and thereby provide specific guidance): substantive rules, authority rules, and procedural rules.

Substantive rules. Rules of truth-telling, confidentiality, privacy, and various rules about forgoing treatment, physician-assisted suicide, informed consent, and the rationing of health care provide more specific guides to action than do abstract principles. Consider a simple example of a rule that sharpens the requirements of the principle of respect for autonomy for certain contexts: "Follow a patient's advance directive whenever it is clear and relevant." To indicate how this rule specifies the principles of respect for autonomy, we may state it more fully as: "Respect the autonomy of patients by following all clear and relevant formulations in their advance directives." This formulation shows how the initial norm remains but becomes specified. (See, further, the section on "specification" below.)

Authority rules. We also defend rules about decisional authority—that is, rules regarding who may and should perform actions. For example, *rules of surrogate authority* determine who should serve as surrogate agents in making decisions for incompetent persons, and *rules of professional authority* determine who, if anyone, should make decisions to override or to accept a patient's decisions if those decisions are medically damaging and poorly considered. Another example appears in *rules of distributional authority* that determine who should make decisions about allocating scarce medical resources.

Authority rules do not delineate substantive standards or criteria for making decisions. However, authority rules and substantive rules do interact. For instance, authority rules are justified, in part, by how well particular authorities can be expected to respect and express substantive rules and principles.

Procedural rules. We also defend rules that establish procedures to be followed. Procedures for determining eligibility for scarce medical resources and procedures for reporting grievances to higher authorities are typical examples. We often resort to procedural rules when we run out of substantive rules and when authority rules are incomplete or inconclusive. For example, if substantive or authority rules are inadequate to determine which patients should receive scarce medical resources, we resort to procedural rules such as first-come-first-served, queuing, and lottery. (See Chapter 6.)

Rights, Virtues, Emotions, and Other Moral Considerations

Our framework of principles and rules, as outlined above, does not mention the rights of persons, the character and virtues of the agents who perform actions, or moral emotions. These aspects of the moral life all merit attention in a comprehensive theory, and all will receive attention in Chapters 2, 8, or 9. Rights, virtues, and emotional responses are as important as principles and rules for a comprehensive vision of the moral life. For example, an ethics of virtue helps us see why good moral choices often depend more on character than principles, and it also allows us to assess a person's moral character in a richer way than does an ethics of principles and rules. Chapter 2 examines these important considerations as they apply to biomedical ethics.

The Prima Facie Nature of Moral Norms

Principles, rules, and rights are not unbending standards that disallow compromise. Although "a person of principle" is sometimes regarded as strict and unyielding, we must specify principles for various circumstances and weigh them against other moral norms.

W. D. Ross's distinction between *prima facie* and *actual* obligations is basic for our analysis. *A prima facie* obligation must be fulfilled unless it conflicts on a particular occasion with an equal or stronger obligation. This type of obligation is always binding *unless* a competing moral obligation overrides or outweighs it in a particular circumstance. Some acts are at once prima facie wrong and prima facie right, because two or more norms conflict in the circumstances. Agents must then determine what they ought to do by finding an actual or overriding (in contrast to prima facie) obligation. That is, they must locate what Ross called "the greatest balance" of right over wrong. Agents can determine their *actual* obligations in such situations by examining the respective weights of the competing prima facie obligations (the relative weights of all competing prima facie norms). What agents ought to do is, in the end, determined by what they ought to do *all things considered*.[14]

For example, imagine that a psychiatrist has confidential medical information about a patient who happens also to be an employee in the hospital where the psychiatrist practices. The employee is seeking advancement in a stress-filled position, but the psychiatrist has good reason to believe this advancement would be devastating for both the employee and the hospital. The psychiatrist has several duties in these circumstances, including confidentiality, nonmaleficence, and beneficence. Should the psychiatrist break confidence in light of the other duties? Could the psychiatrist handle this matter by making thin disclosures only to a hospital administrator and not to the personnel office? Are such disclosures consistent with a psychiatrist's general commitment to rules of medical confidentiality? Addressing these questions through a process of moral deliberation and justification is required to establish an agent's actual duty in the face of conflicting prima facie duties.

No moral theorist or professional code of ethics has successfully presented a system of moral rules free of conflicts and exceptions, but this fact is not cause for either skepticism or alarm. Ross's distinction between prima facie and actual obligations conforms closely to our experience as moral agents and provides indispensable categories for biomedical ethics. Almost daily we confront situations in which we must choose among plural and conflicting values in our personal lives, and we must balance several considerations. Some choices are moral, many nonmoral. For example, our budget may require that we choose between buying books and buying a train ticket to see our parents. Not having the books will be an inconvenience and a loss, while not visiting home will make our parents unhappy. The choice is not easy, perhaps, but usually we can think through the alternatives, deliberate, balance, and reach a conclusion. The moral life presents many similar circumstances of choice.

Specifying Principles and Rules

Our four clusters of principles do not constitute a general moral theory. They provide only a framework for identifying and reflecting on moral problems. The framework is spare, because prima facie principles do not contain sufficient content to address the nuances of many moral circumstances. We therefore need to examine how to specify and balance these abstract principles.

The Nature and Value of Specification

Practical moral problems often require that we make our general norms specific for a particular context or range of cases.[15] If the principles discussed in this book are to have sufficient content for practical applications, we must be able to specify that content to indicate why and how cases properly fall under the principles.[16] Specification is a process of reducing the indeterminateness of abstract norms and providing them with action-guiding content. For example, without further specification, "do no harm" is an all-too-bare starting point for thinking through problems, such as assisted suicide and euthanasia. It will not adequately guide action when norms conflict.

A reasonably typical example of specification arises when psychiatrists do forensic evaluations of patients in a legal context. In such cases, psychiatrists cannot always obtain an informed consent and, therefore, risk violating their obligations to respect autonomy. Yet informed consent is a basic rule of medical practice (see Chapter 3). A simple specification aimed at handling this problem—though we do not say it is the best specification—appears in the following provision in the "Ethical Guidelines for the Practice of Forensic Psychiatry" of the American Academy of Psychiatry and the Law: "The informed consent of the subject of a forensic evaluation is obtained when possible. Where consent is not required, notice is given to the evaluee of the nature of the evaluation. If the evaluee is not competent to give consent, substituted consent is obtained in accordance with the laws of the jurisdiction."[17] This specification indicates how psychiatrists can adequately discharge their various moral obligations.

A second, more extended example of specification involves the oft-cited rule "Doctors should put their patients' interests first." A fact of life in modern medicine in some countries is that patients sometimes can afford the best treatment strategy only if their physicians falsify information on insurance forms or at least thinly spread the truth. A proper interpretation of the rule of patient-priority does not imply that a physician should act illegally by lying or distorting the description of a patient's problem on an insurance form. Rules against deception, on the one hand, and for patient-priority, on the other, are not categorical demands, and they stand in need of specification.

A survey of practicing physicians' attitudes toward deception illustrates how some physicians reconcile their dual commitment to patients and to nondeception. Dennis H. Novack and several colleagues used a questionnaire to obtain physicians' responses to four difficult ethical problems that potentially could be resolved by deception. In one scenario, a physician recommends an annual screening mammography for a 52-year-old woman who protests that last year her insurance company would not cover the test and she had to pay herself, although she could not afford it. A secretary suggests that the patient's insurance company would cover the costs of the mammography if the physician stated the reason as "rule out cancer" rather than "screening mammography," although the latter alone was the reason in this case. Almost 70% of the physicians responding to this survey indicated that they would put "rule out cancer," but 85% of this group also insisted that their act would not involve "deception."[18]

We can interpret these physicians' decisions as crude attempts to specify rules against deception. Most physicians in the study apparently did not operate with the definition of deception favored by the researchers ("to deceive is to make another believe what is not true, to mislead"). Perhaps the physicians believed that deception involves withholding information from or misleading someone who has a *right* to that information, and also believed that an insurance company with unjust policies of coverage has no right to accurate information. Or perhaps they believed that "deception" occurs when one person unjustifiably misleads another, and that it was justifiable to mislead the insurance company in these circumstances. Another possibility is that these physicians understood the rule against deception to prohibit only self-serving actions.

These physicians apparently would not agree on how to specify rules against deception or rules requiring that patients' interests take priority. This survey provides an example of eliminating an apparent dilemma without either "applying" or "balancing" norms. Each of the proposed specifications would resolve the conflict (or, perhaps better, would *dissolve* it), but each specification is debatable. To say that a problem or conflict is resolved or dissolved is here only to say that norms have been made sufficiently determinate in content that, when cases fall under them, we can decide what ought to be done. Yet a *proposed* specification may fail to provide the most adequate or justified resolution.

Specification is an attractive strategy for hard cases of moral conflict as long as the specification can be justified. Many already-specified rules will need further specification to handle new circumstances of conflict. Progressive specification often must occur to handle the variety of problems that arise, gradually reducing the dilemmas and conflicts that abstract principles lack sufficient content to resolve. Adding substance through specification is essential for decision-making in clinical and research ethics and for developing both institutional rules and public policies. All moral norms are, in principle, subject to such specification. They need this further content, because, as Henry Richardson puts it, "the complexity of the moral phenomena always outruns our ability to capture them in general norms."[19]

Limitations of the Method of Specification

Overconfidence in specification can lead to a dogmatic certainty similar to that found in the pronouncements of some professional associations. Despite its strengths, the method of specification has many limitations.

Some moral conflict is inevitable and cannot always be avoided or eliminated by even tightly knit specifications. In any given problematic or dilemmatic case, several competing specifications may constitute possible resolutions, which would return us to conflicts of the sort that drove us to specification in the first place. Even if a specification eliminates contingent conflict, it may be arbitrary, lack impartiality, or fail for other reasons. Nothing in the model of specification suggests that we can avoid judgments that balance different principles or rules in the very act of specifying them.

We therefore must connect specification as a method with a larger model of justification that will support some specifications over others. We will develop this model in Chapter 9.

Balancing Principles and Rules

Principles, rules, and rights require *balancing* no less than *specification*. We need both methods because each addresses a dimension of moral principles and rules: *range and scope,* in the case of specification, and *weight or strength,* in the case of balancing. Specification entails a substantive refinement of the range and scope of norms, whereas balancing consists of deliberation and judgment about the relative weights or strength of norms. Balancing is especially important for reaching judgments in individual cases, and specification is especially useful for policy development.

The Relative Weight of Norms

The metaphor of larger and smaller weights moving a scale up and down graphically depicts the balancing process, but it may also obscure what happens in the process of balancing by suggesting a purely intuitive or subjective assessment. Justified acts of balancing entail that good reasons be provided, not merely that an agent is intuitively satisfied.

Suppose a physician encounters an emergency case that would require her to extend an already long day, making her unable to keep a promise to take her son to the library. She will then engage in a process of deliberation that leads her to consider how urgently her son needs to get to the library, whether they could go later to the library, whether another physician could handle the case, and so on. If she determines to stay deep into the night with the patient, this obligation will have become overriding because she would have, in the circumstances, a good and sufficient reason for her action. For instance, a life may hang in the balance, and she alone has the knowledge to deal adequately with the full array of circumstances. Canceling her evening with her son, distressing as it is, could be justified by this good and sufficient reason for doing what she does.

One way of viewing this process of balancing brings it close to and perhaps merges it with specification. As David DeGrazia and Henry Richardson have pointed out to us, the articulated reasons offered in an act of balancing can be viewed as a specification of norms that incorporates those reasons. In our example, the physician's reasons can be generalized for similar cases: "If a patient's life hangs in the balance and the attending physician alone has the knowledge to deal adequately with the full array of the circumstances, then the physician's conflicting domestic obligations must yield." Even if we do not always state judgments of balancing in the form of a specification, might they not be incorporated into such a form?

Merging specification and balancing in this way has merits, but it seems too neat and too sweeping to handle all situations of balancing and specification. Balancing does often eventuate in specification, but it need not; and specification often involves balancing, but it also might only add details or fill out the commitments of a principle. It also seems pointless or unduly complicated to engage in specification in many circumstances. For example, in individual cases of balancing harms of treatment against the benefits of treatment for incompetent patients, the cases are often unique or so exceptional that it is perilous to generalize a conclusion. (See Chapters 4 and 5 on balancing the principle of nonmaleficence and principles of beneficence.) As noted previously, balancing is particularly useful for case analysis, as specification is for policy development. Accordingly, we do not propose to merge the two methods.

Although all moral norms are subject to balancing as well as specification, some specified norms are virtually absolute, and therefore usually escape the need for balancing. Examples include prohibitions of cruelty and torture, where these actions are defined as gratuitous infliction of pain and suffering.[20] More interesting are norms that are intentionally formulated with the goal of including all legitimate exceptions. An example is, "Always obtain oral or written informed consent for medical interventions with competent patients, *except* in emergencies, in forensic examinations, in low-risk situations, or when patients have waived their right to adequate information." This norm clearly needs interpretation—including an analysis of what constitutes an informed consent, an emergency, a waiver, a forensic examination, and a low risk—but this rule would be absolute if it were correct that all legitimate exceptions had successfully been incorporated in its formulation.

However, if such rules exist, they are rare. Moreover, in light of the enormous range of possibilities for contingent conflicts among rules, even the firmest rules are better construed as evolving rather than finished products. If professional medical associations, health care institutions, and government bureaus had more often taken this lesson to heart, we would have been spared many stubbornly imperious pronouncements in recent biomedical ethics.

Conditions that Restrict Balancing

As a response to criticisms that the model of balancing is too intuitive and open-ended—lacking in a commitment to firm principles—we can list a few conditions that reduce the amount of intuition involved. The following conditions must be met to justify infringing one prima facie norm in order to adhere to another. (To the extent these conditions themselves incorporate norms, the norms are also prima facie, not absolute.)

1. Better reasons can be offered to act on the overriding norm than on the infringed norm (e.g., if persons have a *right*, their interests generally deserve a special place when balancing those interests against the interests of persons who have no comparable right.)

2. The moral objective justifying the infringement must have a realistic prospect of achievement.
3. The infringement is necessary in that no morally preferable alternative actions can be substituted.
4. The infringement selected must be the least possible infringement, commensurate with achieving the primary goal of the action.
5. The agent must seek to minimize any negative effects of the infringement.
6. The agent must act impartially in regard to all affected parties; that is, the agent's decision must not be influenced by morally irrelevant information about any party.

Though some of these conditions will appear to be obvious and noncontroversial, in our experience they often are not observed in moral deliberation and would lead to very different actions were they observed. For example, some proposals to use life-extending technologies against the objections of patients or their surrogates seem to violate (2) by endorsing certain actions in which no realistic prospect exists of achieving the goals of a proposed medical intervention. Typically, this occurs when health professionals regard the intervention as legally required, but in some cases, it occurs merely as a matter of traditional practice or out of a sense of standards of practice.

Even more commonly violated is condition (3). Actions are frequently performed without serious consideration of the range of alternative actions that might be performed. As a result, agents fail to identify morally preferable alternatives. For example, in animal care and use committees, a common conflict involves the obligation to approve a good scientific protocol and the obligation to protect animals against unnecessary suffering. The protocol is typically approved if it proposes a standard form of anaesthesia. However, standard forms of anaesthesia are often not the best way to protect the animal, and further inquiry is needed to determine the best anaesthetic for the interventions proposed. In our schema of conditions, it is *unjustifiable* to approve the protocol or to conduct the experiment without this additional inquiry, which affects conditions (4) and (5) as well as (3).

Finally, consider this example: The principle of respect for autonomy and the principle of beneficence (which includes acts of preventing harm to others) sometimes conflict in the AIDS epidemic. Respect for autonomy sets a prima facie barrier to the mandatory testing of people who are at risk of HIV infection and whose actions may put others at risk, and yet society has a prima facie obligation to act to prevent harm to those at risk. The two prima facie principles conflict, but to justify overriding respect for autonomy, one must show that the mandatory testing of certain individuals is necessary to prevent harm and has a reasonable prospect of preventing harm. If it meets these conditions, mandatory testing will still need to pass the least-infringement test (4), and agents must seek to reduce the negative effects (5), such as the consequences that individuals fear from testing. As we will see in Chapter 7, many (but not all) proposed forms of mandatory testing cannot be justified, because other available alternatives would have a higher probability of success without infringing personal autonomy.[21]

Accordingly, we think the above six conditions are morally demanding. When conjoined with requirements of coherence that we propose in Chapter 9, these minimal conditions should help us achieve a reasonable measure of protection against purely intuitive or subjective judgments. We could try to introduce further criteria or safeguards, such as, "rights override non-rights" and "liberty principles override non-liberty principles," but these rules are certain to fail in various circumstances in which rights claims and liberty interests are relatively minor. Honesty about the process of balancing and overriding compels us to return to our earlier discussion of dilemmas and to acknowledge that in some circumstances we will not be able to determine which moral norm is overriding.

The Acceptability of Moral Diversity and Moral Disagreement

Even conscientious and reasonable moral agents who work diligently at moral reasoning sometimes disagree with other equally conscientious persons. They may disagree about whether disclosure to a fragile patient is appropriate, whether religious values about brain death have a central place in secular bioethics, whether physician-assisted suicide should be legalized, and hundreds of other issues in biomedical ethics. Such disagreement does not indicate moral ignorance or moral defect. We simply lack a single, entirely reliable way to resolve all disagreements.

This fact returns us to the questions about morality in the broad sense that opened this chapter. Neither morality nor ethical theory has the resources to provide a single solution to every moral problem. Moral disagreement can emerge because of (1) factual disagreements (e.g., about the level of suffering that an action will cause), (2) scope disagreements about who should be protected by a moral norm (e.g., whether fetuses or animals are protected), (3) disagreements about which norms are relevant in the circumstances, (4) disagreements about appropriate specifications, (5) disagreements about the weight of the relevant norms in the circumstances, (6) disagreements about appropriate forms of balancing, (7) the presence of a genuine moral dilemma, and (8) insufficient information or evidence.

Different parties may emphasize different principles or assign different weights to principles even when they do not disagree over which principles are relevant. Such disagreement may persist even among morally serious persons who conform to all the demands that morality makes upon them. Moreover, when evidence is incomplete and different sets of evidence are available to different parties, one individual or group may be justified in reaching a conclusion that another individual or group is justified in rejecting. Even when both parties have incorrect beliefs, each party may be justified in holding those beliefs. We cannot hold persons to a higher standard in practice than to make judgments conscientiously in light of the relevant norms and the available and relevant evidence. (See, further, our account of justification in Chapter 9, where we argue that we cannot know whether a moral disagreement is irresolvable until we have examined competing views using a proper method of justification. A declaration of irresolvable conflict is premature without a serious attempt at resolution through an appropriate model of justification. Sometimes we will discover that apparent moral disagreement is resolvable or that it rests on factual disagreement.)

These facts about the moral life may discourage those who must deal with practical problems, but the phenomenon of reasoned moral disagreement provides no basis for skepticism about morality or about moral thinking. Indeed, it offers a reason for taking morality seriously and using the best tools that we have to carry our moral projects as far as we can. We should not forget that we frequently obtain near-complete agreement in our moral judgments and that we have the thin universal basis for morality considered earlier in this chapter. The fact of unresolvable disagreement in some cases does not undermine an expectation that, in most cases, the common morality and other aspects of moral traditions afford us with adequate content to reach agreement or at least an acceptable compromise.

Even when cultural practices and individual beliefs vary, and disagreements are unresolvable, people still may not *fundamentally* disagree about the ultimate moral standards that underlie their judgments. Two cultures or individuals may agree about a fundamental principle of morality, yet disagree about how to interpret or apply that principle in a particular situation. For example, individuals might differ over an appropriate set of actions to protect human subjects of research, not because they have a different set of norms, but because they hold different factual views about risks to subjects. They might invoke identical norms in supporting policies to protect subjects, and yet end up recommending different policies because of their different beliefs about facts. Similarly, controversies over compulsory screening for AIDS may turn on factual claims about HIV transmission, about uses of the information gained through screening, about the number of persons at risk, and about alternative ways to reduce risks (e.g., through teaching safer-sex practices).

When moral disagreements arise, a moral agent can—and often should—defend his or her decision without disparaging or reproaching others who reach different decisions. Recognition of legitimate diversity (by contrast to moral violations that call for criticism) is exceedingly important when we evaluate the actions of others. What one person should do may not be what other persons should do, even when they face the same problem. Similarly, what one institution or government should do may not be what another institution or government should do. From this perspective, individuals and societies legitimately construct different requirements that comprise part of the moral life (consistent with what we have called morality in the broad sense), and we may not be able to judge one as better than another.[22]

Conclusion

In this chapter we have initiated a defense of what is sometimes called the *four-principles approach* to biomedical ethics[23] and is increasingly called *principlism*.[24] The four principles derive from considered judgments in the common morality and medical traditions, both of which form our starting point in this volume. Our goal in later chapters is to develop, specify, and balance these principles. Both the choice of principles and the content ascribed to the principles derive from our attempt to put the common morality and medical traditions into a coherent package.

Thus far, we have only briefly mentioned moral character, the moral virtues, and the moral emotions. This range of topics is the subject of the next chapter.

Notes

1. These distinctions should be used with caution. Metaethics frequently takes a turn toward the normative, as our discussion of the justification of moral standards later in this chapter indicates. Likewise, normative ethics relies on metaethics. Just as no sharp distinction should be drawn between practical ethics and general normative ethics, so no clear line should be drawn to distinguish normative ethics and metaethics.

2. See, for example, Alan Gewirth, *The Community of Rights* (Chicago: University of Chicago Press, 1996); Carl P. Wellman, *The Proliferation of Rights: Moral Progress or Empty Rhetoric?* (Boulder, CO: Westview Press, 1999); Ronald Dworkin, *Taking Rights Seriously* (Cambridge, MA: Harvard University Press, 1977); Elizabeth Wolgast, *Equality and the Rights of Women* (Ithaca, NY: Cornell University Press, 1980); and Judith Jarvis Thomson, *The Realm of Rights* (Cambridge, MA: Harvard University Press, 1990).

3. Talcott Parsons, *Essays in Sociological Theory*, rev. ed. (Glencoe, IL: The Free Press, 1954), p. 372.

4. The American Medical Association Code of Ethics of 1847 was largely adapted from Thomas Percival's *Medical Ethics; or a Code of Institutes and Precepts, Adapted to the Professional Conduct of Physicians and Surgeons* (Manchester, England: S. Russell, 1803). See Donald E. Konold, *A History of American Medical Ethics 1847–1912* (Madison, WI: State Historical Society of Wisconsin, 1962), chs. 1–3; and Chester Burns, "Reciprocity in the Development of Anglo-American Medical Ethics," in *Legacies in Medical Ethics*, ed. Chester Burns (New York: Science History Publications, 1977).

5. Jay Katz, ed., *Experimentation with Human Beings* (New York: Russell Sage Foundation, 1972), pp. ix–x.

6. Omnibus Budget Reconciliation Act of 1990. Public Law 101–508 (Nov. 5, 1990), §§ 4206, 4751. See 42 USC, scattered sections.

7. See Will Kymlicka, "Moral Philosophy and Public Policy: The Case of New Reproductive Technologies," in *Philosophical Perspectives on Bioethics*, ed. L. W. Sumner and Joseph Boyle (Toronto: University of Toronto Press, 1996); Dennis Thompson, "Philosophy and Policy," *Philosophy and Public Affairs* 14 (Spring 1985): 205–18; and a symposium on "The Role of Philosophers in the Public Policy Process: A View from the President's Commission," with essays by Alan Weisbard and Dan Brock, in *Ethics* 97 (July 1987): 775–95.

8. See John Lemmon, "Moral Dilemmas," *Philosophical Review* 71 (1962): 139–58; Walter Sinnott-Armstrong, *Moral Dilemmas* (Oxford: Basil Blackwell, 1988); Daniel Statman, "Hard Cases and Moral Dilemmas," *Law and Philosophy* 15 (1996): 117–48; H. E. Mason, "Responsibilities and Principles: Reflections on the Sources of Moral Dilemmas," in *Moral Dilemmas and Moral Theory*, ed. H. E. Mason (New York: Oxford University Press, 1996).

9. William R. Bascom, *African Dilemma Tales* (The Hague: Mouton, 1975), p. 145 (relying on anthropological research by Roland Fletcher).

10. See Christopher W. Gowans, ed., *Moral Dilemmas* (New York: Oxford University Press, 1987); Walter Sinnot-Armstrong, *Moral Dilemmas* (Oxford: Basil Blackwell, 1988); and Edmund N. Santurri, *Perplexity in the Moral Life: Philosophical and Theological Considerations* (Charlottesville, VA: University Press of Virginia, 1987).

11. For treatments of the problem of a moral residue, see Thomas E. Hill, Jr, "Moral Dilemmas, Gaps, and Residues: A Kantian Perspective"; Walter Sinnott-Armstrong, "Moral Dilemmas and Rights;" and Terrance C. McConnell, "Moral Residue and Dilemmas"—all in *Moral Dilemmas and Moral Theory*, ed. Mason.

12. Alternative accounts in biomedical ethics express some reservations about these principles. See numerous essays in *Principles of Health Care Ethics*, ed. Raanan Gillon and Ann Lloyd (London: John Wylie & Sons, 1994); K. Danner Clouser and Bernard Gert, "A Critique of Principlism," *The Journal of Medicine and Philosophy* 15 (April 1990): 219–36; K. Danner Clouser, "Common Morality as an Alternative to Principlism," *Kennedy Institute of Ethics Journal* 5 (1995): 219–36.

13. Thomas Percival, *Medical Ethics*. See note 4 above.

14. See W. D. Ross, *The Right and the Good* (Oxford: Clarendon Press, 1930), esp. pp. 19–36; and *The Foundations of Ethics* (Oxford: Clarendon Press, 1939).

15. Henry S. Richardson, "Specifying, Balancing, and Interpreting Bioethical Principles," *Journal of Medicine and Philosophy* 25 (2000): 285–307 and "Specifying Norms as a Way to Resolve Concrete Ethical Problems," *Philosophy and Public Affairs* 19 (Fall 1990): 279–310. See also David DeGrazia, "Moving Forward in Bioethical Theory: Theories, Cases, and Specified Principlism," *Journal of Medicine and Philosophy* 17 (1992): 511–39; and DeGrazia and Tom L. Beauchamp, "Philosophical Foundations and Philosophical Methods," in *Methods of Bioethics*, ed. D. Sulmasy and J. Sugarman (Washington, DC: Georgetown University Press, 2001).

16. As R. M. Hare notes, "any attempt to give content to a principle involves specifying the cases that are to fall under it. . . . Any principle, then, which has content goes some way down the path of specificity." *Essays in Ethical Theory* (Oxford: Clarendon Press, 1989), p. 54.

17. As revised October, 1991, p. 2.

18. Dennis H. Novack, et al., "Physicians' Attitudes Toward Using Deception To Resolve Difficult Ethical Problems," *Journal of the American Medical Association* 261 (May 26, 1989): 2980–85. We return to these problems in Chapter 7.

19. Richardson, "Specifying Norms," p. 294. ("Always" in this formulation should per-

haps be understood to mean "in principle always." Specification may, in some cases, reach a final form.)

20. Other prohibitions, such as rules against murder, are absolute only because of the meaning of their terms. For example, to say "murder is categorically wrong" is to say "unjustified killing is unjustified."

21. See James F. Childress, "Mandatory HIV Screening and Testing," in *Practical Reasoning in Bioethics* (Bloomington and Indianapolis, IN: Indiana University Press, 1997), ch. 6. For a sensitive attempt to balance the rights and interests of HIV-infected surgeons and dentists against the rights and interests of their patients—an attempt that reaches conclusions similar to ours about balancing and overriding—see Norman Daniels, "HIV-infected Health Care Professionals: Public Threat or Public Sacrifice?" *The Milbank Quarterly* 70 (1992): 3–42, esp. 26–32.

22. Cf. Walter Sinnott-Armstrong, *Moral Dilemmas*, pp. 216–27; and D. D. Raphael, *Moral Philosophy* (Oxford: Oxford University Press, 1981), pp. 64–65.

23. See the essays in Gillon and Lloyd, eds. *Principles of Health Care Ethics*.

24. See, for example, B. Gert, C. M. Culver, and K. D. Clouser, *Bioethics: A Return to Fundamentals* (New York: Oxford University Press, 1997), ch. 4; Clouser and Gert, "A Critique of Principlism," pp. 219–36; Earl Winkler, "Moral Philosophy and Bioethics: Contextualism versus the Paradigm Theory," in L. W. Sumner and J. Boyle, eds. *Philosophical Perspectives on Bioethics*; John D. Arras, "Principles and Particularity: The Roles of Cases in Bioethics," *Indiana Law Journal* 69 (1994): 983–1014; Susan M. Wolf, "Introduction: Gender and Feminism in Bioethics," in Wolf, ed. *Feminism & Bioethics* (New York: Oxford University Press, 1996); Jeffrey Blustein, "Character-Principlism and the Particularity Objection," *Metaphilosophy* 28 (1997): 135–55; and Richard B. Davis, "The Principlism Debate: A Critical Overview," *Journal of Medicine and Philosophy* 20 (1995): 85–105. We discuss several of the issues presented in these articles in Chapter 9.

2

Moral Character

In Chapter 1, we concentrated on the analysis and justification of acts and policies. We featured the language of ethical principles, rules, obligations, and rights. In this chapter, we concentrate on the *moral virtues* and *moral character*. Whereas ethics grounded in principles emphasizes action, character ethics or virtue ethics emphasizes the agent who performs actions.[1] We also extend our analysis to the domain of *moral ideals*. These categories complement the analysis in the previous chapter without undermining principles and rules.

Often, what counts most in the moral life is not consistent adherence to principles and rules, but reliable character, good moral sense, and emotional responsiveness. Even specified principles and rules do not convey what occurs when parents lovingly play with and nurture their children or when physicians and nurses exhibit compassion, patience, and responsiveness in encounters with patients and families. Our feelings and concerns for others lead us to actions that cannot be reduced to instances of rule-following, and we all recognize that morality would be a cold and uninspiring practice without various emotional responses and heart-felt ideals that reach beyond principles and rules.

Moral Virtues

Some philosophers have criticized a heavy emphasis on the virtues. They see the virtues as lacking order and as difficult to unify in a systematic fashion. Though we accept the view that principles and virtues are very different in nature and are taught very differently, we believe that we can bring some order to standards of virtue. Some forms of order emerge directly from the connection between moral virtues and moral principles and rules. In addition, the goals and structure of medicine, health care, and research themselves give some order to the virtues in biomedical ethics.[2]

We begin by analyzing the concept of virtue and considering the special status of the virtues. We then examine virtues in professional roles and explicate five focal virtues that are of particular importance in medicine, health care, and research.

The Concept of Virtue

A *virtue* is a trait of character that is socially valuable,[3] and a *moral virtue* is a morally valuable trait of character. It is not sufficient that social groups approve a trait and regard it as moral for it to be morally virtuous. A claim or perception of moral virtue must have the support of moral reasons. Communities sometimes disvalue persons who act virtuously or admire persons for their meanness and churlishness. Moral virtue, then, is more than whatever is socially approved.

Some define "moral virtue" as a disposition to act or a habit of acting in accordance with moral principles, obligations, or ideals.[4] For example, they might understand the moral virtue of nonmalevolence as the trait a person has of abstaining from causing harm to others when it would be wrong to harm them. However, this definition unjustifiably derives virtues wholly from principles and fails to capture the importance of motives in the virtuous person's actions. We care morally about people's motives, and we care especially about their *characteristic* motives, that is, the motives deeply embedded in their character. Persons who are motivated in this manner by sympathy and personal affection, for example, meet our approval, whereas others who act the same way, but from motives of personal ambition, might not.

Imagine a person who discharges a moral obligation *because* it is an obligation, but who intensely dislikes being placed in a position in which the interests of others override his or her own interests. This person does not feel friendly toward or cherish others, and he or she respects their wishes only because obligation requires it. This person can nonetheless perform a morally right action and have a disposition to perform that action. But if the motive is improper, a critical moral ingredient is missing; and if a person *characteristically* lacks this motivational structure, a necessary condition of virtuous character is absent. The act may be right and the actor blameless, but neither the person nor the act is *virtuous*. In short, people may be disposed to do what is right, intend to do it, and do it, while also yearning to avoid doing it. Persons who characteristically perform morally right actions from such a motivational structure are not morally virtuous even if they always perform the morally right action.

Aristotle drew an important (although underdeveloped) distinction between right action and proper motive, which he also analyzed in terms of the distinction between external performance and internal state. An action can be right without being virtuous, he maintained, but an action can be virtuous only if performed from the right state of mind. Both right action and right motive are present in a virtuous action: "The agent must . . . be in the right state when he does [the actions]. First, he must know [that he is doing virtuous actions]; second, he must decide on them, and decide on them for themselves; and third, he must also do them from a firm and unchanging state," including the right state of emotion and desire. "The just and temperate person is not the one who [merely] does these actions, but the one who also does them in the way in which just or temperate people do them."[5]

We can conclude our analysis of the nature of virtue by incorporating Aristotle's observations. In addition to being properly motivated, a virtuous person will experience appropriate feelings, such as sympathy and regret—even when the feelings are not motives and no action can result from the feelings. However, some virtues have no clear link to either motives or feelings. Moral discernment and moral integrity—two virtues treated later in this chapter—are examples. Here psychological properties other than feelings are paramount. We will integrate these virtues into our analysis later in the chapter.

The Special Status of the Virtues

Some writers in character ethics maintain that the language of obligation is *derivative* from what they view as the more basic language of virtue. They think that a person disposed by character to have good motives and desires provides the basic model of the moral person and that this model determines obligations.[6] They regard this model as more important than a model of action-from-obligation, because right motives and character tell us more about moral worth than do right actions performed under the prod of obligation.

This position is attractive, because we are often more concerned about the character and motives of persons than about the conformity of their acts to rules. When a friend performs an act of "friendship," we expect it not to be motivated entirely from a sense of obligation to us, but because the person has a desire to be friendly, feels friendly, wants to keep friends in good cheer, and values friendship. The friend who acts only from obligation lacks the virtue of friendliness, and, absent this virtue, the relationship lacks moral merit.[7]

Some writers in biomedical ethics also argue that the attempt in obligation-oriented theories to replace the virtuous judgments of health care professionals with rules, codes, or procedures will not produce better decisions and actions.[8] Rather than using institutional rules and government regulations to protect subjects in research, they claim that the most reliable protection is the presence of an "informed, conscientious, compassionate, responsible researcher."[9] From this perspective, character is more important than conformity to rules, and virtues should be inculcated and cultivated over time through educational interactions, role models, and the like.

This conclusion provides a significant reason for incorporating the virtues into biomedical ethics and into medical and nursing education, but it needs elaboration. A morally good person with the right configuration of desires and motives is more likely than others to understand what should be done, more likely to perform attentively the acts required, and even more likely to form and act on moral ideals. A person we trust is one who has an ingrained motivation and desire to perform right actions. Thus, the person we will recommend, admire, praise, and hold up as a moral model is the person disposed by character to be generous, caring, compassionate, sympathetic, fair, and the like.

A person's character informs our judgment of that person and our assessment of his or her actions. If a virtuous person makes a mistake in judgment, thereby performing a morally wrong act, he or she would be less blameworthy than an habitual offender who performed the same act. In his chronicle of life under the Nazi SS in the Jewish ghetto in Cracow, Poland, Thomas Keneally describes a physician faced with a grave dilemma: either inject cyanide into four immobile patients or abandon them to the SS, who were at that moment emptying the ghetto and had already demonstrated that they would brutally kill all captives and patients. This physician, Keneally reports, "suffered painfully from a set of ethics as intimate to him as the organs of his own body."[10] Here is a person of the highest moral character and virtue, motivated to act rightly and even heroically, yet who at first had no idea what was the morally right action. Ultimately, with uncertainty and reluctance, the physician elected active euthanasia (using 40 drops of hydrocyanic acid) without the consent or knowledge of the four doomed patients—an act almost universally denounced by the canons of professional medical ethics. Even if one thinks that the physician's act was wrong and blameworthy—a judgment we reject—no one could reasonably make a judgment of blame or demerit directed at the physician's motives or character. Having already risked death by choosing to remain at his patients' beds in the hospital rather than take a prepared escape route, this physician is a moral hero who over time displayed an extraordinary moral character.

Judgments of agents' praiseworthiness and blameworthiness are significantly tied to agents' motives, which serve as signs of their character. However, in contrast to radical forms of character ethics, we do not hold that the merit in an action resides in motive or character alone. The action must be appropriately gauged to bring about the desired results and must conform with relevant principles and rules. For example, the physician or nurse who is appropriately motivated to help a patient but who acts incompetently in seeking the desired result does not act in a praiseworthy manner.

Virtues in Professional Roles

Character consists of a set of stable traits (virtues) that affect a person's judgment and action. Although we each have a different set of character traits, all persons with normal capacities can cultivate the traits that are centrally important in morality. Most such traits incorporate a complex structure of beliefs, motives, and emotions. In professional life, the traits that deserve to be encouraged and admired often derive from role responsibilities. Accordingly, we begin with an analysis of virtues in professional and institutional roles and practices.

Virtues in Roles and Practices

Professional roles are generally tied to institutional expectations and professional practices. These roles incorporate virtues as well as obligations. Roles internalize conventions, customs, and procedures of teaching, nursing, doctoring, and the like. Each organized body of professional practices has a history that sustains a tradition and requires professionals to cultivate certain virtues. Standards of virtue incorporate criteria of professional merit, and possession of these virtues disposes a person to act in accordance with the objectives of the practices.[11]

Roles and practices in medicine and nursing embody social expectations as well as standards and ideals internal to these professions. However, the traditional virtues in these professions derive primarily from health care relationships.[12] The particular virtues we analyze below are compassion, discernment, trustworthiness, integrity, and conscientiousness. In later chapters, we treat other key virtues—such as respectfulness, nonmalevolence, benevolence, justice, truthfulness, and faithfulness—during discussions of corresponding principles and rules.

To illustrate the difference between professional standards of moral character and professional standards that define technical skills, we begin with an instructive study of surgical error. Charles L. Bosk's *Forgive and Remember: Managing Medical Failure* presents an ethnographic study of the way two surgical services in "Pacific Hospital" handle medical failure, especially failures by surgical residents.[13] Bosk found that both surgical services distinguish, at least implicitly, between several different forms of error or mistake. The first is *technical*: The professional discharges role responsibilities conscientiously, but his or her technical training or information falls short of what the task requires. Every surgeon can be expected to make this sort of mistake occasionally. The second sort of error is *judgmental*: A conscientious professional develops and follows an incorrect strategy. These errors are also to be expected. Attending surgeons forgive momentary technical and judgmental errors but remember them in case a pattern develops indicating that a surgical resident lacks the technical and judgmental skills to be a competent surgeon.

The third sort of error is *normative*: A physician committing this kind of error violates a norm of conduct, particularly by failing to discharge moral obligations conscientiously. At this point, a moral judgment about the person is considered appropriate. Bosk contends that among surgeons technical and judgmental errors are subordinated in importance to these moral errors, because every conscientious person can be expected to make "honest errors" or "good faith errors." However, moral errors are profoundly serious whenever a pattern indicates a defect of moral character.

Bosk's study and related examples in medicine, nursing, and research help us appreciate how persons of high moral character acquire a reservoir of good will in assessments of the praiseworthiness or blameworthiness of their actions. If a conscientious surgeon and another surgeon who is defective in conscientiousness make the same technical or judgmental errors, the conscientious surgeon is not likely to be subjected to moral blame to the same degree as is the other surgeon.

The Virtues in Alternative Professional Models

Professional virtues were historically integrated with professional obligations and ideals in codes of health care ethics. Insisting that the medical profession's "prime objective" is to render service to humanity, an American Medical Association (AMA) code in effect from 1957 to 1980 urged the physician to be "upright" and "pure in character and . . . diligent and conscientious in caring for the sick." It also endorsed the virtues that Hippocrates commended: modesty, sobriety, patience, promptness, and piety. However, in contrast to its first code in 1847, the AMA over the years has deemphasized virtues in its codes. The references that remained in the 1957 version were perfunctory and marginal, and the 1980 version eliminated all traces of the virtues except for the admonition to "expose those physicians deficient in character or competence."

Different models of the role of health care professionals suggest different primary virtues. For example, if medicine is conceived in paternalistic terms, the physician's virtues differ from those drawn from a conception of medicine as a contract. In a paternalistic model, virtues of benevolence, care, and compassion are dominant.[14] In other models, especially an autonomy model, the virtue of respectfulness is more prominent.

Thomas Percival, who wrote the most influential treatise on medical ethics in the last two centuries, provides a classic example of an attempt to establish the proper set of virtues in medicine. Starting from the assumption that the patient's best medical interest is the proper goal of medicine, Percival reached conclusions about the physician's proper traits of character. Because of the dependence of patients, he counseled physicians that professional authority should direct medicine's understanding of its virtues, which, for Percival, were invariably tied to responsibility for the patient's medical welfare.[15]

Virtues of nurses similarly reflect different conceptions of the nursing profession and its role-responsibilities. In the traditional model, the nurse, as "hand-

maiden" of the physician, was counseled to cultivate the passive virtues of obedience and submission. In contemporary models, active virtues are more prominent. For example, if the nurse's role is viewed as one of advocacy for patients,
prominent virtues will include respectfulness, considerateness, justice, persis-
tence, and courage.[16] Attention to patients' rights and preservation of the nurse's
integrity dominate contemporary models. Even if the same virtue—conscientiousness, for example—appears in competing models, its content may be specified differently.

Questions also arise about the conditions under which certain virtues eventuate in unworthy and condemnable actions. For example, virtues such as loyalty,
courage, kindness, and benevolence at times lead persons to act inappropriately
and unacceptably. As we discuss in Chapter 7, the physician who acts kindly and
loyally by not reporting the incompetence of a fellow physician acts improperly.
Our criticism of a physician's failure to report professional misconduct does not
suggest that loyalty and kindness are not virtues, only that the virtues need to be
accompanied by an understanding of what is right and good, and of what deserves our kindness, generosity, and the like.[17] Virtues warranting caution, for
example, include loyalty, courage, respectfulness, tenderness, generosity, and pa-
triotism. All of these virtues can be misdirected by obedience, zeal, or excessive
devotion.

Five Focal Virtues

We cannot here assess each of the many virtues that are important to the virtuous health professional, but we can analyze a few central virtues, in particular,
compassion, discernment, trustworthiness, integrity, and conscientiousness. They
may not be the cardinal virtues (an idea that has never been made very clear in
moral writings), but they are widely acknowledged in biomedical ethics and they
help us focus on the character of health professionals.

Compassion

The virtue of compassion is a trait that combines an attitude of active regard for
another's welfare with an imaginative awareness and emotional response of deep
sympathy, tenderness, and discomfort at another's misfortune or suffering.[18]
Compassion presupposes sympathy, has affinities with mercy, and is expressed
in acts of beneficence that attempt to alleviate the misfortune or suffering of another person. Unlike integrity, which is focused on the self, compassion is focused on others.

Compassion need not be restricted to others' pain, suffering, disability, and
misery, but in health care, these conditions are the typical sources of compassionate responses. Using the language of sympathy, eighteenth-century philoso-

pher David Hume pointed to a typical circumstance of compassion in health care, together with a psychological explanation of how it arises:

> Were I present at any of the more terrible operations of surgery, 'tis certain, that even before it begun, the preparation of the instruments, the laying of the bandages in order, the heating of the irons, with all the signs of anxiety and concern in the patient and assistants, wou'd have a great effect upon my mind, and excite the strongest sentiments of pity and terror. No passion of another discovers itself immediately to the mind. We are only sensible of its causes or effects. From *these* we infer the passion: And consequently *these* give rise to our sympathy.[19]

Physicians and nurses who express no emotion in their behavior often fail to provide what patients most need. The physician or nurse lacking altogether in the appropriate display of compassion has a moral weakness, although he or she may also display other important moral qualities, including integrity, trustworthiness, and discernment. However, compassion also may cloud judgment and preclude rational and effective responses. In one reported case, a long-alienated son wanted to continue indefinitely a futile and painful treatment in an intensive-care unit (ICU) for his near-comatose father in order to have time to "make his peace" with his father. Although the son understood that his alienated father had no cognitive capacity, the son wanted to work through his sense of regret. Some hospital staff argued that the patient's grim prognosis and pain, combined with the needs of others waiting to receive care in the ICU, justified stopping the treatment (as had been requested by the patient's close cousin and informal guardian). But another group in the unit viewed this case as an appropriate act of compassion toward the son, who, they thought, should have time to express his farewells and regrets in order to make himself feel better about his father's death. The first group, by contrast, viewed compassion as misplaced because of the patient's prolonged agony and dying; in effect, it believed that the second group's compassion prevented clear thinking about primary obligations to this and other patients.[20]

Many writers in the history of ethical theory, most notably Spinoza and Kant, have advanced a cautious approach to compassion. They have maintained that a passionate (even a compassionate) engagement with others frequently blinds reason and impartial reflection. Health care professionals understand and appreciate this phenomenon. Constant contact with suffering can overwhelm and even paralyze a compassionate physician or nurse. Impartial judgment gives way to impassioned decisions and emotional burnout sometimes occurs. To counteract this problem, medical and nursing education is designed to inculcate detachment as well as compassion. The language of *detached concern* and *compassionate detachment* occasionally appears in health care ethics expressly to identify a complex characteristic of the good physician or good nurse.

However, misplaced compassion or excessive emotional involvement only serves as a warning, not as grounds for emotional withdrawal. Emotional responses need not be irrational or impulsive. They are often controlled and voluntary. When compassion appropriately motivates and expresses good character, it has a role in ethics alongside impartial reason and dispassionate judgment.

Discernment

The virtue of discernment brings sensitive insight, acute judgment, and understanding to action. Discernment involves the ability to make judgments and reach decisions without being unduly influenced by extraneous considerations, fears, personal attachments, and the like.

Some analyses closely associate discernment with practical wisdom (*phronesis*, to use Aristotle's term). A person of practical wisdom knows which ends to choose, knows how to realize them in particular circumstances, and carefully selects from among the range of possible actions, while keeping emotions within proper bounds. In Aristotle's aforementioned model, the practically wise person understands how to act with the right intensity of feeling, in just the right way, at just the right time, with a proper balance of reason and desire.[21]

More generally, the person of discernment is disposed to understand and perceive what circumstances demand in the way of human responsiveness. For example, a discerning physician will see when a despairing patient needs comfort rather than privacy, and vice versa. If comfort is the right choice, the discerning physician will find the right type and level of consolation in order to be helpful rather than intrusive. If a rule guides the behavior in a particular case, seeing *how* to follow the rule involves a form of discernment that is independent of seeing *that* the rule applies.[22]

The virtue of discernment thus involves understanding both *that* and *how* principles and rules are relevant in a variety of circumstances. It requires attention and sensitivity attuned to the demands of particular contexts. Acts of respect for autonomy and beneficence will vary in different contexts, and the ways in which clinicians manifest these principles and virtues in the care of patients will be as different as the ways in which devoted parents care for their children. Understanding that one's action should express a balance of moral principles, such as respect for autonomy and beneficence, itself exhibits a complex form of discernment. Discernment is often manifest through a creative response in meeting responsibilities, which principles and rules structure but do not fully determine.

Trustworthiness

Trustworthiness is another prominent virtue. Trust is a confident belief in and reliance upon the moral character and competence of another person. Trust entails a confidence that another will act with the right motives and in accordance with appropriate moral norms.[23] Such trust is often the most important ingredient in a patient's choice of one physician rather than another, and a physician's perceived lack of trustworthiness may be the primary reason for a patient's decision to switch to another physician.

Traditional ethical theories rarely mention trustworthiness. However, Aristotle took note of one aspect of trust and trustworthiness. He maintained that when relationships are voluntary and among intimates, by contrast to legal relationships among strangers, it is appropriate for the law to forbid lawsuits for harms that occur. Aristotle reasoned that, in intimate relationships, "dealings with one another as good and trustworthy," rather than "bonds of justice," hold persons together. The former bond he regarded as strictly a matter of character.[24]

It is hard to fault this assessment. At the same time, trust is a fading ideal in contemporary health care institutions. For centuries, health care professionals managed to keep trust at center stage, even when they had far less effective treatments to offer patients than today's professionals do. Recently, the centrality of trust has declined, as is evidenced by the dramatic rise in medical malpractice suits and adversarial relations between health care professionals and the public. Overt distrust has been engendered by mechanisms of managed care, for example, and by the incentives some health care organizations create for physicians to limit the amount and kinds of care they provide to patients. Talk has increased of the need for ombudsmen, patient advocates, legally binding "directives" to physicians, and the like.

Among the contributing causes of the erosion of trust are the loss of intimate contact between physicians and patients, the increased use of specialists, and the growth of large, impersonal, and bureaucratic medical institutions.[25] These factors undermine interactions that over time could foster knowledge of the professional's or the patient's character and could provide an adequate basis for trust. Physicians also now wonder whether they can trust many of their patients, especially if an injury occurs and litigation looms as a possibility. As a consequence, many physicians and patients welcome mutually agreed–upon rules and signed documentation of mutual decisions; and many physicians practice defensive medicine.

Integrity

Some writers claim that the primary virtue in health care is integrity.[26] We justify many actions or refusals to act on grounds that we would sacrifice our integrity if we acted otherwise. Health care professionals sometimes refuse to comply with the requests of patients or with the decisions of their colleagues on grounds that to do so would compromise or sacrifice their core beliefs. Later, we analyze these appeals to integrity as they appear in invocations of conscience; at present, we confine our attention to the virtue of integrity.

The value of moral integrity is beyond serious dispute, but what we *mean* by the term is less clear. In its most general sense, *moral integrity* means soundness, reliability, wholeness, and integration of moral character. In a more restricted sense, *moral integrity* means fidelity in adherence to moral norms. Accordingly, the virtue of integrity represents two aspects of a person's character. The first is a coherent integration of aspects of the self—emotions, aspirations, knowledge, and so on—so that each complements and does not frustrate the others. The second is the character trait of being faithful to moral values and standing up in their defense when necessary.

Problems in maintaining integrity sometimes arise not from straightforward moral conflict, but from demands that persons abandon personal goals and projects. Persons can feel violated by having to abandon their projects and commitments in order to pursue goals set by others. Sometimes, very demanding moral principles, such as the principle of utility, constrain personal undertakings, because the welfare of other persons constantly makes a moral claim on how we live our lives. Morality, so conceived, will inevitably deprive us of the liberty to structure and integrate our lives as we see fit. If one has structured one's life around specific goals that are ripped away by the agendas of others, a loss of personal integrity occurs just as certainly as if one's moral fiber were ripped away by others' coercive actions.

Persons can lack moral integrity in several respects (e.g., through hypocrisy, insincerity, bad faith, and self-deception). These vices represent a break in the connections among a person's moral convictions, emotions, and actions. Perhaps the most common deficiency is the lack of sincerely held, fundamental moral convictions, but no less important is the failure to act on professed moral beliefs.

Individual conscience and personal commitments sometimes confront especially wrenching conflicts in the health care setting. For example, some medical practitioners with religious commitments to the sanctity of life find it morally difficult to participate in decisions not to do everything possible to prolong life. To them, participating in removing ventilators and intravenous fluids from patients, even from patients with an advance directive, would violate their integrity. Their evaluative commitments may create morally difficult situations in which they must either compromise on their fundamental commitments or withdraw from the care of the patient in question. Yet, compromise seems, by definition, what a person of integrity cannot do; such a person must not sacrifice his or her deep moral commitments. Does this mean that action involving compromise is inconsistent with maintaining integrity? Will it turn out on close inspection that moral integrity in modern health care is little more than a dogmatic insistence that one's cherished values are higher than others' values?[27]

Modern health care facilities cannot entirely eliminate problems of staff disagreements, but persons with the virtues of patience, humility, and tolerance can ameliorate these problems. Situations that compromise integrity can usually be avoided if participants recognize the indeterminateness and fallibility of their own moral views and respect others' perspectives. Participants in a dispute may seek to use a consultative institutional process, such as a hospital ethics committee, if available. A moral climate of mutual respect together with channels of reasoned recourse in institutions can usually prevent people from feeling that their integrity has been compromised.

However, it would be morally bad advice to recommend that the person of integrity can and should always negotiate and compromise in a circumstance of institutional confrontation. There is something ennobling and admirable about the person who refuses to compromise beyond a certain moral threshold. To compromise below the threshold of integrity is simply to lose it.

Conscientiousness

We can extend some of these points about integrity and compromise by examining the virtue of conscientiousness. An individual acts conscientiously if he or she is motivated to do what is right because it is right, has tried with due diligence to determine what is right, intends to do what is right, and exerts an appropriate level of effort to do so. Like other virtues, conscientiousness is significant for both ordinary morality and moral ideals.

Conscience and conscientiousness. Many people view conscience as a faculty of or authority for moral decision-making. Slogans such as "Let your conscience be your guide" suggest that conscience is the final authority in moral justification. However, such an account fails to capture the nature of either conscience or conscientiousness. We can see why by examining the following case (derived from Bernard Williams): Having recently completed his Ph.D. in chemistry, George has not been able to find a job. His family has suffered from his failure: They are short of money; his wife has had to take additional work; and their small children have been subjected to considerable strain, uncertainty, and instability. An established chemist can get George a position in a laboratory that pursues research in chemical and biological warfare. Despite his perilous financial and familial circumstances, George feels that he cannot accept this position because of his conscientious opposition to chemical and biological warfare. The older chemist notes that the research will continue no matter what George decides. Furthermore, if George does not take this position, it will be offered to another young man who would probably pursue the research with great vigor. Indeed, the older chemist confides, his concern about this other candidate's nationalistic fervor and uncritical zeal for research in chemical and biological warfare, in part, led him to recommend George for the job. George's wife is puzzled and hurt by George's reaction, since she sees nothing wrong with the research. She is mainly concerned about their children's problems and the instability of their family.[28] Nonetheless, George forgoes this opportunity to help his family and prevent a destructive fanatic from obtaining the position, because his conscience stands in the way.

Conscience, in this example, is not a special moral faculty or a self-justifying moral authority. It is a form of self-reflection on and judgment about whether one's acts are obligatory or prohibited, right or wrong, good or bad. It is an internal sanction that comes into play through critical reflection. This sanction often appears as a bad conscience—in the form of painful feelings of remorse, guilt, shame, disunity, or disharmony—as the individual recognizes his or her acts as wrong. A conscience that sanctions in this way does not signify bad moral character. Indeed, this form of conscience is likely to occur in persons of strong moral character.[29] For example, kidney donors have been known to say, "I had to do it. I couldn't have backed out, not that I had the feeling of being trapped, because the doctors offered to get me out. I just had to do it."[30] Such poignant statements indicate that, for the individuals in question, some ethical standards are sufficiently fundamental and powerful that violating them would diminish integrity and result in guilt or shame.[31]

When people claim that their actions are conscientious, they sometimes feel compelled by conscience to resist demands made by others. They may claim that if they were to perform a particular act (e.g., providing an illegal drug to a patient), they would violate their conscience and compromise their integrity. In particularly troublesome cases, agents may even act out of character in order to perform what they judge to be the morally appropriate action. For example, a normally cooperative and cheerful person might angrily protest another's decision. Such moral indignation and outrage are sometimes warranted. In cases involving serious wrongdoing, the conscientious agent will resist the temptation to set aside what he or she believes to be right. Instructive examples include military physicians who believe they have to answer first to their consciences and cannot plead "superior orders" when commanded by a superior officer to commit what they believe to be a moral wrong.

Conscientious objection. Conflicts of conscience sometimes emerge in health care because people regard as unethical some role obligation or official order that descends from a hierarchical structure of authority. In cases of refusal, the individual need not rebuke others or obstruct them from performing an act, but only say, "Not through me."[32] Occasionally, this situation arises for physicians when a patient refuses a procedure in a context the physician views as medically unconscionable or requests a procedure the physician finds morally objectionable, such as amniocentesis for sex selection or an untested cancer therapy. If a physician wishes to withdraw, his or her conscientious convictions should be respected, and he or she should be free to withdraw—assuming that the requested actions are not among the general responsibilities of physicians. A patient's right of autonomy should not be purchased at the price of the physician's parallel right. These observations hold for other health professionals as well.

The Relationship of Moral Virtues and Moral Principles

There is a rough, though imperfect, correspondence between virtues and principles. The following (radically incomplete) list illustrates the correspondence between a few select virtues and principles or rules.

Principles	*Corresponding Virtues*
Respect for Autonomy	Respectfulness
Nonmaleficence	Nonmalevolence
Beneficence	Benevolence
Justice	Justice (or Fairness)

Rules	*Corresponding Virtues*
Veracity	Truthfulness
Confidentiality	Confidentiality
Privacy	Respect for privacy
Fidelity	Faithfulness

Ideals of Action	*Corresponding Ideals of Virtue*
Exceptional forgiveness	Exceptional forgiveness
Exceptional generosity	Exceptional generosity
Exceptional compassion	Exceptional compassion
Exceptional kindness	Exceptional kindness

We could expand this list to include many additional action-guides and virtues, but such a schema of correspondence would be misleading. Many virtue-standards do not directly correspond to action-guides in the kind of one-to-one correspondence indicated above. Not every moral virtue has a corresponding moral principle of obligation. For example, concern, compassion, caring, sympathy, courage, modesty, and patience are all virtues that do not correspond to norms of obligation. Many virtues have no corresponding norms of obligation because virtues and obligations do not function in the same way in the moral life. Typical examples are cautiousness, integrity (in the sense of consistently upholding and standing firm in one's values), cheerfulness, unpretentiousness, sincerity, appreciativeness, cooperativeness, and commitment. These virtues often have no corresponding moral obligations, but they often have corresponding moral ideals—a topic to which we now turn.

Moral Ideals

There are two levels of moral standards: ordinary moral standards and extraordinary moral standards. The first level is limited to standards in the common morality that pertain to everyone. These standards form the moral minimum. They include obligations specified in moral principles and rules, as well as the virtues that we expect all moral agents to possess (e.g., virtues of faithfulness, trustworthiness, and honesty). The second level is a morality of aspiration in which individuals adopt moral ideals that do not hold for everyone. This level does not require impartiality and permits agents to pursue the moral objectives they choose. Other persons can praise and admire those who fulfill these ideals, but they cannot blame or criticize those who do not pursue them. Persons who do not accept these ideals are not bound by them and cannot be criticized for not adopting them.

With the addition of moral ideals, we now have four categories of moral action: (1) actions that are right and obligatory (such as truth-telling); (2) actions that are wrong and prohibited (such as murder); (3) actions that are optional and morally neutral (neither wrong nor obligatory); and (4) actions that are optional but morally meritorious and praiseworthy. We concentrated on the first two in Chapter 1, occasionally mentioning the third. We will now focus exclusively on the fourth.

Supererogatory acts. Supererogation is a category of moral ideals pertaining principally to actions.[33] The etymological root of *supererogation* means paying or performing beyond what is owed or, more generally, doing more than is required. Supererogation has four defining conditions, which specify category 4 above. First, a supererogatory act is optional; it is neither required nor forbidden by common-morality standards. Second, supererogatory acts exceed what the common morality expects or demands. Third, supererogatory acts are intentionally undertaken to promote the welfare of others. Fourth, supererogatory acts are morally good and praiseworthy in themselves (not merely undertaken from good intentions).

Despite the first condition, individuals do not always consider the quality of their actions (or their characters) to be morally optional. Many heroes and saints describe their actions in the language of *ought, duty,* and *necessity*: "I had to do it." "I had no choice." "It was my duty." The point of this language is to express a personal sense of obligation. The agent accepts, as a pledge or assignment of personal responsibility, a personal norm that lays down what ought and must be done, despite the fact that it is not obligatory in the common morality or in a professional tradition. At the end of Albert Camus's *The Plague*, Dr. Rieux decides to make a record of those who fought the pestilence. It is to be a record, he says, of "what *had to be done* . . . despite their personal afflictions, by all who, while unable to be saints but refusing to bow down to pestilences, strive their utmost to be healers."[34] These healers accept major risks and thereby exceed the obligations of both the common morality and their professional tradition.

Supererogatory acts typically would be morally required were it not for some abnormal adversity or risk present in the particular circumstances, but the individual elects not to invoke the exemption introduced by the abnormal adversity or risk.[35] If persons have the strength of character that enables them to resist extreme adversity or assume additional risk in order to fulfill their own conception of their obligations, then it makes sense to accept their view that they are under a self-imposed obligation. The hero who says, "I was only doing my duty," is, from this perspective, speaking correctly, as one who accepts a standard of moral excellence. Such a person does not make a mistake in regarding the action as personally required, and can view failure as grounds for guilt, although no one else is free to so evaluate the act.

Not all supererogatory acts are exceptionally arduous, costly, or risky in the way this analysis may suggest. Examples of less demanding forms of supererogation include generous gift-giving, volunteering for public service, forgiving another's costly error, exceptional kindness, and complying with requests made by other persons when these exceed the obligatory requirements of the common morality or professional morality. Many everyday actions exceed obligation without reaching the highest level of supererogation. For example, a nurse may put in extra hours of work and return to the hospital to visit patients without becoming a saint or hero.

Often we are uncertain whether an action exceeds obligation, because the boundaries are ill-defined. For example, what is a nurse's role obligation to desperate, terminally ill patients who cling to the nurse for comfort in their few remaining days? If the obligation is that of spending 40 hours a week in conscientiously fulfilling a job description, then the nurse exceeds that obligation by a few off-duty visits to patients for an extra hour after work. If the obligation is simply to help patients overcome burdens and meet a series of challenges, then a nurse who does this while also displaying exceptional patience, fortitude, and friendliness exceeds the demands of obligation. There are also many cases of health care professionals living up to what would ordinarily be a role obligation (e.g., standard care of a patient), but where they make a sacrifice or accept a risk that exceeds what is ordinarily faced in such care (e.g., in risky care for HIV-infected patients).

In some special relationships between parties—involving, for example, debts of gratitude, close kinship, and commitments of loyalty—acts that would otherwise be optional become obligatory. This is not surprising because, as we will now see, the distinction between the obligatory and the nonobligatory is not as sharp as many writers have suggested.

The Continuum from Obligation to Supererogation

Contemporary ethical theories commonly classify anything in the domain of rule-governed behavior as either an obligation or beyond obligation (the latter being the pursuit of an exceptional but optional ideal). However, some actions do not fit neatly into these categories because they fall between the two levels. Appeals to the common morality cannot determine whether these actions are morally required or morally elective. This problem is compounded in professional ethics, because professional roles engender obligations that do not bind persons who do not occupy these roles. From this perspective, the two "levels" of the obligatory and the supererogatory lack sharp boundaries both in the common morality and in professional ethics.

The continuum from strict obligation to the highest ideals. We distinguish in the moral life between actions that are strictly obligatory, others that are borderline, and still others that are not obligatory. These distinctions suggest a continuum running from strict obligation (the core demands in the common morality) through weaker obligations (the periphery of ordinary expectations in the common morality, such as the obligation to be thorough in evaluating another's performance) and on to the domain of the morally nonrequired, including lower-level supererogation (e.g., kindly assisting a visitor lost in a hospital's corridors). From this perspective, an absence of charitableness or generosity is a defect in the moral life, even if not a failure of obligation. The continuum ends with higher-level supererogation (for example, heroic acts of self-sacrifice). A continuum exists on each level and across their boundaries. The following table represents these categories and the continuum:

Obligation		Beyond Obligation (Supererogation)	
Strict obligation	Weak obligation	Ideals beyond the obligatory	Saintly and heroic ideals
[1]	[2]	[3]	[4]

This continuum moves from the strictest obligation to the most arduous and elective moral ideal. The horizontal line represents a continuum with rough rather than sharply defined breaks; the vertical line divides the general categories, but also does not represent a sharp break. The horizontal line expresses a continuum within as well as between the four lower categories.

Joel Feinberg argues that supererogatory acts are "located on an altogether different scale than" obligations.[36] The above table suggests that this comment is correct in one respect and misleading in another. The right half of the table is not scaled by obligation at all, whereas the left half is. In this respect, Feinberg's comment is correct. However, the full horizontal line is connected by a single scale of moral value in which the right is continuous with the left. For example, obligatory acts of beneficence and supererogatory acts of beneficence are on the same scale because they are morally of the same kind. The domain of supererogatory ideals is continuous with the domain of principles of obligation by exceeding those obligations in accordance with the several defining conditions of supererogation listed previously.

The place of ideals in biomedical ethics. Many beneficent actions by health care professionals straddle the territory marked in the above table between "Obliga-

tion" and "Beyond Obligation" (in particular, between (2) and (3)). Matters become more complicated when we distinguish professional obligations from obligations incumbent upon everyone. Many moral *obligations* in health care are moral *ideals* from the perspective of the common morality. Many duties in medicine and nursing are profession-relative, rather than obligations either in the common morality or in other forms of professional practice. Some are role-obligations even when not formally stated in professional codes. For example, the expectation that physicians and nurses will encourage and cheer patients is a profession-imposed obligation, but not one incorporated in a professional code.

Some customs in the medical community are more ambiguous, such as the belief that physicians and nurses have an obligation to efface self-interest and take risks in attending to patients. One issue is the nature of "obligations" to care for patients with HIV when the risk of transmission is significant. Proposed policies have been controversial, and professional codes and medical association pronouncements have varied extensively.[37] We probably cannot resolve such issues without considering the level of risk that professionals are expected to assume and setting a threshold beyond which the level of risk is so high as to be optional rather than obligatory. The unresolved character of this problem should help us appreciate why some medical associations urge their members to exhibit the virtue of courage and treat HIV-infected patients, why other associations advise their members that treatment is optional,[38] and why still others with particularly high expectations insist that both virtue and obligation converge to the conclusion that health care professionals should set aside self-interest to care for such patients and that the health care professions should take actions to ensure that such patients receive appropriate care.[39]

It is doubtful that health care professionals fail to discharge moral obligations when they fall short of the latter high standards of obligation, even if obligations are measured exclusively by role obligations. Confusion arises because of the indeterminate boundaries of obligations both in the common morality and in the community of health professionals.

Moral Excellence

Aristotelian ethical theory has long insisted that moral excellence is closely connected to virtues and moral ideals. We will draw on this Aristotelian tradition and on our prior analysis of moral ideals and supererogation for an account of moral excellence.[40]

The Place of Moral Excellence

We begin with four reasons that prompt us to attend to this subject. First, we hope to overcome an undue imbalance in contemporary ethical theory, which often focuses narrowly on the moral minimum of obligations while largely ignoring supererogation and moral ideals.[41] This concentration on minimal obligations has diluted the moral life, including our expectations for ourselves, our close associates, and health professionals. If we expect only the moral minimum, we have lost an ennobling sense of excellence in character and performance.

A second reason connects to the first. We aspire to overcome a certain skepticism in contemporary ethical theory about high ideals in the moral life. This skepticism is evident in some of our best writers, including some who have influenced the present authors and some who have produced influential works in character ethics (e.g., Susan Wolf, Philippa Foot, Bernard Williams, and Thomas Nagel). The thrust of their concern is that high moral ideals must compete with many other goals and responsibilities in life, and these ideals may demand too much morally or may lead persons to neglect other matters worthy of attention, including personal projects, family relationships, friendships, and experiences that broaden outlooks.[42]

We do not wholly reject this view, but these writings suggest that high moral ideals are only one of life's major considerations and that moral excellence is no more valuable or worthwhile than hobbies, recreation, and other "agent-relative" projects. Lost is the Aristotelian aspiration to an admirable life of moral achievement. Consequently, the accepted model of a moral person is uninspiring and devoid of moral challenge for earnest and reflective persons. As John Stuart Mill once noted, "The contented man, or the contented family, who have no ambition to make any one else happier, to promote the good of their country or their neighborhood, or to improve themselves in moral excellence, excite in us neither admiration nor approval."[43]

Our third reason concerns what we call in Chapter 8 the criterion of comprehensiveness in an ethical theory. Recognizing moral excellence will allow us to incorporate a broad range of moral virtues and forms of supererogation beyond the obligations and virtues that comprise ordinary morality. We can include virtues such as tactfulness, courage, patience, hospitality, and what Aristotle called "greatness of soul" without maintaining that these virtues are conditions of morality that everyone is somehow required to meet or that there are *principles* of patience, hospitality, courage, and the like. These vital aspects of the moral life merit inclusion in a comprehensive account.

Finally, a model of moral excellence merits pursuit because it indicates what is worthy of our aspiration. Morally exemplary lives provide developed ideals that help guide and inspire us to higher goals and morally better lives. Such models exemplify high moral aspiration and achievement and illustrate why excellence is important in the moral life, alongside moral principles and virtues.

Aristotelian Ideals

Aristotle maintained that we acquire virtues much as we do skills, such as carpentry, playing a musical instrument, and cooking. Obligations play a less central role in this account, because the theory turns on the level of effort and commitment involved, as well as on depth in the development of character. Consider, for example, a person who undertakes to expose scientific fraud in an academic institution. It is easy to frame this action as a matter of obligation, especially if the institution has a policy on fraud; but suppose this person's reports to superiors are ignored, and eventually her job is in jeopardy and her family receives threats. At some point, we likely would say that she has fulfilled her obligations and is not morally required to pursue the matter further. However, we would praise her for doing so. Her continued efforts to bring about institutional reform would then take on heroic dimensions.

An Aristotelian theory could frame this situation in terms of the person's level of commitment, the perseverance and endurance shown, the resourcefulness and discernment in marshalling evidence, and the courage, as well as the decency and diplomacy displayed in confronting superiors, and the like.

Here an analogy to educational goals illustrates why setting goals beyond the moral minimum is central to the Aristotelian framework. Most of us are trained to aspire to an ideal of education. We are taught to prepare ourselves as best we can. No educational aspirations are too high unless they exceed our abilities and thus cannot be attained. If we reach only an ordinary educational level, we frequently consider this achievement a matter of disappointment and regret. In the midst of fulfilling our aspirations, we sometimes expand our goals beyond what we had originally planned. We think of getting another degree, learning another language, or reading widely beyond our specialized training. We do not say, however, that we have an *obligation* to achieve as high a level of education as we can achieve.

The Aristotelian model for ethics is analogous. Moral character and moral achievement are functions of self-cultivation and aspiration. Each individual should aspire to a level as elevated as his or her ability permits. Just as persons vary in the quality of their performances in athletics and medical practice, so too in the moral life some persons are more capable than others and deserve more acknowledgment, praise, and admiration. Some persons are so advanced morally that what they believe they can achieve is different from what those who are less morally developed can expect to achieve. One's goals of moral excellence enlarge as moral development advances.

It is both simplistic and morally undesirable to distinguish sharply between ordinary moral requirements and extraordinary ideals. What persons should strive to achieve when at lower levels of moral development is different from what they should attempt at more advanced levels of development (though everyone is, of course, bound to the moral minimum). Wherever a person is on the continuum of development, there will be a goal of moral excellence that exceeds what he or she has already achieved. What we ought to do, then, is to follow a moving target of moral excellence.

This analysis explains why, in Aristotelian ethics, ideals rather than principles of obligation take center stage. Our account is suited for persons with the will to aspire, not for persons who merely want to know what social obligations require. For example, the investigator who uses human subjects of research might ask (as is typical in protocol review), "What am I obligated to do to protect human subjects?" The presumption is that once this question has been addressed, the researcher can then accept a burden of moral obligation and proceed with the research. But on the Aristotelian model, this question and answer are only starting points. The more important question is, "How could I conduct this research in order to maximally protect and minimally inconvenience subjects, commensurate with achieving the objectives of the research?" Not to address this question at all indicates that one is morally less serious than one could be.

The Aristotelian model does not expect perfection, only that persons strive toward perfection. The model might seem impractical, but a fairer assessment is that moral ideals are practical instruments. As *our* ideals, they motivate us in a way that basic obligations may not, and they also set out a path that we can climb in stages, with a renewable sense of progress and achievement.

Exceptional Moral Excellence: Saints, Heroes, and Others

Extraordinary persons often function as models of excellence whose examples we aspire to follow. Among the many types of models, the moral hero and the moral saint are the most celebrated, and deservedly so.

The term "saint" has a long history within religious, especially Christian, traditions, but it also has a secular use, just as "hero" does. Other-directedness, altruism, and benevolence are prominent features of the moral saint.[44] Saints do their duty and realize their ideals where most people would fail to do so because of inclination, desire, or self-interest. Saintliness requires regular fulfillment of duty and realization of ideals over time; it demands consistency and constancy. We cannot make a final judgment about a person's moral saintliness until the record is complete.[45] By contrast, a person may become a moral hero through one exceptional action, such as accepting extraordinary risk while discharging duty or realizing ideals. The hero resists fear and the desire for self-preservation in undertaking risky actions that most people would eschew. However, the hero may lack the constancy that distinguishes the saint.

Many persons who serve as our moral models, or from whom we draw moral inspiration, are not so advanced morally that they qualify as saints or heroes (although we sometimes incorrectly label them saints and heroes). We often learn about virtuous conduct from persons with a limited repertoire of exceptional virtues, such as exceedingly conscientious health professionals.

Consider, for example, John Berger's biography of an English physician, John Sassall, who chose to practice medicine in a poverty-ridden, culturally deprived country village in a remote region of northern England. Under the influence of works by Joseph Conrad, Sassall chose this village from an "ideal of service" that reached beyond "the average petty life of self-seeking advancement." Sassall was aware that he would have almost no social life and that the villagers had few resources with which to pay him, to develop their community, and to attract better medicine, but he focused on their needs rather than his own. Progressively, Sassall grew morally as he interacted with members of the community. He developed a deep understanding of, and profound respect for, the members of the village and learned how to attend to them as whole human beings. He became a person of exceptional caring, devotion, discernment, conscientiousness, and patience when taking care of the villagers. His moral character grew and deepened year after year in caring for them. They, in turn, trusted him under the most adverse and personally difficult circumstances.[46]

From exemplary lives like that of John Sassall and from our previous analysis, we can extract four criteria of moral excellence and then test these criteria against our experience of other exceptional persons.[47] First, Sassall is faithful to a *worthy moral ideal* that he keeps constantly before him in making judgments and performing actions. In his case, the ideal is deeply devoted service to a poor and needy community. Second, he has a *motivational structure* that conforms closely to our earlier description of the motivational patterns of virtuous persons, which include being prepared to forgo benefits to themselves in the service of a moral ideal. Third, he has an *exceptional moral character*; that is, he possesses moral virtues that dispose him to perform supererogatory actions to an exceptional extent.[48] Fourth, he is a *person of integrity*—both of moral integrity and of a deep personal integrity—and thus is not overwhelmed by distracting conflicts or personal desires in making judgments and performing actions.

These four conditions appear to be sufficient conditions of moral excellence. They are also relevant (but not sufficient) conditions of moral saintliness and moral heroism. John Sassall, exceptional as he is, is neither a saint nor a hero. To achieve this elevated status, he would have to satisfy additional conditions. Sassall is not a person who faces either deep adversity (though he faces modest adversity), extremely difficult tasks, or a high level of risk, and these are typically the sorts of conditions that contribute to making a person a saint or a hero.

Examples of prominent moral saints include St. Francis, Mother Theresa, and Albert Schweitzer. Examples of prominent moral heroes include soldiers, political prisoners, and ambassadors who take substantial risks to save endangered persons by such acts as falling on hand grenades and resisting political tyrants. Scientists and physicians who experiment on themselves in order to generate knowledge that can benefit others are also sometimes heroes. There are many examples: Daniel Carrion injected blood into his arm from a patient with verruga peruana (an unusual disease marked by many vascular eruptions of the skin and mucous membranes as well as fever and severe rheumatic pains), only to discover that it had given him a fatal disease (Oroya fever). Werner Forssman performed the first heart catheterization on himself, walking to the radiological room with the catheter sticking into his heart.[49] More recently, a French researcher, Dr. Daniel Zagury, injected himself with an experimental AIDS vaccine, maintaining that his act was "the only ethical line of conduct."[50]

A person can qualify as a moral hero or a moral saint only if he or she meets some combination of the above-listed four conditions of moral excellence, together with other conditions noted above. While it is not clear that a person needs to satisfy all four conditions to be a moral hero, a person must satisfy all of them to qualify as a moral saint. This appraisal does not imply that moral saints are more valued or more admirable than moral heroes. We simply propose conditions of moral excellence that are more stringent for saints than for heroes. We will not consider whether these conditions might point to another and still higher form of moral excellence: the combination of saint and hero in one person. There have been such extraordinary persons, and we could make a case that some of these extraordinary figures are more excellent than others. But at this level of exemplariness, such fine distinctions seem gratuitous.

Physician David Hilfiker's *Not All of Us Are Saints* offers another instructive model of very exceptional but not saintly or heroic conduct in medicine—in his case resulting from his efforts to practice "poverty medicine" in Washington, D.C.[51] His decision to leave a rural medical practice in the Midwest to provide medical care to the very poor, including the homeless, reflected both a desire and a felt obligation to help, based in part on religious convictions. Many of the health problems he encountered stemmed from an unjust social system, in which his patients had limited access to health care and to other basic social goods that contribute significantly to health. He experienced severe frustration as he encountered immovable social and institutional barriers to providing poverty medicine, and as he tried to balance institutional goals and rules with the care of patients who were often difficult and uncooperative. His frustrations generated stress, depression, and hopelessness, all of which weighed heavily on him, along with his vacillating feelings and attitudes, including anger, pain, impatience, and guilt. One day, his wellspring of compassion exhausted by his sense of endless needs and personal limitations, he failed to respond as he felt he should have in a particular case—he had "reached his limit for this particular day." He continues: "Like those whom on another day I would criticize harshly, I harden myself to the plight of a homeless man and leave him to the inconsistent mercies of the city police and ambulance system. Numbness and cynicism, I suspect, are more often the products of frustrated compassion than of evil intentions."

Hilfiker realized that he is "anything but a saint." He also considered the label "saint" to be inappropriate for people, like himself, who have a safety net to protect them. Having accepted the Mother Teresa model of selfless giving and sacrificial service, and blaming himself for his "selfishness," he redoubled his efforts in the face of frustrations and failures. He saw patients after the clinic closed, strained to be pleasant in such circumstances, stopped for curbside consultations, and the like; but he recognized "the gap between who I am and who I would like to be," and he considered that gap "too great to overcome." He then abandoned "in frustration the attempt to be Mother Teresa," observing that "there are few Mother Teresas, few Dorothy Days who can give everything to the poor with a radiant joy." Yet he managed to continue to find ways to work compassionately and effectively, within the limits set by available personal, social, institutional, and technological resources. He arrived at the answer that "every good doctor anywhere must come to: I can offer myself and my presence as a healer." Hilfiker is unwilling to consider himself a hero or his actions heroic, yet he insists that many of the people with whom he works "are heroes, people who struggle against all odds and survive; people who have been given less than nothing, yet find ways to give."

Our understanding of moral saints and moral heroes is very difficult to capture with clarity. The model of moral saintliness is extremely demanding and arduous, and may produce conflicts with other important goals. For instance, if saints embody the motive to be morally perfect, they may not appreciate that high standards of nonmoral excellence are also worthy of pursuit. Furthermore, the hero may not be a person of prudent or balanced judgment. For example, we praise "heroic" efforts by clinicians to provide medical care, but what they provide in some cases may be disproportionate to the probable benefits to the recipients. Questions also arise about whether some heroic actions on balance should not be performed, because they are too risky or threaten other obligations.

Such questions have deeply affected debates about the acceptability of moral heroism in living organ donation—a topic to which we turn in conclusion.

Living Organ and Tissue Donation

Because of the shortage of cadaveric organs for transplantation, as well as the advantages of living donors in many cases, living donations have become more and more common in the United States. There were slightly more than 10,000 acts of organ donation in 1998, and living donors made over 40% of those donations, mainly of kidneys.[52] Transplant teams remove, transfer, and implant the donated organs. They also select the donors, often searching for donors in the needy patient's family, screening prospective donors for compatibility and suitability, offering them an uncommon opportunity to help others, advising them about courses of action, estimating the risks involved, and evaluating those risks as "reasonable," "excessive," and so forth.

In these activities, health care professionals sometimes function as *moral gatekeepers* to determine who may undertake variably risky acts of living donation of organs and tissues for transplantation. Blood donation raises few questions. However, in cases of bone marrow donation and the donation of kidneys or portions of livers or lungs, health care professionals have to consider whether, when, and from whom to invite, accept, and effectuate acts of donation. Living organ donation raises complex ethical issues because the transplant team subjects a healthy person to a major and somewhat risky surgical procedure, with no medical benefit to him or her, in order to provide a medical benefit to someone else. Not every offer to donate tissue or organs for transplantation is heroic, and not every heroic or even nonheroic offer is acceptable. It is appropriate for transplant teams, reflecting societal rules and values, to probe the donor's understanding and voluntariness. It is also appropriate to consider potential donors' motives, at least to the extent of investigating whether financial gain is the motivating factor.

Some commentators urge a system in which the competent prospective donor alone should decide whether donation is worth the risks involved.[53] However, simply letting prospective donors decide or letting transplant teams decide (assuming the potential donor's willingness to donate) is inadequate. Both parties should be involved. Letting the potential donor decide neglects the role of physicians and other health care professionals in effectuating the donation; letting the transplant team decide ignores the prospective donor's moral projects.

Transplant teams have generally been suspicious of living, genetically unrelated donors—not only strangers and acquaintances but often even spouses and friends who are emotionally related donors. This suspicion has various sources, including concerns about donors' motives and worries about their competence to decide and the voluntariness of their decisions, as though such supererogatory actions signal problematic motives, incompetence, or involuntariness. In contrast to professionals' attitudes,[54] a majority of the public holds that the gift of a kidney to a stranger is reasonable and proper and that the transplant team should accept it.[55]

Although this gap in perspectives in part reflects different conceptions of reasonable risk, the offer to donate a kidney by a friend, acquaintance, or stranger typically does not involve such high risks that questions should automatically emerge about the donor's competence, voluntariness, and motivations. From 1989 to 1998, the annual percentage of genetically unrelated kidney donors (those who were not also spouses) increased from 1.9% to 5.3%. In 1997, almost 5% of the 73 living donors of portions of their livers were genetically unrelated to and not married to the recipient.[56] Transplant teams may and should decline some heroic offers of organs for moral reasons, even when the donors are competent, their decisions informed and voluntary, and their moral excellence beyond question. For instance, transplant teams would have good grounds to decline a mother's offer to donate her heart to save her dying child, because the donation would involve others in directly causing her death—even though we would rightly praise a mother's sacrifice of her life in other settings (e.g., in trying to save her drowning child).

A more complicated case arose when an imprisoned, 38-year old father who had already lost one of his kidneys wanted to donate his remaining kidney to his 16-year old daughter whose body had already rejected one kidney transplant, in part because of her failure to take her immunosuppressant medication as prescribed.[57] The family insisted that medical professionals and ethics committees had no right to examine, let alone reject, the father's act of donation. However, questions arose about the voluntariness of the father's offer (in part because he was in prison), about the risks to him (a substantial number of patients without kidneys do not thrive on dialysis), about the probable success of the transplant because of his daughter's problems with the first one, and about the costs to the prison system (approximately \$40,000 to \$50,000 a year for dialysis).

The society and health care professionals should start with the presumption that living organ donation, in contrast to some tissue donation, is praiseworthy but optional, even if living donors view their acts as obligatory. As moral gatekeepers, transplant teams need to subject their criteria for selecting living donors to careful and public scrutiny in order to ensure that they do not inappropriately use their own values about sacrifice, risk, and the like, as the basis for their judgments. For example, legitimate concerns about professional bias arise because of the disparities between male and female kidney donation. In 1998, almost 58% of the living kidney donors were female. Studies indicate that, when asked, males and females tend to donate at about the same rates, even though males tend to view their acts of donation as extraordinary and heroic, while females tend to view them as mere extensions of their basic obligations.[58] More research is needed to determine whether the current gender disparities in living kidney donation involve biases either in patient offers or in professional requests, or both.

Conclusion

In this chapter we have moved beyond principles, rules, obligations, and rights. Virtues, ideals, and aspirations of moral excellence support and enrich the moral framework developed in the previous chapter. Ideals transcend obligations and rights, and many virtues dispose persons to act in accordance with principles and rules as well as ideals. Next, we will discuss particular principles and rules in great detail.

Notes

1. For two influential anthologies, see *Midwest Studies in Philosophy Volume XIII—Ethical Theory: Character and Virtue*, ed. Peter A. French, Theodore E. Uehling, Jr., and Howard K. Wettstein (Notre Dame, IN: University of Notre Dame Press, 1988); and *Identity, Character, and Morality*, ed. Owen Flanagan and Amélie Oksenberg Rorty (Cambridge, MA: MIT Press, 1990). For two very different treatments of the Aristotelian perspective, see Nancy Sherman, *The Fabric of Character: Aristotle's The-*

ory of Virtue (Oxford: Clarendon Press, 1989) and Alasdair MacIntyre, *After Virtue: A Study in Moral Theory*, 2d ed. (Notre Dame, IN: University of Notre Dame Press, 1984) and *Dependent Rational Animals: Why Human Beings Need the Virtues* (Chicago: Open Court, 1999). Other valuable collections of essays include Roger Crisp and Michael Slote, eds., *Virtue Ethics* (Oxford: Oxford University Press, 1997); Roger Crisp, ed., *How Should One Live? Essays on the Virtues* (Oxford: Oxford University Press, Clarendon Press, 1996); Daniel Statman, ed., *Virtue Ethics: A Critical Reader* (Washington, DC: Georgetown University Press, 1997); and Ellen Frankel Paul, Fred D. Miller, Jr., and Jeffrey Paul, eds., *Virtue and Vice* (Cambridge: Cambridge University Press, 1998).

2. Compare, for instance, the list of virtues presented by Edmund D. Pellegrino and David C. Thomasma in *The Virtues in Medical Practice* (New York: Oxford University Press, 1993). They list fidelity to trust, compassion, phronesis, justice, fortitude, temperance, integrity, and self-effacement.

3. This is not the broadest possible sense of "Virtue," inasmuch as machines, tools, horses, and the like are often said to have virtues. Some writers more tightly restrict the meaning of virtue than we do. For example, Aristotle required that virtue involve habituation rather than a natural character trait [*Nicomachean Ethics*, trans. Terence Irwin (Indianapolis, IN: Hackett Publishing Co., 1985), 1103^{a}18–19]. Thomas Aquinas (relying on a formulation by Peter Lombard) additionally held that virtue is a good quality of mind by which we live rightly and therefore cannot be put to bad use. See *Treatise on the Virtues* (from *Summa Theologiae*, I–II), Question 55, Arts. 3–4.

4. This definition is the primary use reported in the Oxford English Dictionary (O.E.D). It is defended by Alan Gewirth, "Rights and Virtues," *Review of Metaphysics* 38 (1985): 751, and R. B. Brandt, "The Structure of Virtue," in *Midwest Studies in Philosophy* 13 (1988): 76. Edmund Pincoffs presents a definition of virtue in terms of desirable dispositional qualities of persons, in *Quandaries and Virtues: Against Reductivism in Ethics* (Lawrence, KS: University Press of Kansas, 1986), pp. 9, 73–100. We accepted a definition similar to these in the first two editions of this book, for which we were criticized by John Waide, "Virtues and Principles," *Philosophy and Phenomenological Research* 48 (1988): 455–72. See further Julia Driver, "The Virtues and Human Nature," in *How Should One Live?: Essays on the Virtues*, ed. Crisp, pp. 111–29.

5. *Nicomachean Ethics*, 1105^{a}17–33, 1106^{b}21–23; cf. 1144^{a}14–20 (trans. Terence Irwin).

6. See Philippa Foot, *Virtues and Vices* (Oxford: Basil Blackwell, 1978); Gregory Trianosky, "Supererogation, Wrongdoing, and Vice," *Journal of Philosophy* 83 (1986): 26–40; and Jorge L. Garcia, "The Primacy of the Virtuous," *Philosophia* 20 (1990): 69–91.

7. See Diane Jeske, "Friendship, Virtue, and Impartiality," Philosophy and Phenomenological Research 57 (1997): 51–72; and Michael Stocker, "The Schizophrenia of Modern Ethical Theories," *Journal of Philosophy* 73 (1976): 453–66.

8. Gregory Pence notes that almost any health professional can successfully evade a system of rules. Therefore, we should create a climate in which health professionals "desire not to abuse their subjects." Gregory Pence, *Ethical Options in Medicine* (Oradell, NJ: Medical Economics Co., 1980), p. 177.

9. Henry K. Beecher, "Ethics and Clinical Research," *New England Journal of Medicine* 274 (1966): 1354–60.

10. Thomas Keneally, *Schindler's List* (New York: Penguin Books, 1983), pp. 176–80.

11. This analysis is influenced by Alasdair MacIntyre, *After Virtue*, esp. pp. 175–80, and Dorothy Emmet, *Rules, Roles, and Relations* (New York: St. Martin's Press, 1966).

12. A similar thesis is defended in dissimilar ways in Edmund D. Pellegrino, "Toward a Virtue-Based Normative Ethics for the Health Professions," *Kennedy Institute of Ethics Journal* 5 (1995): 253–77, and "The Virtuous Physician and the Ethics of Medicine," in *Virtue and Medicine*, ed. Earl Shelp (Dordrecht, the Netherlands: D. Reidel, 1985), pp. 237–56. See also John Cottingham, "Medicine, Virtues and Consequences," in *Human Lives: Critical Essays on Consequentialist Bioethics*, ed. David S. Oderberg (New York: Macmillan, 1997).

13. Charles L. Bosk, *Forgive and Remember: Managing Medical Failure* (Chicago: University of Chicago Press, 1979). Bosk also recognizes a fourth type of error: "quasi-normative errors" based on the attending's special protocols.

14. In one paternalistic conception of the physician's role, arrogance is seen as a virtue that is preferable to the virtue of humility. See Franz J. Ingelfinger, "Arrogance," *New England Journal of Medicine* 303 (December 25, 1980): 1507–11.

15. Thomas Percival, *Medical Ethics; or a Code of Institutes and Precepts, Adapted to the Professional Conduct of Physicians and Surgeons* (Manchester, England: S. Russell, 1803), pp. 165–66. This book formed the substantive basis of the first AMA code.

16. For models of nursing, see Dan W. Brock, "The Nurse-Patient Relation: Some Rights and Duties," in *Nursing: Images and Ideals*, ed. Stuart F. Spicker and Sally Gadow (New York: Spring Publishing Co., 1980), pp. 102–24; and Gerald Winslow, "From Loyalty to Advocacy: A New Metaphor for Nursing," *Hastings Center Report* 14 (June 1984): 32–40. See also Betty J. Winslow and Gerald Winslow, "Integrity and Compromise in Nursing Ethics," *Journal of Medicine and Philosophy* 16 (1991): 307–23.

17. Rosalind Hursthouse and other philosophers have argued that virtue ethics functions to guide actions. While she thinks it unreasonable to expect virtue ethics to resolve moral dilemmas, Hursthouse claims that this is actually a strength of this type of theory and a more accurate representation of the moral life. See her "Normative Virtue Ethics," in *How Should One Live?: Essays on the Virtues*, ed. Crisp, pp. 19–36; "Applying Virtue Ethics" in *Virtues and Reasons*, ed. Hursthouse, Gavin Lawrence, and Warren Quinn (New York: Oxford University Press, 1995), pp. 57-75; and her *On Virtue Ethics* (New York: Oxford University Press, 1999). See also Nancy Sherman, *Making a Necessity of Virtue: Aristotle and Kant on Virtue* (New York: Cambridge University Press, 1997).

18. See Lawrence Blum, "Compassion," in *Explaining Emotions*, ed. Amélie Oksenberg Rorty (Berkeley: University of California Press, 1980) and David Hume, *A Dissertation on the Passions*, Sect. 3, §§ 4–5 (London, 1772), pp. 208–09.

19. David Hume, *A Treatise of Human Nature*, ed. David Norton and Mary Norton (Oxford: Oxford University Press, 2000), 3.3.1.7.

20. Baruch Brody, "Case No. 25. 'Who is the patient, anyway': The difficulties of compassion," in *Life and Death Decision Making* (New York: Oxford University Press, 1988), pp. 185–88.

21. Aristotle, Nicomachean Ethics, trans. Terence Irwin (Indianapolis, IN: Hackett Publishing Co., 1985), 1106^b15–29, 1141^a15–1144^b17.

22. Some writers in biomedical ethics maintain that persons of discernment (when they are also conscientious, compassionate, etc.) afford greater protection against moral wrongdoing in medicine than do frameworks of rules and regulations. See Leon R. Kass, "Ethical Dilemmas in the Care of the Ill," *Journal of the American Medical Association* 244 (October 17, 1980): 1811; and Henry K. Beecher, "Ethics and Clinical Research," *New England Journal of Medicine* 274 (1966): 1354–60.

23. See the instructive analyses in Annette Baier's "Trust and Antitrust" and two later essays on trust in her *Moral Prejudices* (Cambridge: Harvard University Press, 1994);

54 PRINCIPLES OF BIOMEDICAL ETHICS

Philip Pettit, "The Cunning of Trust," *Philosophy and Public Affairs* 24 (1995): 202–25; and H. J. N. Horsburgh, "The Ethics of Trust," *Philosophical Quarterly* 10 (October 1960): 343–54.

24. Aristotle, *Eudemian Ethics*, 1242^{b}23-1243^{a}13, in *The Complete Works of Aristotle*, ed. Jonathan Barnes (Princeton, NJ: Princeton University Press, 1984).

25. For a discussion of the erosion of trust in medicine, see David Mechanic, "Public Trust and Initiatives for New Health Care Partnerships," *Milbank Quarterly* 76 (1998): 281–302, and his "Changing Medical Organization and the Erosion of Trust," *Milbank Quarterly* 74 (1996): 171–89.

26. Brody, *Life and Death Decision Making,* p. 35.

27. For useful discussions of this question, see Martin Benjamin and Joy Curtis, *Ethics in Nursing,* 3d ed. (New York: Oxford University Press, 1992), pp. 105–8; and Winslow and Winslow, "Integrity and Compromise in Nursing Ethics," pp. 307–23.

28. Williams, "A Critique of Utilitarianism," in J. J. C. Smart and Williams, *Utilitarianism: For and Against* (Cambridge: Cambridge University Press, 1973), pp. 97–98.

29. We have here drawn on two sources: Hannah Arendt, *Crises of the Republic* (New York: Harcourt, Brace, Jovanovich, Inc., 1972), p. 62; and John Stuart Mill, *Utilitarianism,* ch. 3, pp. 228–29; and *On Liberty,* ch. 3, p. 263, in *Collected Works of John Stuart Mill,* vols. 10, 18 (Toronto: University of Toronto Press, 1969, 1977).

30. Carl H. Fellner, "Organ Donation: For Whose Sake?," *Annals of Internal Medicine* 79 (October 1973): 591.

31. See Larry May, "On Conscience," *American Philosophical Quarterly* 20 (1983): 57–67. See also C. D. Broad, "Conscience and Conscientious Action," in *Moral Concepts,* ed. Joel Feinberg (Oxford: Oxford University Press, 1970), pp. 74–79, and Childress, "Appeals to Conscience," *Ethics* 89 (1979): 315–35.

32. See Bernard Williams, *Moral Luck: Philosophical Papers* 1973–1980 (Cambridge: Cambridge University Press, 1981), esp. p. 50.

33. Our analysis is indebted to David Heyd, *Supererogation: Its Status in Ethical Theory* (Cambridge: Cambridge University Press, 1982) and "Tact: Sense, Sensitivity, and Virtue," *Inquiry* 38 (1995): 217–231. We are also indebted to J. O. Urmson, "Saints and Heroes," *Essays in Moral Philosophy,* ed. A. I. Melden (Seattle, WA: University of Washington Press, 1958), pp. 198–216. Other analyses that have influenced our views include John Rawls, *A Theory of Justice* (Cambridge, MA: Harvard University Press, 1971; revised edition 1999), pp. 116–17, 438–39, 479–85 (1999: 100–01, 385–86, 420–25); Joel Feinberg, "Supererogation and Rules," in *Ethics,* ed. Judith J. Thomson and Gerald Dworkin (New York: Harper & Row, 1968), pp. 391–411; Roderick M. Chisholm, "Supererogation and Offense: A Conceptual Scheme for Ethics," *Ratio* 5 (June 1963): 1–14; Millard Schumaker, *Supererogation: An Analysis and Bibliography* (Edmonton, Canada: St. Stephen's College, 1977); and Gregory Mellema, *Beyond the Call of Duty: Supererogation, Obligation, and Offence* (Albany, NY: State University of New York Press, 1991).

34. Albert Camus, *The Plague,* trans. Stuart Gilbert (New York: Alfred A. Knopf, Inc., 1988), p. 278.

35. The formulation in this sentence relies in part on Rawls, *A Theory of Justice,* p. 117 (1999: 100).

36. Feinberg, "Supererogation and Rules," *Ethics* 71 (1961): 397.

37. See Bernard Lo, "Obligations to Care for Persons with Human Immunodeficiency Virus," *Issues in Law & Medicine* 4 (1988): 367–81; Doran Smolkin, "HIV Infection, Risk Taking, and the Duty to Treat," *Journal of Medicine and Philosophy* 22 (1997):

55–74; John Arras, "The Fragile Web of Responsibility: AIDS and the Duty to Treat," *Hastings Center Report* 18 (April/May 1988): S10–S20; Georgene G. Eakes and JoAnne B. Lewis, "Should Nurses be Required to Administer Care to Patients with AIDS?" *Nurse Educator* 16 (1991): 36–38; Association of Nurses in AIDS Care, "Position Paper: Duty to Care," *Journal of the Association of Nurses in AIDS Care* 2 (1991): 44; Minnesota Medical Association, Committee on Ethics and Medical–Legal Affairs, "A Physician's Ethical and Legal Obligations to Treat HIV-Infected Patients: A Report," *Minnesota Medicine* 75 (1992): 27–31; and William P. Schecter, "Surgical Care of the HIV-Infected Patient: A Moral Imperative," *Cambridge Quarterly of Healthcare Ethics* 1 (1992): 223–28.

38. See George J. Annas, "Legal Risks and Responsibilities of Physicians in the AIDS Epidemic," *Hastings Center Report* 18 (April/May 1988): 26S–32S; and American Medical Association, Council on Ethical and Judicial Affairs, "Ethical Issues Involved in the Growing AIDS Crisis," *Journal of the American Medical Association* 259 (March 4, 1988): 1360–61.

39. Health and Public Policy Committee, American College of Physicians and Infectious Diseases Society of America, "The Acquired Immunodeficiency Syndrome (AIDS) and Infection with the Human Immunodeficiency Virus (HIV)," *Annals of Internal Medicine* 108 (1988): 460–61; Norman Daniels, "Duty to Treat or Right to Refuse?," *Hastings Center Report* 21 (March/April 1991): 36–46; Edmund Pellegrino, "Altruism, Self-interest, and Medical Ethics," *Journal of the American Medical Association* 258 (1987): 1939; and Pellegrino, "Character, Virtue, and Self-Interest in the Ethics of the Professions," *Journal of Contemporary Health Law and Policy* 5 (1989): 53–73, esp. 70–71.

40. We do not claim to be presenting a distinctively Aristotelian theory, and we are motivated by objectives that contemporary Aristotelians may or may not share.

41. Urmson recognized part of this problem in "Saints and Heroes," pp. 206, 214. A telling sign of such imbalance is found in contemporary utilitarianism, which as much as any ethical theory makes exceedingly strong demands. Despite some brilliant passages on moral excellence in Mill, there has never been a systematic or even sustained utilitarian treatise on supererogation or conceptions of moral excellence.

42. Several of these sources are cited and criticized in Richard B. Brandt, "Morality and Its Critics," in his *Morality, Utilitarianism, and Rights* (Cambridge: Cambridge University Press, 1992), ch. 5. See further Tracy L. Isaacs and Diane Jeske, "Moral Deliberations, Nonmoral Ends, and the Virtuous Agent," *Ethics* 107 (1997): 486–500.

43. John Stuart Mill, *Considerations on Representative Government*, in *The Collected Works of John Stuart Mill*, vol. 19 (Toronto: University of Toronto Press, 1977), ch. 3, p. 409.

44. For example, Edith Wyschogrod defines a "saintly life" as "one in which compassion for the other, irrespective of cost to the saint, is the primary trait." Wyschogrod, *Saints and Postmodernism: Revisioning Moral Philosophy* (Chicago: University of Chicago Press, 1990), pp. xiii, xxii, et passim.

45. Urmson, "Saints and Heroes."

46. John Berger (and Jean Mohr, photographer), *A Fortunate Man: The Story of a Country Doctor* (London: Allen Lane, the Penguin Press, 1967), esp. pp. 48, 74, 82f, 93f, 123–25, 135. Lawrence Blum pointed us to this book and influenced our perspective on it.

47. Our conditions of moral excellence are indebted to Lawrence A. Blum, "Moral Exemplars," *Midwest Studies in Philosophy* 13 (1988): 204. See also Blum's "Community and Virtue," in *How Should One Live?: Essays on the Virtues*, ed. Crisp.

48. Our second and third conditions are influenced by the characterization of a saint in Susan Wolf's "Moral Saints," *Journal of Philosophy* 79 (1983): 419–39.

49. Jay Katz, ed., *Experimentation with Human Beings* (New York: Russell Sage Foundation, 1972), pp. 136–40.

50. Philip J. Hilts, "French Doctor Testing AIDS Vaccine on Self," *Washington Post*, March 10, 1987, p. A7. For a thorough discussion of self-experimentation in medicine, see Lawrence K. Altman, *Who Goes First?: The Story of Self-Experimentation in Medicine*, 2nd ed. (Berkeley: University of California Press, 1998).

51. David Hilfiker, *Not All of Us Are Saints: A Doctor's Journey with the Poor* (New York: Hill and Wang, 1994). The summaries and quotations that follow come from this book.

52. See *1999 Annual Report of the U.S. Scientific Registry for Transplant Recipients and the Organ Procurement and Transplant Network: Transplant Data: 1989–1998* (Rockville, MD: U.S. Department of Health and Human Services, Health Resources and Services Administration, Office of Special Programs, Division of Transplantation; and Richmond, VA: United Network for Organ Sharing, 1999). For evidence of the relatively low risks of living kidney donation, see John S. Najarian, et al., "20 Years or More of Follow-up of Living Kidney Donors," *The Lancet* 340 (October 3, 1992): 807–10. For a discussion of the risks of living split liver donation, see R. W. Strong and S. V. Lynch, "Ethical Issues in Living Related Donor Liver Transplantation," *Transplantation Proceedings* 28, no. 4 (August 1996): 2366–69; reprinted in *The Ethics of Organ Transplants: The Current Debate*, ed. Arthur L. Caplan and Daniel H. Coelho (Amherst, NY: Prometheus Books, 1998).

53. See Aaron Spital, "Living Organ Donation: Shifting Responsibility," *Archives of Internal Medicine* 151 (February 1991): 234.

54. For the attitudes of nephrologists, transplant nephrologists, and transplant surgeons, see Carol L. Beasley, Alan R. Hull, and J. Thomas Rosenthal, "Living Kidney Donation: A Survey of Professional Attitudes and Practices," *American Journal of Kidney Diseases* 30 (October 1997): 549–57.

55. See Aaron Spital and Max Spital, "Living Kidney Donation: Attitudes Outside the Transplant Center," *Archives of Internal Medicine* 148 (May 1988): 1077–80; and Carl H. Fellner and Shalom H. Schwartz, "Altruism in Disrepute," *New England Journal of Medicine* 284 (March 18, 1971): 582–85.

56. *1999 Annual Report of the U.S. Scientific Registry for Transplant Recipients and the Organ Procurement and Transplant Network: Transplant Data: 1989–1998*. Data were unavailable on about 25% of the 4,273 living kidney donors in 1998 and on ten of the living donors of portions of their livers in 1997. One new version of stranger donation involves the spouse of patient A donating a kidney to patient B in exchange for the spouse of patient B donating a kidney to patient A in cases where the spouses themselves do not match. Lainie Freidman Ross, David T. Rubin, Mark Siegler, et al., Sounding Board: "Ethics of a Paired-Kidney-Exchange Program," *New England Journal of Medicine* 336, No. 24 (June 12, 1997): 1751–55.

57. Evelyn Nieves, "Girl Awaits Father's 2nd Kidney, and Decision by Medical Ethicists," *New York Times*, December 5, 1999, pp. A1, A11.

58. See Roberta G. Simmons, "Psychological Reactions to Giving a Kidney," in *Psychonephrology 1*, ed. Norman B. Levy (New York: Plenum Publishing Co., 1981), p. 235.

PART II

3

Respect for Autonomy

Respect for the autonomous choices of persons runs as deep in common morality as any principle, but little agreement exists about its nature, scope, or strength. We use the concept of autonomy in this chapter to examine individuals' decision-making in health care and research, especially informed consent and refusal. This account is essential to our objectives in subsequent chapters, which fill out and qualify the principle of respect for autonomy.

Although we begin our discussion of principles of biomedical ethics with respect for autonomy, our order of presentation does not imply that this principle has priority over all other principles. A misguided criticism of our account is that the principle of respect for autonomy overrides all other moral considerations. This we firmly deny. We aim to construct a conception of respect for autonomy that is not excessively individualistic (neglecting the social nature of individuals and the impact of individual choices and actions on others), not excessively focused on reason (neglecting the emotions), and not unduly legalistic (highlighting legal rights and downplaying social practices).

The Nature of Autonomy

The word *autonomy*, derived from the Greek *autos* ("self") and *nomos* ("rule," "governance," or "law"), originally referred to the self-rule or self-governance of independent city-states. *Autonomy* has since been extended to individuals and has acquired meanings as diverse as self-governance, liberty rights, privacy, individual choice, freedom of the will, causing one's own behavior, and being one's own person. Clearly autonomy is not a univocal concept in either ordinary English or contemporary philosophy and needs to be refined in light of particular objectives.

Personal autonomy is, at a minimum, self-rule that is free from both controlling interference by others and from limitations, such as inadequate understanding, that prevent meaningful choice.[1] The autonomous individual acts freely in accordance with a self-chosen plan, analogous to the way an independent government manages its territories and sets its policies. A person of diminished autonomy, by contrast, is in some respect controlled by others or incapable of deliberating or acting on the basis of his or her desires and plans. For example, prisoners and mentally retarded individuals often have diminished autonomy. Mental incapacitation limits the autonomy of the retarded person, whereas coercive institutionalization constrains the autonomy of prisoners.

Virtually all theories of autonomy agree that two conditions are essential for autonomy: (1) *liberty* (independence from controlling influences) and (2) *agency* (capacity for intentional action). However, disagreement exists over the meaning of these two conditions and over whether additional conditions are needed. Later in this chapter, we analyze autonomy in terms of three more precise conditions that build on these two general conditions.

Theories of Autonomy

Some theories of autonomy feature the traits of the *autonomous person*, which include capacities of self-governance, such as understanding, reasoning, deliberating, and independent choosing. However, the focus in this chapter on decision-making leads us to concentrate on *autonomous choice* rather than general capacity for governance. Even autonomous persons with self-governing capacities sometimes fail to govern themselves in particular choices because of temporary constraints caused by illness or depression, or because of ignorance, coercion, or other conditions that restrict their options. An autonomous person who signs a consent form without reading or understanding the form is qualified to act autonomously, but fails to do so. Similarly, some persons who are generally not incapable of autonomous decision-making can, at times, make autonomous choices. For example, some patients in mental institutions who are unable to care for themselves and have been declared legally incompetent may make some autonomous choices, such as stating preferences for meals, refusing medications, and making telephone calls to acquaintances.

Some writers maintain that autonomy is a matter of having the capacity to reflectively control and identify with one's basic (first-order) desires or preferences through higher-level (second-order) desires or preferences.[2] For example, an alcoholic may have a desire to drink, but also a higher-order desire to stop drink-ing. An autonomous person, in this account, is one who has the capacity to ra-tionally accept, identify with, or repudiate a lower-order desire independently of others' manipulation of that desire. Such acceptance or repudiation of first-order desires at the higher level (that is, the capacity to change one's preference struc-ture) constitutes autonomy.

Serious problems confront this theory. Acceptance or repudiation of a desire can be motivated by an overriding desire that is simply *stronger*, not more *ra-tional* or *autonomous*. Second-order desires can be caused by potent first-order desires or by a condition such as alcohol addiction that is antithetical to auton-omy. If second-order desires (decisions, volitions, etc.) are generated by prior de-sires or commitments, then the process of identifying with one desire rather than another does not distinguish autonomy from nonautonomy. The second-order de-sires would not be significantly different from first-order desires.

This theory needs more than a convincing account of second-order preferences: It needs a way for ordinary persons to qualify as deserving respect for their au-tonomy, even when they have not reflected on their preferences at a higher level. Few choosers, and also few choices, would be autonomous if held to the stan-dards of higher-order reflection in this theory, which in effect presents an aspi-rational ideal of autonomy. No theory of autonomy is acceptable if it presents an ideal beyond the reach of normal choosers.

Instead of depicting an ideal of this sort, our analysis will be closely tied to nonideal moral requirements of "respect for autonomy." We analyze autonomous action in terms of normal choosers who act (1) intentionally, (2) with under-standing, and (3) without controlling influences that determine their action. The first of these three conditions of autonomy is not a matter of degree: Acts are ei-ther intentional or nonintentional. However, acts can satisfy both the conditions of understanding and absence of controlling influences to a greater or lesser ex-tent. Actions, therefore, can be autonomous by degrees, as a function of satisfy-ing these two conditions to different degrees. For both conditions, a broad continuum exists on which autonomy goes from being fully present to being wholly absent. Many children and many elderly patients, for example, exhibit various degrees of understanding and independence found on this continuum and thus varying degrees of autonomous action.[3]

For an action to be autonomous in this account, it needs only a substantial de-gree of understanding and freedom from constraint, not a full understanding or a complete absence of influence. To restrict adequate decision-making by pa-tients and research subjects to the ideal of fully or completely autonomous decision-making strips their acts of any meaningful place in the practical world, where people's actions are rarely, if ever, fully autonomous. A person's appreci-ation of information and independence from controlling influences in the con-text of health care need not exceed, for example, a person's information and independence in making a financial investment, hiring a new employee, buying a house, or selecting a university. Such consequential decisions must be *substantially* autonomous, but not necessarily *fully* autonomous.

The line between what is substantial and what is insubstantial often appears arbitrary. However, thresholds marking substantially autonomous decisions can be carefully fixed in light of specific objectives, such as meaningful decision-making. Patients and research subjects can achieve substantial autonomy in their decisions, just as substantially autonomous choice occurs in other areas of life, such as buying a house or choosing a university to attend. Accordingly, appropriate criteria of substantial autonomy are best addressed in a particular context.

Autonomy, Authority, and Community

Some theorists have argued that autonomous action is incompatible with the authority of states, religious organizations, and other communities that legislate persons' decisions. They maintain that autonomous persons must act on their own reasons and can never submit to an authority or choose to be ruled by others without losing their autonomy.[4] We believe, however, that no fundamental inconsistency exists between autonomy and authority, because individuals can exercise their autonomy in choosing to accept an institution, tradition, or community that they view as a legitimate source of direction. Having welcomed the authority of his or her religious institution, a Jehovah's Witness can refuse a recommended blood transfusion, and a Roman Catholic can choose against an abortion. As we saw in Chapter 1, morality is not a set of personal rules created by individuals. That we share moral principles in no way prevents them from being *our* principles. Individuals autonomously accept moral notions that derive from cultural traditions. Rules or codes of professional ethics are also not an individual's invention, and they, too, are compatible with the exercise of autonomy.

We encounter many problems of autonomy in medical contexts because of the patient's dependent condition and the medical professional's authoritative position. On some occasions, authority and autonomy are incompatible, but not because the two *concepts* are incompatible. Conflict arises because authority has not been properly delegated or accepted. In these instances, the patient's autonomy may be compromised because the physician has assumed an unwarranted degree of authority over his or her patient.

Some critics of the prominent role of autonomy in biomedical ethics charge that it focuses too narrowly on the self as independent and rationally controlling. They question the model of an independent, rational will that is inattentive to emotions, communal life, reciprocity, and the development of persons over time. For instance, some feminist critics view moral theories that focus on autonomous agents and actions as unrealistic and even pernicious, particularly if they place a supreme and overriding value on autonomy and interpret it in masculine ways.[5]

However, in recent years some feminists have sought both to affirm autonomy and to revise individualistic or atomistic conceptions of autonomy through ideas of "relational autonomy" that center on the conviction that "persons are socially embedded and that agents' identities are formed within the context of social relationships and shaped by a complex of intersecting social determinants, such as race, class, gender, and ethnicity." These accounts maintain that "oppressive socialization and oppressive social relationships" can impair autonomy, for instance, through forming an agent's desires, beliefs, emotions, and attitudes, through thwarting the development of the capacities and competencies essential for autonomy, and through various restrictions and limitations on the range of options for action.

We support calls for overturning oppressive socialization and relationships, and note that they promote relational autonomy and do not reject autonomy altogether.[6]

The Triumph or Failure of Autonomy?

Some writers lament in different ways the "triumph of autonomy" in American bioethics. They charge that autonomy's proponents force choices on patients, though many patients do not want to receive information about their condition or to make their own decisions. For instance, Carl Schneider claims that proponents of autonomy, whom he labels "autonomists," are less concerned with what patients *do want* than with what, from the point of view of autonomy, they *should want*." Schneider attempts to correct these views by appealing to human experience and empirical research, including quantitative studies of medical care, studies in medical sociology, psychological research, and the memoirs of patients and their families. After reviewing certain empirical studies, Schneider concludes that, "while patients largely wish to be informed about their medical circumstances, a substantial number of them [especially the elderly and the very sick] do not want to make their own medical decisions, or perhaps even to participate in those decisions in any very significant way."[7]

While it is true that some writers in bioethics seem to affirm a duty of medical decision-making by patients,[8] we do not. We defend a principle of respect for autonomy with a correlative *right* to choose (not a mandatory *duty* to choose).[9] Several recent empirical studies of the sort cited by Schneider also seem to misunderstand how autonomous choice functions in a theory such as ours and how it should function in clinical medicine. In one study, U.C.L.A. researchers examined the differences in the attitudes of elderly subjects (sixty-five years or older) from different ethnic backgrounds toward (1) disclosure of the diagnosis and prognosis of a terminal illness, and (2) decision-making at the end of life.[10] The researchers summarize their main findings, based on 800 subjects (200 from each ethnic group): "Korean Americans (47%) and Mexican-Americans (65%)

were significantly less likely than European Americans (87%) and African Americans (88%) to believe that a patient should be told the diagnosis of metastatic cancer. Korean Americans (35%) and Mexican Americans (48%) were less likely than African-Americans (63%) to believe that a patient should be told of a terminal prognosis and less likely to believe that the patient should make decisions about the use of life-supporting technology (28% and 41% vs. 60% and 65%). Korean-Americans and Mexican-Americans tended to believe that the family should make decisions about the use of life support." Ethnicity was the primary factor correlated with attitudes toward disclosure and decision-making. Secondary factors were years of education and personal experience with illness and withholding or withdrawing treatment.

Investigators in this study stress that "belief in the *ideal* of patient autonomy is far from universal" (our emphasis), and they contrast that ideal with a "family-centered model" that focuses on an individual's web of relationships and tends to place a higher value on "the harmonious functioning of the family than on the autonomy of its individual members." However, this analysis may be misleading. The investigators themselves conclude that "physicians should ask their patients if they wish to receive information and make decisions or if they prefer that their families handle such matters."[11] Far from abandoning or supplanting the commitment to respect individual autonomy, this recommendation accepts its central condition that the choice is rightly the patient's. Even if the patient delegates that right to someone else, the choice to delegate is itself autonomous.

In a second study, this time of Navajo values and ways of thinking regarding the disclosure of risk and medical prognoses, two researchers sought to learn how health care providers "should approach the discussion of negative information with Navajo patients" in order to provide "more culturally appropriate medical care."[12] Frequent conflicts emerge, according to these researchers, between autonomy and the traditional Navajo conception that "thought and language have the power to shape reality and to control events." According to the traditional conception, telling a Navajo patient who has recently been diagnosed with a disease about the potential complications of that disease may actually produce those complications, because "language does not merely describe reality, language shapes reality." Traditional Navajo patients may "regard the discussion of negative information as potentially harmful." They expect a "positive ritual language" that promotes or restores health.

One middle-aged Navajo nurse reported that a surgeon had explained the risks of bypass surgery to her father in such a way that he refused to undergo the procedure: "The surgeon told him that he may not wake up, that this is the risk of every surgery. For the surgeon it was very routine, but the way that my Dad received it, it was almost like a death sentence, and he never consented to the surgery." Because of this characteristic Navajo discomfort with information about risks, the researchers found "ethically troublesome" those policies that, in com-

pliance with the Patient Self-Determination Act, attempt to "expose all hospitalized Navajo patients to the idea, if not the practice, of advance care planning."

These two studies—and numerous other studies over the last several years—
enrich our understanding of diverse cultural beliefs and values that affect what
particular communities and individuals hold and do. However, several of these
studies reflect a misinterpretation of what the principle of respect for autonomy
and many laws and policies propose. They mistakenly view their results as op-
posing, rather than enriching, the principle of respect for autonomy.

A more adequate interpretation of respecting autonomy will put these problems to rest. There is a fundamental obligation to ensure that patients have the
right to choose, as well as the right to accept or to decline information. Forced
information, forced choice, and evasive disclosure are inconsistent with this obligation. From this perspective, there is a tension between the two studies discussed
above. One study recommends inquiring in advance to ascertain patients' preferences regarding information and decision-making, while the other suggests (ten-
uously) that even being informed of a right to decide may be harmful. The tricky
practical question is whether it is possible to inform patients of their rights to
know and to decide without compromising their systems of belief and value or
otherwise disrespecting them. Health professionals should always inquire in general terms about their patients' wishes to receive information and to make decisions, and they should never assume that because a patient belongs to a particular
community, he or she affirms that community's world view and values. The fundamental requirement is to respect a particular person's autonomous choices. Respect for autonomy is not a mere *ideal* in health care; it is a professional
obligation. Autonomous choice is a *right*, not a *duty* of patients.

The Principle of Respect for Autonomy

To respect an autonomous agent is, at a minimum, to acknowledge that person's
right to hold views, to make choices, and to take actions based on personal values and beliefs. Such respect involves respectful *action*, not merely a respectful
attitude. It also requires more than noninterference in others' personal affairs. It
includes, at least in some contexts, obligations to build up or maintain others'
capacities for autonomous choice while helping to allay fears and other conditions that destroy or disrupt their autonomous actions. Respect, on this account,
involves acknowledging decision-making rights and enabling persons to act autonomously, whereas disrespect for autonomy involves attitudes and actions that
ignore, insult, or demean others' rights of autonomy.

Why is such respect owed to persons? In Chapter 8, we examine two philosophers who have influenced contemporary interpretations of respect for autonomy:
Immanuel Kant and John Stuart Mill. Kant argued that respect for autonomy
flows from the recognition that all persons have unconditional worth, each hav-

ing the capacity to determine his or her own moral destiny.[13] To violate a person's autonomy is to treat that person merely as a means, that is, in accordance with others' goals without regard to that person's own goals. Mill was primarily concerned about the "individuality" of autonomous agents. He argued that society should permit individuals to develop according to their convictions, as long as they do not interfere with a like expression of freedom by others; but he also insisted that we sometimes are obligated to seek to persuade others when they have false or ill-considered views.[14] Mill's position requires both not interfering with and actively strengthening autonomous expression, whereas Kant's entails a moral imperative of respectful treatment of persons as ends in themselves. In their different ways, these two philosophies both support the principle of respect for autonomy.

This principle can be stated as a negative obligation and as a positive obligation. As a *negative* obligation: *Autonomous actions should not be subjected to controlling constraints by others.* The principle asserts a broad, abstract obligation that is free of exceptive clauses, such as, "We must respect individuals' views and rights *so long as their thoughts and actions do not seriously harm other persons.*" This principle of respect for autonomy needs specification in particular contexts to become a practical guide to conduct, and appropriate specification will, in due course, incorporate valid exceptions. Part of this process of specification will appear in rights and obligations of liberty, privacy, confidentiality, truthfulness, and informed consent (several of which receive sustained attention in Chapter 7).

As a *positive* obligation, this principle requires respectful treatment in disclosing information and fostering autonomous decision-making. In some cases, we are obligated to increase the options available to persons. Many autonomous actions could not occur without others' material cooperation in making options available. Respect for autonomy obligates professionals in health care and research involving human subjects to disclose information, to probe for and ensure understanding and voluntariness, and to foster adequate decision-making. As some contemporary Kantians declare, the demand that we treat others as ends requires that we assist persons in achieving their ends and foster their capacities as agents, not merely that we avoid treating them solely as means to our ends.[15]

Temptations sometimes arise in health care for physicians and other professionals to foster or perpetuate patients' dependency, rather than to promote their autonomy. But discharging the obligation to respect patients' autonomy requires equipping them to overcome their sense of dependence and achieve as much control as possible and as they desire. These positive obligations of respect for autonomy derive, in part, from the special fiduciary obligations that health care professionals have to their patients and researchers to their subjects.

Because of various ways in which these negative and positive sides of respect for autonomy function in the moral life, they are capable of supporting many more specific moral rules. (Other principles, such as beneficence and nonmalef-icence, sometimes help justify some of these same rules.) Examples include the following:

1. Tell the truth.
2. Respect the privacy of others.
3. Protect confidential information.
4. Obtain consent for interventions with patients.
5. When asked, help others make important decisions.

Respect for autonomy has only prima facie standing and can sometimes be overridden by competing moral considerations. Examples include the following: If our choices endanger the public health, potentially harm others, or require a scarce resource for which no funds are available, others can justifiably restrict our exercises of autonomy. The principle of respect for autonomy does not by it-self determine what, on balance, a person ought to be free to know or do or what counts as a valid justification for constraining autonomy. For example, in Case 2 (see Appendix), a patient with an inoperable, incurable carcinoma asks, "I don't have cancer, do I?" The physician lies, saying, "You're as good as you were ten years ago." This lie denies the patient information he may need to determine his future course of action, thereby infringing the principle of respect for autonomy. Though controversial, the lie on balance may be justified (in this context by a principle of beneficence).

Our obligations to respect autonomy do not extend to persons who cannot act in a sufficiently autonomous manner (and cannot be rendered autonomous) be-cause they are immature, incapacitated, ignorant, coerced, or exploited. Infants, irrationally suicidal individuals, and drug-dependent persons are examples. Those who vigorously defend rights of autonomy in biomedical ethics, as do the pres-ent authors, do not deny that many forms of intervention are justified if persons are substantially nonautonomous and cannot be rendered autonomous for spe-cific decisions. We will return to this problem of using respect for autonomy as a canopy to protect nonautonomous persons in this chapter's final section (and in Chapter 5, where we discuss justifiable paternalistic interventions).

Complexities in Respecting Autonomy and Consent/Refusal

Varieties of autonomous consent. The basic paradigm of autonomy in health care, research, politics, and other contexts is *express* consent. However, this paradigm captures only one form of consent. Another form is *tacit* consent, which is ex-pressed silently or passively by omissions. For example, if residents of a long-term-care facility are asked whether they object to having the time of dinner changed by one hour, a uniform lack of objection constitutes consent (assuming the residents understand the proposal and the need for their consent). Similarly, *implicit* or *implied* consent is inferred from actions. Consent to one medical procedure is often implicit in a specific consent to another procedure, and voluntarily seeking treatment at a teaching hospital may imply consent to various roles for physicians, nurses, and others in training. *Presumed* consent is generally held to be another variety, although if consent is presumed on the basis of what we know about a particular person's choices or values, it reduces to either implied or express consent. By contrast, if consent is presumed on the basis of a general theory of human goods or of the rational will, the moral situation is more problematic. Consent should refer to an individual's actual choices, not to presumptions about the choices the individual would or should make.

Consider two situations in which non-express forms of consent—namely, implicit consent and presumed consent—are sometimes deemed morally relevant, even though their connection to autonomous choice is tenuous. In current debates about organ procurement, concern exists that requirements of express consent by the decedent while alive or by the family after a relative's death impair rather than facilitate collection of needed organs. Several countries have adopted what is variously called "presumed," "tacit," or "implicit consent" for solid organs, and several states in the United States have done likewise for corneas (in specified situations, such as mandatory autopsy). The moral rationale for the medical examiner's removal of corneas where decedents have not registered their opposition is typically tacit consent. However, if no evidence of tacit consent exists—for example, if the decedents were unaware of the law—then the practice either falls under another form of consent or simply expropriates organs without regard to consent. It is difficult to see how consent to donation is implicit in the decedent's actions while alive, and presumed consent based on a theory of human goods is not bona fide consent. Thus, the principle of respect for autonomy is sometimes unjustifiably invoked through fictions of consent that are misleading and dangerous. (A related and also risky overextension of consent language refers to a cadaveric source of organs for transplantation as a "donor" when he or she never "donated," that is, never chose to donate.)

Another controversy about non-express forms of consent appears in the testing of hospital admittees for antibodies to the human immunodeficiency virus (HIV), which causes AIDS. If a newly admitted hospital patient gives express consent when asked for permission to perform an HIV-antibody test, the staff is authorized to proceed. If a patient is silent when told the test will be performed unless he or she objects, silence constitutes valid tacit consent, as long as understanding and voluntariness are present. But if the question is not asked, the patient's failure to object to the test cannot be presumed to be a consent without additional information.

Suppose, to alter the case, that a patient has given consent for *routine blood tests*. Do health care professionals now have the patient's valid consent for an *HIV test*? Here the appeal might be to a specific consent implicit in the general consent to blood tests (or to admission to the hospital). There are reasons to be suspicious of this claim, because, as we shall now see, express consent is the only appropriate consent in these circumstances. Even if a patient's blood has already been drawn with consent, the HIV test carries psychological and social risks. For a seropositive individual, the psychological risks include anxiety and depression, and the social risks include stigma, discrimination, and breaches of confidentiality.[16] Because of these potential consequences, hospitals are not justified in testing patients for HIV antibodies without express consent. Although appeals to fictions such as deemed consent are common, it is more defensible to argue straightforwardly that a patient's autonomy, liberty, privacy, or confidentiality can be *justifiably overridden* to obtain information about an individual's HIV-antibody status in order to protect a health care provider who has been exposed to the risk of infection.

The varieties of consent we have examined point to a fundamental question that pervades this chapter: Who should seek what kind of consent from whom and for what? The principle of respect for autonomy does not entail that in health care and research only first-person, express, informed consent is applicable. Other varieties of consent may have their place. The question concerns when each form of consent is acceptable. For instance, debates about training health professionals in intubation procedures by using newly dead patients and about genetic research on anonymous tissue samples that have been stored following diagnostic or therapeutic procedures center on whether any consent is required at all and, if so, from whom and in what form.[17]

Consents and refusals over time. Beliefs and choices shift over time. Moral and interpretive problems arise when a person's present choices contradict his or her prior choices, which in some cases were explicitly designed to prevent future changes of mind from affecting an outcome. In one case, a 28-year-old man decided to terminate chronic renal dialysis because of his restricted lifestyle and the burdens on his family. He had diabetes, was legally blind, and could not walk because of progressive neuropathy. His wife and physician agreed to provide medication to relieve his pain and further agreed not to put him back on dialysis, even if he requested this action under the influence of pain or other bodily changes. (Increased amounts of urea in the blood, which result from kidney failure, can sometimes lead to altered mental states, for example.) While dying in the hospital, the patient awoke complaining of pain and asked to be put back on dialysis. The patient's wife and physician decided to act on the patient's earlier request not to intervene, and he died four hours later.[18] Although their decision was understandable, respect for autonomy suggests that the spouse and physician should have put the patient back on dialysis to flush the urea out of his blood stream and thereby determine if he had autonomously revoked his prior choice. If the patient later indicated that he had not revoked his prior choice, he could have refused again, thereby providing the caregivers with increased assurance about his settled preferences.

A key question in this and many other cases is whether people have autonomously revoked their prior decisions. Discerning whether particular actions are autonomous may depend, in part, on whether they are in character or out of character. Consider, for example, a woman's sudden and unexpected decision to discontinue dialysis even though she has displayed considerable courage and zest for life despite years of disability. The abrupt and unexpected change is evidence, but not necessarily decisive evidence, that her decision may not be adequately autonomous. Actions are more likely to be substantially autonomous if they are in character (e.g., when a committed Jehovah's Witness refuses a blood transfusion), but acting in character is not a necessary condition of autonomy. At most, actions that are out of character can raise caution flags that warn others to seek explanations and probe more deeply into whether the actions are autonomous.

Another factor in some cases is a patient's anticipated future approval of a course of action to which he or she cannot or will not now consent. Sometimes physicians and other health professionals believe, with good reason, that if they can get a patient through a particular crisis, he or she will be glad to be alive or to have reached another level of function. In a well-known case, Donald (Dax) Cowart received treatment against his wishes for severe burns and was subsequently glad to be alive and did not want to end his life. Nonetheless, he has steadfastly refused to ratify or provide retrospective approval for the physicians' and other health professionals' actions on the grounds that they wrongfully denied his right to make his own choice, whether that choice was shortsighted or not.[19]

Future or "deferred consent"—which means consent to another's action after it has already occurred—is not consent in a meaningful sense. It is merely an anticipated outcome that reassures health professionals that they are acting in the patient's best interests. Such "consent" becomes even more problematic in research. In a typical situation, researchers have been unable to determine which medications and procedures will most effectively treat severe head injuries, but it is impossible to obtain the injured person's consent upon arrival in an emergency room—and often impossible to get his or her family's permission in the time available. A patient's subsequent or deferred consent is an autonomous authorization that continues what has already been started, but it does not retroactively authorize the research's initiation.[20]

Problems about personal identity and continuity. Related issues arise about whether and to what extent we should honor the prior decisions and projects of persons who have died. For example, concerns exist about proper respect for the dead in autopsy, transplantation, research, and medical education, including dissection. Other issues surround advance directives by patients who can be expected to survive, but never to regain competence. Underlying theoretical issues concern personal identity and continuity of the self over time. Stated in an extreme form, the problem is that later selves can evolve to be so different from earlier selves that they are, in effect, two different people. If so, it appears unfair for self 1 to bind self 2 through an advance directive (e.g., when severe dementia produces radical changes).[21] A radical discontinuity thesis set out to protect a second self is attractive in the case of many vulnerable patients, but its plausibility and relevance in ethics diminish when we try to envision ways to mark the point of discontinuity in order to draw the line between different selves and to determine thereby when advance directives become inapplicable. As with respect for prior wishes of the now-deceased, we are, except in rare cases, obligated to respect the previously expressed autonomous wishes of the now severely nonautonomous person because of our respect for the autonomy of the person who made the decision.

The Capacity for Autonomous Choice

Many patients and potential subjects are not competent to give a valid consent. Inquiries about competence focus on whether patients or potential subjects are capable, psychologically or legally, of adequate decision-making. Competence in decision-making is closely connected to autonomous decision-making, as well as to the validity of consent. Several commentators distinguish judgments of capacity from judgments of competence on the grounds that health professionals assess capacity and incapacity, whereas courts determine competence and incompetence. However, as Thomas Grisso and Paul Appelbaum note, this distinction breaks down in practice: "When clinicians determine that a patient lacks decision-making capacity, the practical consequences may be the same as those attending a legal determination of incompetence."[22]

The Gatekeeping Function of Competence Judgments

Competence judgments serve a gatekeeping role in health care by distinguishing persons whose decisions should be solicited or accepted from persons whose decisions need not or should not be solicited or accepted. Health professionals' judgments of a person's incompetence may lead them to override that person's decisions, to turn to informal surrogates for decision-making, to ask the court to appoint a guardian to protect his or her interests, to seek involuntary institutionalization, and the like. When a court establishes legal incompetence, it appoints a surrogate decision maker with either partial or plenary (full) authority over the incompetent individual. Physicians and other health professionals do not have the authority to declare patients incompetent as a matter of law, but, within limits, they often have the de facto power to override or constrain patients' decisions about care. Their judgments about incompetence are rarely challenged in court.[23]

Competence judgments have the distinctive *normative* role of qualifying or disqualifying persons for certain decisions or actions, but these judgments are sometimes incorrectly presented as *empirical* findings. For example, a person who appears irrational or unreasonable to others might fail a psychiatric test, and so be declared incompetent. The test is an empirical measuring device, but normative judgments determine how to use the test to sort persons into the two classes of competent and incompetent. The judgments are normative because they concern how persons ought to be or may permissibly be treated.

The Concept of Competence[24]

Some commentators hold that we lack a single acceptable *definition* of competence and a single acceptable *standard* of competence. They contend that no nonarbitrary *test* exists to distinguish between competent and incompetent persons. However, *definitions, standards*, and *tests* should be kept distinct. We confine attention for the moment to the problem of definition.

A single core meaning of the word *competence* applies in all contexts. That meaning is "the ability to perform a task."[25] By contrast to this core meaning, the *criteria* of particular competencies vary from context to context because the criteria are relative to specific tasks. The criteria for someone's competence to stand trial, to raise dachshunds, to write checks, or to lecture to medical students are radically different. The competence to decide is therefore relative to the particular decision to be made. A person should rarely be judged incompetent with respect to every sphere of life. We usually need to consider only some type of competence, such as the competence to decide about treatment or about participation in research. These judgments of competence and incompetence affect only a limited range of decision-making. For example, a person who is incompetent to decide about financial affairs may be competent to decide to participate in medical research or able to handle simple tasks easily while faltering before complex ones. Competence is therefore best understood as specific rather than global: It depends not only on a person's abilities but also on how that person's abilities match the particular decision-making task he or she confronts.

Competence may vary over time and be intermittent. Many persons are incompetent to do something at one point in time but competent to perform the same task at another point in time. Judgments of competence about such persons can be complicated by the need to distinguish categories of illness that result in chronic changes of intellect, language, or memory from those characterized by rapid reversibility of these functions, as in the case of transient ischemic attack, transient global amnesia, and the like. In some of the latter cases, competence varies from hour to hour. If a patient's level of competence cannot be established at first, it is appropriate to evaluate that patient's understanding, deliberative capacity, and coherence over time.

Intermittent competence and specific competence are evident in the following case. A woman involuntarily hospitalized because of periods of confusion and loss of memory is competent most of the time to perform ordinary tasks. However, a court must determine whether health professionals can provide this legally incompetent patient with an alternative medical therapy suitable to her condition.[26] In such cases, a declaration of *specific incompetence* may prevent vague generalizations that exclude persons from all forms of decision-making.

These conceptual observations have practical significance. The law has traditionally presumed that a person who is incompetent to manage his or her estate is also incompetent to vote, make medical decisions, get married, and the like. Such laws were usually designed to protect *property* rather than persons, and so were ill-suited to medical decision-making. Their global sweep, based on a total judgment of the person, has at times extended too far. In one classic case, a physician argued that a patient was incompetent to make decisions because of epilepsy,[27] although in fact many persons who suffer from epilepsy are competent in most contexts. Such judgments defy much that we now know about the etiology of various forms of incompetence, even in hard cases of mentally retarded individuals, psychotic patients, and patients with uncontrollably painful afflictions. In addition, persons who are incompetent by virtue of dementia, alcoholism, immaturity, and mental retardation present radically different types and problems of incompetence.

Sometimes a competent person who is generally able to select means appropriate to reach his or her goals will act incompetently in a particular circumstance. Consider the following actual case of a patient who is hospitalized with an acute disk problem and whose goal is to control back pain. The patient has decided to manage the problem by wearing a brace, a method she has used successfully in the past. She believes strongly that she should return to this treatment modality. This approach conflicts, however, with her physician's unwavering and insistent advocacy of surgery. When the physician—an eminent surgeon who alone in her city is suited to treat her—asks her to sign the surgical permit, she is psychologically unable to refuse. The patient's hopes are vested in this assertive and, in her view, powerful and authoritative physician. Her illness increases both her hopes and her fears, and, in addition, she has a passive personality. In these circumstances, it is psychologically too risky for her to act as she desires. Even though she is competent to choose in general, she is not competent to choose on this occasion because she lacks the capacity.

This analysis indicates that the concept of competence in decision-making has close ties to the concept of autonomy. Patients or subjects are competent to make a decision if they have the capacity to understand the material information, to make a judgment about the information in light of their values, to intend a certain outcome, and to communicate freely their wishes to care givers or investigators. Law, medicine, and, to some extent, philosophy presume a context in which the characteristics of the competent person are also the properties possessed by the autonomous person. Although *autonomy* and *competence* are different in meaning (*autonomy* meaning self-governance; *competence* meaning the ability to perform a task or range of tasks), the criteria of the autonomous person and of the competent person are strikingly similar. Two plausible hypotheses resulting from this similarity are that an autonomous person is (necessarily) a competent person (for making decisions) and that judgments about whether a person is competent to authorize or refuse an intervention should be based on whether that person can choose autonomously in particular circumstances.

Persons are more and less able to perform a specific task to the extent that they possess a certain level or range of abilities, just as persons are more and less intelligent and athletic. For example, in the emergency room, an experienced and knowledgeable patient is likely to be more qualified to consent to a procedure than a frightened, inexperienced patient. This ability continuum runs from full mastery through various levels of partial proficiency to complete ineptitude. It is confusing to view this continuum in terms of degrees of *competency*. For practical and policy reasons, we need threshold levels below which a person with a certain level of abilities is incompetent.[28] Not all competent persons are equally able and not all incompetent persons equally unable, but competence determinations sort persons into these two basic classes, and thus treat persons as either competent or incompetent for specific purposes. Above the threshold, we treat persons as equally competent; below the threshold we treat them as equally incompetent. Gatekeepers test to determine who is above and who is below the threshold. Where we draw the line will depend on the particular tasks involved.[29]

Standards of Competence

Questions about competence often center on standards for its determination—that is, the conditions a competence judgment must satisfy. Standards of competence feature mental skills or capacities closely connected to the attributes of autonomous persons, such as cognitive skills and independence of judgment. In criminal law, civil law, and clinical medicine, standards for competence cluster around various abilities to comprehend and process information and to reason about the consequences of one's actions. In medical contexts, for example, a person is usually considered competent if able to understand a therapeutic or research procedure, to deliberate regarding its major risks and benefits, and to make a decision in light of this deliberation. If a person lacks any of these capacities, then his or her competence to decide, consent, or refuse is thrown into doubt.

Troublesome questions arise about how to classify persons who merely have a diminished capacity to understand, deliberate, or decide. Some patients have a significant capacity to understand, deliberate, and reach conclusions, and yet, because they fall below the threshold, are not competent. For example, some religious fanatics and psychotic patients have fictitious and delusional beliefs that drive their actions; yet they have a wide range of capacities to understand, deliberate, and decide. Another example is found in patients with a low IQ as a result of meningitis at an early age. These patients may still have a significant capacity to decide about an intervention such as intubation or catheterization.

The following case illustrates some difficulties encountered in attempts to judge competence. A man who generally exhibits normal behavior patterns is involuntarily committed to a mental institution as the result of bizarre self-destructive behavior (pulling out an eye and cutting off a hand). This behavior results from his unusual religious beliefs. He is judged incompetent, despite his generally competent behavior and despite the fact that his peculiar actions follow "reasonably" from his religious beliefs.[30] We cannot interpret this troublesome case in terms of intermittent competence. While analysis in terms of limited competence might at first appear plausible, such an analysis entails that persons with unorthodox or bizarre religious beliefs are less than competent, even if they reason clearly in light of their beliefs. This approach is morally perilous and fails as a policy (without specific and careful qualification).

Rival standards of incompetence. The following schema expresses the range of *in*abilities currently required by competing standards of *in*competence.[31] These standards range progressively from one requiring the least ability to the other end of the spectrum.

1. Inability to express or communicate a preference or choice
2. Inability to understand one's situation and its consequences
3. Inability to understand relevant information
4. Inability to give a reason
5. Inability to give a rational reason (although some supporting reasons may be given)
6. Inability to give risk/benefit-related reasons (although some rational supporting reasons may be given)
7. Inability to reach a reasonable decision (as judged, for example, by a reasonable person standard)

These standards cluster around three kinds of abilities or skills. Standard 1 looks for the simple ability to state a preference—a noticeably weak standard. Standards 2 and 3 probe for abilities to understand information and to appreciate one's situation. Standards 4–7 look for the ability to reason through a consequential life decision, although only standard 7 restricts the range of acceptable outcomes of a reasoning process. These standards have been and still are used, either alone or in combination, in order to determine incompetence.[32]

Testing for incompetence. A clinical need exists to select one or more of these general standards and to turn it into an operational test of incompetence that establishes passing and failing grades. Dementia rating scales, mental status exams, and similar devices test for factors such as time-and-place orientation, memory, understanding, and coherence. These tests are clinical assessments that are generally administered when incompetence is suspected. Although these tests are empirical, normative judgments underlie each test. The following ingredients involve normative judgments:[33]

1. Establishing the relevant abilities for competence
2. Fixing a threshold level of the abilities in item 1
3. Accepting an empirical test for item 2.

More specifically, for any test accepted under item 3, it is an empirical question whether someone possesses the requisite level of abilities, but this question can only be asked and answered if other criteria have already been fixed under items 1 and 2. Institutional rules or traditions establish these criteria, which, nevertheless, should be open to further review and modification. Even established criteria could have been different and can shift over time.

Physicians and other health professionals informally assess patients' competence in various interactions. However, good reasons often support an independent assessment of competence, especially when the usual assessors may have a conflict of interest. With regard to potential research subjects who have mental disorders that may affect their decision-making capacity, and who are being considered for research that involves greater than minimal risk, the U.S. National Bioethics Advisory Commission (NBAC) has recommended that researchers indicate to Institutional Review Boards (IRBs) *who* will conduct the capacity assessment and *which methods* they will employ. Because of its concerns about assessors' potential conflicts of interest, NBAC recommends that IRBs require that "an independent, qualified professional assess the potential subject's capacity to consent," unless investigators can provide good reasons for an alternative method.[34]

The Sliding-Scale Strategy

Properties of autonomy and of mental and psychological capacity are not the only criteria used in fashioning competence standards. Many policies use pragmatic criteria of efficiency, feasibility, and social acceptability to determine whether a person is competent or has given a valid authorization. For example, age has conventionally been used as an operational criterion of valid authorization. Established thresholds of age vary in accordance with a community's standards, with the degree of risk involved, and with the importance of the prospective benefits. Such criteria are used to protect immature or mistake-prone persons against making decisions that fail to promote their best interest. From this perspective, standards of competence should be connected closely to levels of experience, maturity, responsibility, and welfare.

Some writers offer a sliding-scale strategy to realize this goal. They argue that, as an intervention in medicine increases the risks for patients, we should raise the level of ability required for a judgment of competence to elect or refuse the intervention. As the consequences for well-being become less substantial, we should lower the level of capacity required for competence. The sliding-scale approach allows standards of competence in decision-making to slide with risk. For example, Grisso and Appelbaum present a "competence balance scale." An "autonomy" cup is suspended from the end of one arm of this scale, and a "protection" cup is suspended from the other; the fulcrum is set initially to give more weight to the "autonomy" cup. The balancing judgment depends "on the balance of (1) the patient's abilities in the face of the decisional demands, weighed against (2) the probable gain-risk status of the patient's treatment choice, (3) when the fulcrum is set to favor autonomy."[35] If a serious risk, such as death is present, then we need a stringent standard of competence; if a low or insignificant risk is present, then we may use a relaxed or lower standard of competence. Thus, the same person—a child, for example—might be competent to decide whether to take a tranquilizer but incompetent to decide whether to authorize an appendectomy.[36]

Such a sliding-scale strategy is attractive in many ways. A decision about which standard to use to determine competence for decision-making depends on several factors, and these factors are often risk-related. All methods for setting standards of incompetence encounter difficult questions about whether to emphasize respecting the patient's autonomy or protecting the patient from harm—a moral rather than a medical choice. If an institution is especially concerned about preventing abuses of autonomy, it might accept standard 1 in the section above on "Rival Standards of Incompetence" as the only valid standard of incompetence, or perhaps it would accept only standards 1, 2, and 3. But if its primary concern is that sick patients receive the best medical treatment possible, it might hold that patients who have any of the seven inabilities is incompetent. Those who accept a stringent standard of competence (such as 6 and 7) will place patients' welfare or medical interests and safety above their autonomy interests.

The sliding-scale strategy rightly recognizes that our interests in ensuring good outcomes legitimately contribute to the way that we inquire about and create standards for judging persons competent or incompetent. If the consequences for welfare are grave, our need to be able to certify that the patient possesses the requisite capacities increases; but if little in the way of welfare is at stake, we might lower the level of capacity required for decision-making. For example, if a patient with a reversible dementia needs enteral nutrition to recover, a powerful reason exists for protecting that patient against rash or imprudent decision-making and thus for adopting a rigid standard of competence. However, the standard of competence might be relaxed if the dementia were irreversible, the illness were terminal, and the physician's primary purpose in using enteral nutrition were simply to make the patient comfortable.

The sliding-scale strategy is generally a sound protective device. However, it will create confusion about the nature of both competence judgments and competence itself because of its conceptual and moral difficulties. This strategy suggests that a person's *competence* to decide is contingent on the decision's importance or upon some harm that might follow from the decision—a dubious thesis. A person's competence to decide whether to participate in cancer research does not depend upon the decision's consequences. As risks increase or decrease, we can legitimately increase or reduce the rules, procedures, or measures we use to *ascertain* whether someone is competent; but in formulating what we are doing, we need to distinguish between a person's competence and our modes of ascertaining that person's competence.[37]

Leading proponents of the sliding-scale strategy hold just the reverse—namely, that *competence* itself varies with risk. According to the most meticulous and convincing proponents of this strategy, Allen Buchanan and Dan Brock,

> Because the appropriate level of competence properly required for a particular decision must be adjusted to the consequences of acting on that decision, no single standard of decision making competence is adequate. Instead, the level of competence appropriately required for decision making varies along a full range from low/minimum to high/maximal. . . . The greater the risk relative to other alternatives . . . the greater the level of communication, understanding, and reasoning skills required for competence to make that decision. . . . [38]

This account is conceptually and morally perilous. It is correct to say that the threshold level of competence to decide will rise as the complexity or difficulty of a task increases (deciding about spinal fusion, say, as contrasted with deciding whether to take a minor tranquilizer). However, the level of competence to decide does not rise as the risk of an outcome increases. It is confusing to blend a decision's complexity or difficulty with the risk at stake. No basis exists for believing that risky decisions require more ability at decision-making than less risky decisions. To the contrary, a solid basis exists for believing that many non-risky decisions require more ability at decision-making than many risky decisions. For persons whose competence is in question, it also seems disrespectful of their autonomy to say, in effect, "You are competent to decide what to do with your children, what to do with your financial affairs, and whether to be in this hospital, but you are not competent to refuse to be intubated or catheterized because of the increased risk."[39]

We can avoid these problems by recognizing that the level of *evidence* for determining competence should vary according to risk, while competence itself varies only along a scale of difficulty in decision-making. For instance, some statutes have required a higher standard of evidence for competence in making than in revoking advance directives, and the National Bioethics Advisory Commission recommended a higher standard of evidence of competence to consent to participate in most research than to object to participation.[40] Whereas Brock and Buchanan insist that the level of decision-making competence itself belongs on a sliding scale from low to high in accordance with risk, we recommend placing only the required *standards of evidence* for determining decision-making competence on a sliding scale.

The Meaning and Justification of Informed Consent

Since the Nuremberg trials, which presented horrifying accounts of medical experimentation in concentration camps, consent has been at the forefront of biomedical ethics. The term *informed consent* did not appear until a decade after these trials (held in the late 1940s), and it did not receive detailed examination until the early 1970s. In recent years, the focus has shifted from the physician's or researcher's obligation to *disclose* information to the quality of a patient's or subject's *understanding* and *consent*. The forces behind this shift of emphasis were autonomy-driven. Throughout this section, we note how standards of informed consent have evolved through the regulation of research, case law governing medical practice, changes in the patient–physician relationship, and ethical analysis.

The Justification of Informed Consent Requirements

Virtually all prominent medical and research codes and institutional rules of ethics now hold that physicians and investigators must obtain the informed consent of patients and subjects prior to any substantial intervention. Throughout the early history of concern about research subjects, consent requirements appeared primarily as a way to minimize the potential for harm. Reducing risk and avoiding unfairness and exploitation still function as reasons for many professional, regulatory, and institutional controls. However, since the mid-1970s, the primary justification advanced for requirements of informed consent has been to protect autonomous choice, a loosely defined goal that is often buried in broad discussions of protecting the rights of patients and research subjects.[41] Historically, we can claim little beyond the fact that a general, inchoate societal demand has emerged for the protection of patients' and subjects' rights, particularly their autonomy rights.

The Meanings and Elements of Informed Consent

Some commentators attempt to reduce the idea of informed consent to shared decision-making between doctor and patient, so that *informed consent* and *mutual decision-making* are synonymous.[42] They do not claim that *informed consent* has this meaning in ordinary language or law, but rather that it *should* have this meaning. However, informed consent cannot be reduced to shared decision-making. Informed consent is obtained and will continue to be obtained in many contexts of research and medicine in which shared decision-making is a misleading model. For example, a patient may have already decided in an informed manner what he or she wants prior to seeing a health professional. It is critically important to distinguish informational exchanges through which patients elect medical interventions from acts of approving and authorizing those interventions. Shared decision-making is a worthy ideal in medicine, but it neither defines nor displaces informed consent.

Two meanings of "informed consent."[43] Two different senses of "informed consent" appear in current literature and practices. In the first sense, informed consent is analyzable through the account of autonomous choice presented earlier in this chapter: An informed consent is an individual's *autonomous authorization* of a medical intervention or of participation in research. In this first sense, a person must do more than express agreement or comply with a proposal. He or she must *authorize* something through an act of informed and voluntary consent. In the classic case of *Mohr v. Williams*, a physician obtained Anna Mohr's consent to an operation on her right ear. While operating, the surgeon determined that the left ear instead needed surgery. A court found that the physician should have obtained the patient's consent to the surgery on the left ear: "If a physician advises a patient to submit to a particular operation, and the patient weighs the dangers and risks incident to its performance, and finally consents, the patient thereby, in effect, enters into a contract authorizing the physician to operate to the extent of the consent given, but no further."[44] An informed consent in this first sense occurs if and only if a patient or subject, with substantial understanding and in absence of substantial control by others, intentionally authorizes a professional to do something.

In the second sense, informed consent is analyzable in terms of *the social rules of consent* in institutions that must obtain legally or institutionally valid consent from patients or subjects before proceeding with diagnostic, therapeutic, or research procedures. Informed consents are not necessarily autonomous acts under these rules and sometimes are not even meaningful authorizations. *Informed consent* refers here only to an institutionally or legally effective authorization, as determined by prevailing rules. For example, if a mature minor is not legally authorized to consent, he or she may autonomously authorize an intervention without thereby giving an effective consent under existing rules (although some laws give mature minors the right to authorize medical treatments in a limited range of circumstances). Thus, a patient or subject can *autonomously* authorize an intervention, and so give an informed consent in the first sense, without *effectively* authorizing the intervention and thus without giving an informed consent in the second sense.

Institutional rules of informed consent have generally not been judged by the demanding standard of autonomous authorization. As a result, institutions, laws, or courts may impose on physicians and hospitals nothing more than an obligation to warn of risks of proposed interventions. Consent under these circumstances is not bona fide informed consent.[45] This problem arises from the gap between the two senses of informed consent: A physician who obtains a consent under institutional criteria can fail to meet the more rigorous standards of an autonomy-based model.

While it is easy to criticize institutional rules as superficial, health care professionals should not be expected to obtain a consent that satisfies the demands of rigorous autonomy-protecting rules in all circumstances. The latter rules may turn out to be excessively difficult or even impossible to implement. We should evaluate institutional rules not only in terms of respect for autonomy but also in terms of the probable consequences of imposing burdensome requirements on institutions and on professionals. Policies may legitimately account for what is fair and reasonable to require of health care professionals and researchers, the effect of alternative consent requirements on efficiency and effectiveness in delivering health care and advancing science, and the effect of consent requirements on the welfare of patients. Nevertheless, we take it as axiomatic that *the model of autonomous choice* (following the first sense of "informed consent") ought to serve as the benchmark for the moral adequacy of institutional rules.

The elements of informed consent. Some commentators have attempted to define *informed consent* by specifying the elements of the concept, in particular by dividing the elements into an *information* component and a *consent* component. The information component refers to disclosure of information and comprehension of what is disclosed. The consent component refers to both a voluntary decision and an authorization to proceed. Legal, regulatory, philosophical, medical, and psychological literatures tend to favor the following elements as the components of informed consent:[46] (1) competence, (2) disclosure, (3) understanding, (4) voluntariness, and (5) consent. Some writers present these elements as the building blocks for a definition of *informed consent:* One gives an informed consent to an intervention if (and perhaps only if) one is competent to act, receives a thorough disclosure, comprehends the disclosure, acts voluntarily, and consents to the intervention.

This five-element definition is vastly superior to the one-element definition in terms of *disclosure* that courts and medical literature have often proposed.[47] The latter definition is unduly influenced by medical convention and malpractice law. Such a definition incorporates dubious assumptions about medical authority, physician responsibility, and legal theories of liability, all of which focus on the *obligation to make disclosures* rather than the *meaning of informed consent. Disclosure* of information is often less vital in clinical medicine than a health professional's *recommendation* of one or more actions. This is typically the case in direct exchanges between physicians and patients regarding surgery, medications, and the like; but it is also true, for example, of notifications to employees or pensioners by corporate medical divisions after routine surveillance or after a study of hazardous chemicals. Recommendations of treatments or of lifestyle changes, such as smoking cessation, are likely to be more meaningful than information about the results of empirical studies or surveillance.

Despite the qualifications surrounding disclosure, we accept the premise that the above "elements" capture basic notions about informed consent that merit analysis. This chapter treats each of the following seven elements. (The importance of authorization in our analysis leads us to substitute elements 6 and 7 below for "consent," which is listed above as element 5.)

I. Threshold Elements (Preconditions)
    1. Competence (to understand and decide)
    2. Voluntariness (in deciding)

II. Information Elements
    3. Disclosure (of material information)
    4. Recommendation (of a plan)
    5. Understanding (of 3. and 4.)

III. Consent Elements
    6. Decision (in favor of a plan)
    7. Authorization (of the chosen plan)

This list requires some explanation and qualification. First, an informed refusal entails a modification of items under III by turning the categories into Refusal Elements—for example, 6. "Decision (against a plan)." Whenever we use the phrase "informed consent," we include the possibility of informed refusal. Second, consent for research involving human subjects does not necessarily involve a recommendation. If a recommendation is made, it may be quite different from recommendations in clinical medicine. Third, competence is more a presupposition or condition of the practice of obtaining informed consent than an element.

Because this chapter is principally about respect for autonomy rather than informed consent and refusal, our treatment of these elements will extend into several regions of autonomous choice. We will concentrate on elements of general importance for the analysis of both informed consent and autonomy. Having already examined competence, we will now concentrate on disclosure, understanding, and voluntariness, beginning with disclosure.

Disclosure

We have just seen that the obligation to disclose information to patients has often been presented as a necessary, and sometimes as the sole, condition of informed consent. The legal doctrine of informed consent in the United States has been primarily a requirement of disclosure based on a physician's general obligation to exercise reasonable care by providing information. Civil litigation has emerged over informed consent because of injury to one's person or property (measured in terms of monetary damages) that was intentionally or negligently caused by a physician's failure to disclose. The term *informed consent* was born in this legal context. However, from the moral viewpoint, informed consent has less to do with the liability of professionals as agents of disclosure and more to do with the autonomous choices of patients and subjects.

Nevertheless, disclosure remains a pivotal topic. Without an adequate way for professionals to deliver information, many patients and subjects will have an inadequate basis for decision-making. Professionals are generally obligated to disclose a core set of information, including (1) those facts or descriptions that patients or subjects usually consider material in deciding whether to refuse or consent to the proposed intervention or research, (2) information the professional believes to be material, (3) the professional's recommendation, (4) the purpose of seeking consent, and (5) the nature and limits of consent as an act of authorization.[48] If research is involved, disclosures should generally cover the aims and methods of the research, anticipated benefits and risks, any anticipated inconvenience or discomfort, and the subjects' right to withdraw, without penalty, from the research.

Such lists could be expanded almost indefinitely. For example, in one controversial decision, the California Supreme Court held that, when seeking an informed consent, "a physician must disclose personal interests unrelated to the patient's health, whether research or economic, that may affect the physician's professional judgment."[49] Such a disclosure requirement has acquired increased moral significance as conflicts of interest have become more dramatic and problematic in research and managed care. For example, researchers may hold stock in a pharmaceutical company that is sponsoring the research, and physicians may have an investment in the radiological center to which the patient is referred. (We examine conflicts of interest in Chapter 7.)

Standards of Disclosure

Courts in the United States have struggled to determine which norms should govern the disclosure of information. Two competing standards of disclosure have emerged: the professional practice standard and the reasonable person standard. A third, the subjective standard, has also received support, though courts have generally avoided it.

The professional practice standard. The first standard holds that a professional community's customary practices determine adequate disclosure. That is, professional custom establishes the amount and kinds of information to be disclosed. Disclosure, like treatment, is a task that belongs to physicians because of their professional expertise and commitment to the patient's welfare. As a result, only expert testimony from members of this profession could count as evidence that a physician has violated a patient's right to information.

Several difficulties affect this standard, which is sometimes called a *reasonable doctor standard*. First, it is uncertain in many situations whether a customary standard exists for the communication of information in medicine. Second, if custom alone were conclusive, pervasive negligence could be perpetuated with impunity. The majority of professionals could offer the same inadequate level of information or have total discretion to determine the scope of disclosure. Third, it is also questionable whether many physicians have developed skills to determine the information that is in their patients' best interests. The assumption that they have such expertise would rest on empirical studies, but available data cast doubt on it.[50] The weighing of risks in the context of a person's subjective beliefs, fears, and hopes is not an expert skill, and information provided to patients and subjects sometimes needs to be freed from the entrenched values and goals of medical professionals. Finally, and perhaps most compellingly, the professional practice standard subverts the right of autonomous choice. Professional standards in medicine are fashioned for medical judgments, but decisions for or against medical care, which are nonmedical decisions, are rightly the province of the patient.

The reasonable person standard. Although many legal jurisdictions retain the traditional professional practice standard, the reasonable person standard has gained acceptance in over half of the states in the United States. According to this standard, we must determine the information to be disclosed by reference to a hypothetical reasonable person. Whether information is pertinent or material is thus measured by the significance a reasonable person would attach to it in deciding whether to undergo a procedure. In this way, the authoritative determination of informational needs shifts from the physician to the patient, and physicians may be found guilty of negligent disclosures, even if their behavior conforms to recognized professional practice.

Whatever its merits, the reasonable person standard encounters conceptual, moral, and practical difficulties. First, the concepts of "material information" and "reasonable person" have never been carefully defined. Second, questions arise about whether and how the reasonable person standard can be employed in practice. Its abstract and hypothetical character makes it difficult for physicians to use, because they have to project what a reasonable patient would need to know. A related problem emerges from empirical studies regarding whether patients use disclosed information in reaching their decisions. Data collected in one study indicate that although 93% of the patients surveyed believed they benefitted from the information disclosed, only 12% used the information in their decisions to consent.[51]

This study, involving family-planning patients, reached conclusions similar to an earlier study of kidney donors.[52] In both studies, the data indicate that patients generally make their decisions prior to and independent of the process of receiving information. Other studies indicate that patients often deferentially accept physicians' recommendations without carefully weighing risks and benefits,[53] and that many patients would agree to a procedure during their first meeting with a physician (82% of candidates for breast cancer adjuvant therapy in one study[54]).

These data do not always indicate that patients' decisions are uninformed or that disclosed information is irrelevant. The patients may have believed that additional information received from physicians did not alter their prior commitment to a course of action, such as surgery. Nonetheless, these empirical findings raise questions about what should count as material information for the individual patient and whether this information is the same for each patient.

The subjective standard. Finally, the subjective model judges adequacy of information by reference to the specific informational needs of the individual person, rather than the hypothetical "reasonable person." Individual needs can differ, because persons may have unconventional beliefs, unusual health problems, or unique family histories that require a different informational base than the reasonable person needs. For example, a person with a family history of reproductive problems might desire information that other persons would not need or want before becoming involved in research on sexual and familial relations or accepting employment in certain industries. If a physician knows or has reason to believe that a person wants such information, then withholding it may undermine autonomy. At issue is the extent to which a standard should be tailored to the individual patient—that is, made subjective. According to the subjective standard, the physician is obligated to disclose the information a particular patient needs to know, if the physician could reasonably be expected to know that patient's informational needs.[55]

The subjective standard is a preferable *moral* standard of disclosure, because it alone acknowledges persons' specific informational needs. Nevertheless, exclusive reliance on a subjective standard is insufficient for both law and ethics, because patients often do not know what information would be relevant for their deliberations, and a doctor cannot reasonably be expected to do an exhaustive background and character analysis of each patient to determine what information would be relevant.

Intentional Nondisclosure

Some types of research are incompatible with complete disclosure, and in certain clinical situations, physicians claim that nondisclosures benefit the patient. Are such intentional nondisclosures justifiable?

The therapeutic privilege. Legal exceptions to the rule of informed consent allow the health professional to proceed without consent in cases of emergency, incompetency, and waiver. These three exceptive conditions are not controversial. However, a controversial exception appears in the therapeutic privilege, according to which a physician may legitimately withhold information, based on a sound medical judgment that divulging the information would be potentially harmful to a depressed, emotionally drained, or unstable patient. Several harmful outcomes are possible, including endangering life, causing irrational decisions, and producing anxiety or stress.[56] Despite the protected status this doctrine has traditionally enjoyed, U.S. Supreme Court Justice Byron White once vigorously attacked the idea that concerns about increasing a person's anxiety about a procedure provide grounds for an exception to rules of informed consent: "It is the very nature of informed consent provisions that they may produce some anxiety in the patient and influence her in her choice. This is in fact their reason for existence, and . . . it is an entirely salutary reason."[57] White suggested that the legal status of the doctrine of therapeutic privilege is no longer as secure as it once was.

The precise formulation of this therapeutic privilege varies across legal jurisdictions. Some formulations permit physicians to withhold information if disclosure would cause *any* countertherapeutic deterioration in the patient's condition. Other formulations permit the physician to withhold information if and only if the patient's knowledge of the information would have serious health-related consequences (e.g., by jeopardizing the treatment's success or by critically impairing relevant decision-making processes). The narrowest formulation is analogous to a circumstance of incompetence: The therapeutic privilege can be validly invoked only if the physician has sufficient reason to believe that disclosure would render the patient incompetent to consent to or refuse the treatment. To invoke the therapeutic privilege under this condition does not, in principle, conflict with respect for autonomy, because the patient would not be capable of an autonomous decision at the point it would be needed.

Therapeutic use of placebos. The therapeutic use of placebos typically involves intentional deception or incomplete disclosure. A placebo is a substance or intervention that the health care professional believes to be pharmacologically or biomedically inert for the condition being treated. Studies indicate that placebos relieve some symptoms in approximately 35% of patients who suffer from conditions such as angina pectoris, cough, anxiety, depression, hypertension, headache, and the common cold.[58]

Evidence also suggests that the placebo effect—an improvement in the patient after use of a placebo—can sometimes be produced without nondisclosure, incomplete disclosure, or deception. For example, the placebo effect sometimes occurs even if patients have been informed that a substance is pharmacologically inert and have consented to its use. In many cases, placebos appear to work because of the "healing context," which includes the professional's care, compassion, and skill in fostering hope and trust.[59]

Nevertheless, a placebo is less likely to be effective if used with the patient's knowledge. This raises the question of whether nondisclosure of placebo use is morally permissible. In one case, professionals thought that an undisclosed placebo offered the only hope of effective pain treatment. There, a man had undergone several abdominal operations for gallstones, postoperative adhesions, and bowel obstructions, and subsequently experienced chronic pain. He became somewhat depressed, lost weight, had poor personal hygiene, was unkempt, and withdrew socially. After using the addictive drug Talwin (pentazocine) six times a day for more than two years to control pain, he had trouble finding injection sites for the Talwin. He sought help "to get more out of life in spite of pain" and voluntarily entered a psychiatric ward that used relaxation techniques and other behavioral procedures.

In the ward, he successfully reduced his Talwin usage to four times daily, but insisted that no more reductions occur since he believed that this level was necessary to control his pain. His therapists decided to withdraw the Talwin over time without his knowledge by diluting it with increasing proportions of normal saline. He experienced withdrawal symptoms of nausea, diarrhea, and cramps. He thought the cause was Elavil (omitriptyline), which the therapists had introduced to relieve the withdrawal symptoms, again without informing him of the purpose. The physicians gradually increased the intervals between injections of the saline. The man was aware of these changes, but unaware that the injections contained only saline. After three weeks, his therapist informed him of the placebo substitution. After his initial incredulity and anger subsided, the patient asked that the saline be discontinued and self-control techniques continued. When discharged three weeks later, he could control his abdominal pain more effectively with the self-control techniques than he had been able to with Talwin. Six months later, he was still using self-control techniques and had resumed social activities.

The therapists defended their deception on the grounds that they "felt ethically obliged to use a treatment that had a high probability of success." Yet, the therapists continued, "We saw no option without ethical problems. Although it is precarious to justify the means by the end, we felt most obliged to use a procedure designed to help the patient achieve a personally and medically desirable goal." They hinted that their actions did not infringe their patient's autonomy because his autonomy was already compromised by his addiction. They also suggested that they even acted in accord with his autonomous choices by taking account of his own therapeutic goals.[60]

One defense of this last claim appeals to the man's implicit consent when he admitted himself to a ward where adjustment in medication was a clear expectation. He accepted the therapy "to get more out of life." However, what he implicitly consented to when he entered the psychiatric ward is unclear, because we do not know what he understood, and no appeal to implicit consent can be accepted for all maneuvers, because he expressly refused to allow further reduction in his Talwin dosage. A related justification for the undisclosed placebo is that the patient subsequently ratified the therapists' decision to use the placebo when he decided to continue the self-control techniques, rather than returning to Talwin. However, predicted future "consent" is only an expected future approval, not a *consent* and, at best, it rests on evidence about the patient's beliefs or goals.

Even though the therapists saw "no option without ethical problems," they had not exhausted the moral options. One possibility was to obtain the patient's general consent to the administration of several drugs and placebos, as part of the effort to wean him from Talwin and to enable him to develop adequate self-control techniques to manage his pain. Such consent would have obviated the need for specific consent to the placebo substitution. The staff's commitment to behavioral therapy may have blinded them to some aspects of the problem by focusing their attention on correctable behaviors, rather than on the person behind the behaviors. We conclude that the staff's justification is deficient in its appeals to implicit consent and future consent. However, we leave open the possibility that a paternalistic use of placebos of the sort found in this case may be justifiable on other grounds (see Chapter 5).

Withholding information from research subjects. Problems of intentional nondisclosure in clinical practice have parallels in research, where investigators sometimes need to withhold some information from subjects. Occasionally, good reasons support such nondisclosure. Vital research in fields such as epidemiology could not be conducted if consent from subjects were always required to obtain access to medical records. Using those records without consent is often ethically justified (e.g., to establish the prevalence of a particular disease). Such research is sometimes only the first phase of an investigation intended to determine whether a need exists to trace and contact particular individuals who are at risk of disease and obtain their permission for further participation in research. Occasionally, individuals need not be contacted at all, for example, when personal identifiers are stripped from hospital records so that epidemiologists cannot identify the patients. In other circumstances, persons need only to be *notified* in advance about how data being gathered will be used and offered the opportunity to refuse to participate in the research. In short, disclosures, warnings, and opportunities to decline involvement are sometimes legitimately substituted for an informed consent.

Many other forms of intentional nondisclosure in research are difficult to justify, however. For instance, debate arose about a study, designed and conducted by two physicians at the Emory University School of Medicine in Atlanta, to determine the prevalence of cocaine use among patients and the reliability of their self-reports about drug use. Controversy centered on the questions that would most likely elicit accurate answers from a group of men in an Atlanta walk-in, inner-city hospital clinic that serves low-income, predominantly black residents. In this study, which was approved by the institutional human investigations committee, weekday outpatients at Grady Memorial Hospital were "asked to participate in a study about asymptomatic carriage of STDs," for which they would receive ten dollars. Study participants had to be between 18 and 39 years old and sexually active within the previous six months. Eighty-two percent of those asked agreed to participate. The average age of the participants was 29.5 years; 91.6% were black, and 89% were uninsured.

The participants provided informed consent for the sexually transmitted disease study, but not for either the unmentioned piggy-back study of recent cocaine use or for a study of the reliability of self-reports of such use. More specifically, patients were informed that their urine would be tested for STDs, but they were not informed that it would also be analyzed for cocaine metabolites. Of the 415 eligible men who agreed to participate, 39% tested positive for a major cocaine metabolite, although 72% of those with positive urinary assays denied any illicit drug use in the three days prior to sampling. (The metabolite is cleared from the body within three days following single-dose cocaine injection.) In answering questions, subjects with positive urine assays were more likely to admit to "any illegal drug" use (87.5%) than to admit to the more specific "any form of cocaine" use (60.6%) over the prior year. Overall, 42.4% of the 415 participants admitted they had used cocaine within the last year. Researchers concluded:

Our findings underscore the magnitude of the cocaine abuse problem for young men seeking care in inner-city, walk-in clinics. Health care providers need to be aware of the unreliability of patient self-reports of illicit drug use. In this high-risk population, any admission of illicit drug use within the prior year, despite denial of ongoing abuse, should lead physicians to suspect recent use.[61]

The researchers deceived the subjects about some aims and purposes of the research and did not disclose the means that would be used. Investigators thought they faced a dilemma: On the one hand, accurate information was needed about illicit drug use for health care and public policy. On the other hand, obtaining adequate informed consent was difficult, because many potential subjects would either refuse to participate or would offer false information to researchers.

Nonetheless, requirements of informed consent should not have been so easily set aside. Rules requiring consent are designed specifically to protect subjects from manipulation and abuse during the research process. Reports of this cocaine study could easily increase suspicion of medical institutions and professionals and could make patients' self-reports of illegal activities even less reliable.[62] Though informed consent is sometimes unnecessary, this study of cocaine use is not a legitimate example. Investigators should have sought to resolve their dilemma by developing alternative research designs, including sophisticated methods of using questions that can either reduce or eliminate response errors without abridging informed consent.

In general, research cannot be justified if (1) significant risk is involved, and (2) subjects are not informed that they are being placed at risk. This conclusion does not imply that research involving deception can *never* justifiably be undertaken. Relatively risk-free research that requires deception or incomplete disclosure is often warranted in fields such as behavioral and physiological psychology. But deception should be permitted in research only if (1) it is essential to obtain vital information, (2) no substantial risk is involved, (3) subjects are informed that deception or incomplete disclosure is part of the study, and (4) subjects consent to participate under these conditions. We return in Chapter 7 to some needed qualifications to this conclusion in the context of randomized clinical trials.

Understanding

Clinical experience and empirical data indicate that patients and subjects exhibit wide variation in their understanding of information about diagnoses, procedures, risks, and prognoses.[63] Some patients and subjects are calm, attentive, and eager for dialogue, whereas others are nervous or distracted in ways that impair or block understanding. Many conditions limit their understanding, including illness, irrationality, and immaturity.

The Nature of Understanding

No consensus exists about the nature of understanding, but an analysis sufficient for our purposes is that persons understand if they have acquired pertinent information and have justified, relevant beliefs about the nature and consequences of their actions. Such understanding need not be complete, because a grasp of central facts is generally sufficient. Some facts are irrelevant or trivial; others are vital, perhaps decisive. In some cases, a person's lack of awareness of even a single risk or missing fact can deprive him or her of adequate understanding. Consider, for example, the case of *Bang v. Miller Hospital*, in which patient Bang did not intend to consent to a sterilization entailed in prostate surgery.[64] Bang did, in fact, consent to prostate surgery, but without being told that sterilization was an inevitable outcome. (Sterilization is not necessarily an outcome of prostate surgery, but it is inevitable in the specific procedure selected in this case.) Bang's failure to understand this one surgical consequence compromised what was otherwise an adequate understanding and invalidated what otherwise would have been a valid consent.

Patients and subjects usually should understand at least what a health care professional or researcher believes a patient or subject needs to understand in order to authorize an intervention. Diagnoses, prognoses, the nature and purpose of the intervention, alternatives, risks and benefits, and recommendations are typically essential. Patients or subjects also need to share an understanding with professionals about the terms of the authorization before proceeding. Unless agreement exists about the essential features of what is authorized, there can be no assurance that a patient or subject has made an autonomous decision. Even if both physician and patient use a word such as *stroke* or *hernia*, their interpretations will be different if standard medical definitions and conceptions have no meaning for the patient.

Some argue that many patients and subjects cannot comprehend enough information or sufficiently appreciate its relevance to make decisions about medical care or participation in research. Such statements are overgeneralizations, based partially on ideals of full disclosure and full understanding. If we replace this ideal standard with a more acceptable account of understanding relevant information, we can thwart such skepticism. From the fact that actions are never *fully* informed, voluntary, or autonomous, it does not follow that they are never *adequately* informed, voluntary, or autonomous.

Some patients, however, have such limited knowledge bases that communication about alien or novel situations is exceedingly difficult, especially if new concepts and cognitive constructs are required. Studies indicate that these patients' understanding of scientific goals and procedures is likely to be both impoverished and distorted.[65] But even under these difficult situations, enhanced understanding and adequate decision-making are often possible. For instance, professionals may be able to communicate novel and specialized information to lay persons by drawing analogies between this information and more ordinary events familiar to the patient or subject. Similarly, professionals can express risks in both numeric and non-numeric probabilities, while helping the patient or subject to assign meanings to the probabilities through comparison with more familiar risks and prior experiences, such as risks involved in driving automobiles or using power tools.[66]

However, even with these strategies, enabling a patient not only to comprehend but also to appreciate risks and benefits can be a formidable task. For example, many patients confronted with various forms of surgery understand that they will suffer postoperative pain. Nevertheless, their projected expectations of the pain are often inadequate. Many patients cannot, in advance, adequately appreciate the nature of the pain, and many ill patients reach a point at which they can no longer balance with clear judgment the threat of pain against the benefits of surgery. At this point, they find the benefits of surgery overwhelmingly attractive, while devaluing the risks. In one respect, these patients correctly understand basic facts about procedures that involve pain, but, in other respects, their understanding is inadequate.

Empirical studies often fail to provide data that can illuminate how much patients and subjects understand. These studies concentrate on memory and recall—

that is, they focus on what patients or subjects remember about what they were told at the time they made their decisions.[67] By focusing on what patients or subjects later recall, these studies cannot adequately reveal what patients or subjects understood at the time of their consent or refusal.[68] Even though a large majority of patients in one study, when questioned prior to the surgery, understood that there was a risk of death from elective cholecystectomy, over 50% of the same patients did not recall this risk when questioned several weeks following the surgery.[69] However, recall studies do provide a useful reminder that patients and subjects may, at various times, lack the information that gives their continued participation in health care and research moral legitimacy. Many subjects, for example, do not recall that they have the right to withdraw from a trial.[70]

Problems of Information Processing

With the exception of a few limited studies of comprehension, studies of patients' decision-making typically pay little attention to information processing. Too much information can be as much of a problem as too little. Information overload may prevent adequate understanding, and this problem is exacerbated if unfamiliar terms are used or if information cannot be meaningfully organized. Patients and potential subjects also may rely on modes of selective perception, and it is often difficult to determine when words have special meaning for them, when preconceptions distort their processing of the information, and when other biases intrude.

Some studies have uncovered difficulties in processing information about risks, indicating that risk disclosures commonly lead subjects to distort information and promote inferential errors and disproportionate fears of risks. Some ways of framing information are so misleading that both health professionals and patients regularly misconstrue the content. For example, choices between risky alternatives can be heavily influenced by whether the same risk information is presented as providing a gain or an opportunity for a patient, or as constituting a loss or a reduction of opportunity.[71] One study asked radiologists, outpatients with chronic medical problems, and graduate business students to make a hypothetical choice between two alternative therapies for lung cancer: surgery and radiation therapy.[72] The preferences of all three groups were affected by whether the information about outcomes was framed in terms of survival or death. When faced with outcomes framed in terms of probability of *survival*, 25% chose radiation over surgery. However, when the identical outcomes were presented in terms of probability of *death*, 42% preferred radiation. The mode of presenting the risk of immediate death from surgical complications, which has no counterpart in radiation therapy, appears to have made the decisive difference.

These framing effects reduce understanding, with direct implications for autonomous choice. If a misperception prevents a person from adequately understanding the risk of death and this risk is material to the person's decision, then the person's choice of surgery does not reflect a substantial understanding and does not qualify as an autonomous authorization. The lesson to be learned is the need for better understanding of techniques that will enable professionals to communicate the positive and the negative sides of information (e.g., both the survival and the mortality probabilities).

Problems of Nonacceptance and False Belief

Decision-making can be compromised by a breakdown in a person's ability to *accept* information as true or untainted, even if he or she adequately *comprehends* the information. Reliance on recall tests has often obscured the distinction between comprehension of information and acceptance of information. At best, "correct" answers on these tests provide evidence of a person's memory of what the physician or investigator disclosed, not whether the subject correctly interpreted or believed what was disclosed. A false belief can invalidate a patient's or subject's consent even in the presence of suitable disclosure and comprehension. Here are three examples: (1) A patient might falsely and irrationally believe that a doctor will not fill out insurance forms unless he or she consents to a procedure the doctor has suggested. (2) A sufficiently informed patient capable of consent might agree to participate in nontherapeutic research under the false belief that it is therapeutic. (3) A seriously ill patient asked to make a treatment decision might refuse under the false belief that he or she is not ill. Even if the physician recognizes the patient's false belief and adduces conclusive evidence to prove to the patient that the belief is mistaken, and the patient comprehends the information provided, the patient may go on believing that what has been (truthfully) reported is false.

Inconclusive evidence and failure to achieve agreement about the truth or falsity of beliefs complicate these problems. The probabilities and uncertainties that surround many beliefs suggest that we should judge truth claims by the available evidence, which is often subject to different interpretations. More than one standard of evidence may exist, and all evidence must be collected within some framework that determines what qualifies as evidence. If disagreement persists on the criteria for determining the justifiability of beliefs, there will be no adequate basis for determining whether a given belief compromises understanding or simply involves an essentially contestable proposition. This conclusion does not skeptically deny the possibility of knowledge. It only provides a warning that the evidence for thinking that a belief is false may be rationally contestable.

When beliefs are demonstrably false, the question arises whether professionals should force patients and subjects to abandon their beliefs to enable them to reach an informed decision. It seems wrong to say that we should never pressure patients or subjects to change their beliefs or to process information differently.

If ignorance prevents an informed choice, it may be permissible or possibly even obligatory to promote autonomy by attempting to impose unwelcome information. Consider the following case in which a false belief played a major role in a patient's refusal of treatment:[73]

A 57-year-old woman was admitted to the hospital because of a fractured hip. . . . During the course of the hospitalization, a Papanicolaou's test and biopsy revealed stage 1A carcinoma of the cervix. . . . Surgery was strongly recommended, since the cancer was almost certainly curable by a hysterectomy. . . . The patient refused the procedure.

The patient's treating physicians at this point felt that she was mentally incompetent. Psychiatric and neurological consultations were requested to determine the possibility of dementia and/or mental incompetency. The psychiatric consultant felt that the patient was demented and not mentally competent to make decisions regarding her own care. This determination was based in large measure on the patient's steadfast "unreasonable" refusal to undergo surgery. The neurologist disagreed, finding no evidence of dementia. On questioning, the patient stated that she was refusing the hysterectomy because she *did not believe* she had cancer. "Anyone knows," she said, "that people with cancer are sick, feel bad, and lose weight," while she felt quite well. The patient continued to hold this view despite the results of the biopsy and her physicians' persistent arguments to the contrary.

The physician seriously considered overriding the patient's refusal, because sound medical evidence demonstrated that she was unjustified in believing she did not have cancer. As long as this patient continues to hold such a false belief and it is material to her decision, her refusal is not an *informed* refusal. This case illustrates the complexities involved in effective communication: The patient was a poor white woman from Appalachia with a third-grade education. The fact that her treating physician was black turned out to be the major reason for her false belief that she did not have cancer. She would not believe what a black physician told her. However, intense discussions with a white physician and with her daughter eventually corrected her belief and led her to consent to a successful hysterectomy.

The Problem of Waivers

A further problem about understanding arises in waivers of informed consent. In the exercise of a waiver, a patient voluntarily relinquishes the right to an informed consent and relieves the physician from the obligation to obtain informed consent. The patient delegates decision-making authority to the physician—or to someone else—or asks not to be informed. In effect, the patient makes a decision not to make an informed decision.

Some courts have held that "a medical doctor need not make disclosures of risks when the patient requests that he not be so informed,"[74] and some prominent writers in biomedical ethics hold that "rights are always waivable,"[75] including the right to an informed consent. Various studies indicate that perhaps 60% of patients want to know virtually nothing about certain procedures or about the risks of those procedures, that a high percentage would consent without knowledge of risk, and that only a small percentage uses the information provided in reaching their decisions.[76]

It is usually appropriate to recognize waivers of rights because we enjoy discretion over whether to exercise our rights. Contexts of consent seem no exception. For example, if a committed Jehovah's Witness were to inform a doctor that he wished to have everything possible done for him, but did not want to know if transfusions or similar procedures would be employed, it is difficult to construct a moral argument to support the conclusion that he must give a specific informed consent to the transfusions. Nevertheless, a general practice of allowing waivers is dangerous. Many patients have an inordinate trust in physicians, and the general acceptance of waivers of consent in research and therapeutic settings could make patients more vulnerable to those who have conflicts of interest or abbreviate or omit consent procedures for convenience, already a serious problem in health care.

No general solution to these problems about waivers is likely to emerge. Each case or situation of waiver needs to be considered separately. There may, however, be appropriate procedural responses. For example, rules could be developed that disallow waivers except when they have been approved by deliberative bodies, such as institutional review committees and hospital ethics committees. If a committee determined that recognizing a waiver would best protect a person's interest in a particular case, then the waiver could be sustained. This procedural solution could effectively eliminate the problem since it could be responsive to appropriate requests, while disallowing inappropriate ones. Nonetheless, it would be easy to violate autonomy and to fail to discharge our responsibilities by inflexible rules that either permit or prohibit waivers in institutional settings. Close monitoring by review could provide the necessary level of protection for patients, as well as flexibility in deliberation and decision-making.

Voluntariness

We will concentrate in this section on a person's voluntariness in acting. We use the term *voluntariness* narrowly in order to distinguish it from broader uses that make it synonymous with autonomy. Some have analyzed voluntariness in terms of the presence of adequate knowledge, the absence of psychological compulsion, and the absence of external constraints.[77] If we adopted this broad meaning, the voluntariness condition would be equivalent to the complete set of conditions of autonomous action. We therefore hold that a person acts voluntarily to the degree that he or she wills the action without being under the control of another's influence. We consider here only control by other individuals, although conditions such as debilitating disease, psychiatric disorders, and drug addiction can also diminish or void voluntariness.

Control of another person is necessarily an influence, but not all influences are controlling. If a physician orders a reluctant patient to undergo cardiac catheterization and coerces the patient into compliance through a threat of abandonment, then the physician's influence controls the patient. If, by contrast, a physician persuades the patient to undergo the procedure when the patient is at first reluctant to do so, then the physician's actions influence, but do not control, the patient. Many influences are resistible, and some are welcomed rather than resisted. The broad category of influence includes acts of love, threats, education, lies, manipulative suggestions, and emotional appeals, all of which can vary dramatically in their impact on persons.

Forms of Influence

Our analysis focuses on three categories of influence: coercion, persuasion, and manipulation. Coercion occurs if and only if one person intentionally uses a credible and severe threat of harm or force to control another.[78] The threat of force used by some police, courts, and hospitals in acts of involuntary commitment for psychiatric treatment is a typical form of coercion. For a threat to be credible, both parties must believe that the threat maker can effect it, or the threat maker must successfully deceive the person threatened into so believing. A physician in a prison who tells an inmate he *must* submit to sedation may need an accompanying prison guard for the threat to be credible and for coercion to occur. Some threats will coerce virtually all persons (for example, a credible threat to kill the person), whereas others will coerce only a few persons (for example, an employee's threat to an employer to quit a job unless a raise is offered). Whether coercion occurs depends on the subjective responses of the coercion's intended target. However, a subjective response in which persons comply because they *feel* threatened (though no threat has been issued) does not by itself qualify as coercion. Coercion occurs only if a credible and intended threat displaces a person's self-directedness. Coercion voids an act of autonomy; that is, coercion renders even intentional and well-informed behavior nonautonomous.

In *persuasion*, a person must come to believe in something through the merit of reasons another person advances. We do not recognize as a form of persuasion what Paul Appelbaum and Loren Roth label "forceful persuasion," which involves persistent forcefulness and sometimes misleading language. They cite a case of an intern who did not accept a patient's refusal of an X-ray. The intern insisted that he "absolutely must have the film and that [the patient] could not refuse it." The patient then reluctantly agreed.[79] In our usage, neither nonrational nor forceful "persuasion" qualifies as a form of persuasion, because both are actually forms of manipulation.

We assume that influence by appeal to reason—persuasion—is distinguishable from influence by appeal to emotion. In health care, the problem is to distinguish emotional responses from cognitive responses and to determine which are likely to be evoked. Disclosures or approaches that might rationally persuade one patient might overwhelm another whose fear or panic would short circuit reason. A primary goal is to avoid overwhelming a person with frightening information, particularly if that person is psychologically vulnerable.

Manipulation is a generic term for several forms of influence that are neither persuasive nor coercive. The essence of manipulation is swaying people to do what the manipulator wants by means other than coercion or persuasion. In health care, the key form of manipulation is informational manipulation, a deliberate act of managing information that nonpersuasively alters a person's understanding of a situation and thereby motivates him or her to do what the agent of influence intends. Many forms of informational manipulation are incompatible with autonomous decision-making. For example, deception that involves lying, withholding information, and misleading exaggeration to lead persons to believe what is false are all inconsistent with autonomous choice.

Several problems encountered previously in discussing understanding reappear as issues of informational manipulation. For example, clinicians' uses of the therapeutic privilege to withhold information to manipulate patients into consenting to a medically desirable procedure is informational manipulation.[80] The manner in which a health care professional presents information—by tone of voice, by forceful gesture, and by framing information positively ("we succeed most of the time with this therapy") rather than negatively ("we fail with this therapy in 35% of the cases")—can also manipulate a patient's perception and response, and thereby affect understanding and voluntariness.

Nevertheless, one can easily inflate the threat of control by manipulation beyond its actual significance in health care. We typically make decisions in a context of competing influences, such as personal desires, familial constraints, legal obligations, and institutional pressures. These influences need not be controlling to a substantial degree. From the perspective of decision-making by patients and subjects, we need only establish general criteria for the point at which autonomous choice is imperiled, while recognizing that in many cases no sharp boundary separates controlling and noncontrolling influences.

The Obligation to Abstain from Controlling Influence

Patients and subjects welcome many influences, and even unwelcome influences do not always subvert autonomous decision-making. In some cases, professionals are morally blameworthy if they do *not* attempt to persuade resistant patients to pursue treatments that are medically essential, and such persuasion need not violate respect for autonomy. Reasoned argument in defense of an option is itself a form of providing information and is often vital to ensuring understanding. It is never an unjustified form of influence, although in some contexts (for instance, when a patient has justifiably waived his or her right to information), it can be unduly intrusive and therefore unjustifiable.

Coercion and controlling manipulation are occasionally justified, though these occasions are infrequent in medicine (by contrast to police work, where such techniques are more commonly justified). If a physician responsible for a disruptive and childishly noncompliant patient threatens to discontinue treatment unless the patient alters certain behaviors, the physician's mandate may be justified even if coercive. The most difficult problems about manipulation concern not threat and punishment, which are almost always unjustified in health care and research, but rather the effect of rewards, offers, and encouragement.

A classic example of an unjustified offer occurred during the aforementioned Tuskegee syphilis study. Researchers used various offers to stimulate and sustain the subjects' interest in continued participation. These offers included free burial assistance and insurance, free transportation to and from the examinations, and a free stop in town on the return trip. Subjects received free medicines and free hot meals on the days of the examination. The subjects' socioeconomic deprivation made them vulnerable to these overt and unjustified forms of manipulation.[81]

The conditions under which an influence is both controlling and morally unjustified may be clear in theory, but they are often unclear in concrete situations. For example, many patients report feeling severe pressure to enroll in clinical trials, though their enrollment is voluntary.[82] Some difficult cases in health care involve manipulation-like situations in which patients or subjects are in desperate need such that, without a given medication or a source of income, a high probability exists that the person (or some loved one) will be seriously harmed. Attractive offers such as free medication or extra money can leave a person without any meaningful choice. Such a person is constrained by a desperate situation, but not controlled by another's intentional manipulation. Yet some suggest that an offer of great magnitude to a person in desperate need is inherently exploitative. In some circumstances, such an offer is likely to appear to the beneficiary as a threat—for example, if an experimental therapy is the sole therapy and can be obtained only if a person becomes a research subject. However, this sort of offer is sometimes perceived differently. In 1722, Newgate Prison officials offered several inmates their freedom, as an alternative to hanging, if they volunteered to be subjects in an experiment on smallpox inoculation.[83] It might at first seem that they were coerced, because the offer appears to be a disguised threat on the order of "We will hang you unless you become an experimental subject." More plausibly, though, this manipulation-like circumstance involved a welcome offer to desperately needy persons who, without the offer, would be hanged. The prisoners certainly considered the offer to be fortuitous, as these condemned men all survived and were released.

In contrast, influences that ordinarily are resistible can become controlling for abnormally weak, dependent, and surrender-prone patients. For example, contributing to or playing on such patients' desperation, anxiety, boredom, or other emotions or pandering to their hope of more attention and better care can unfairly influence a bedridden person. What a health professional intends as rational persuasion can irrationally influence the patient by attacking his or her vulnerabilities. We do not imply that health professionals routinely manipulate or exploit patients' vulnerabilities, but only that many patients are susceptible to this kind of influence and thus need protection against it.[84]

It is essential to develop and maintain conditions that permit resistance to control in total institutions, whose populations are admitted involuntarily. The threat of exploitation is substantial in these institutions, yet that a person is coercively institutionalized or in a coercive institution need not entail that each decision he or she makes is coerced. There is no reason why prisoners, for example, cannot validly consent to some research if coercive tactics are not involved in enlisting them as subjects and if there are no manipulative offers, such as unduly large payments for excessive risk taking.

Such problems are often subtle in institutions to which persons are admitted voluntarily, but in which rules, policies, and practices can work to compromise autonomous choice. Perhaps nowhere is this compromise more evident than in long-term care. For example, the elderly in nursing homes frequently experience consticted choices, particularly in routine or everyday matters. Many people in nursing homes have already suffered a decline in their ability to carry out personal choices because of physical impairments. This decline in *executional* autonomy need not be accompanied by a decline in *decisional* autonomy, but caregivers in nursing homes often neglect, misunderstand, or override residents' autonomous decisions.[85]

Everyday decisions range over food (when, what kind, how prepared, and how much), roommates (who selects them and how to resolve conflicts), possessions (which to keep and how to protect them), exercise (when, what kind, and with what supervision), sleep (when and how much), clothes (what to wear and when to wash), as well as baths, medications, and restraints. The liberty of competent residents to live their lives in accord with their preferences and life plans must often be balanced against protecting their health, protecting other residents' interests, promoting safety and efficiency in the facility, and allocating limited financial and other resources. Respect for autonomy suggests individualized care in the nursing home setting, but such care can rarely be individualized in the ways we expect outside such institutions.

Consider the following example from a facility named "Mansion Manor." Mrs. Hollinger, who is 76 years old, has encountered difficulty with the nurses's aides about the facility's requirement that residents rise in time for breakfast, which is served at 7:30 a.m. She has never liked breakfast and she now moves slowly after a second stroke. She finds the effort to make it to breakfast almost intolerable. She has been late each morning for two weeks, and the aides say that her late arrival disrupts the feeding of other residents and that she fails to finish her breakfast when she is late because she is a slow eater. The floor nurse warns her, in a manner she finds threatening, that if her tardiness for breakfast continues, she will be put with those who cannot feed themselves in a separate dining room. Mrs. Hollinger's worries about being late for breakfast have begun to cause her trouble in sleeping and have increased her tiredness. The staff has had several earlier conflicts with her, and she charges that the staff "poked around" in her room and removed some of her belongings that were deemed to be unsafe to others who might wander into her room. The staff's animosity makes it difficult to determine whether Mrs. Hollinger's late arrival at breakfast in fact infringes on the rights of others and disrupts institutional order.

The staff's efforts at persuasion are justifiable, but their coercive threat to put her in the separate dining room is not justified unless her actions genuinely pose problems for others or for the institution. The aides could respond that they are not overriding Mrs. Hollinger's autonomy, only respecting it, because she accepted the rules and regulations that restrict liberty when she voluntarily entered the nursing home. Thus, the argument might go, she has an obligation of compliance, not only because of the need for institutional order but also because of her prior consent. However, before this claim can be sustained, we would need to know exactly what Mrs. Hollinger (and her son) were told at the outset about the rules and regulations. They might well have grounds to complain about initial disclosures or about the nursing home's narrow interpretations of its rules and of governmental regulations.[86]

Some contend that respect for autonomy demands too much of nursing homes and other long-term-care facilities. They propose to replace this principle by a communitarian perspective that employs "negotiated consent" rather than informed consent and that stresses mutual responsibilities rather than individual rights.[87] However, this alternative is risky without explicit protections against violations of autonomy and specification of the proper role of surrogate decision makers.

A Framework of Standards for Surrogate Decision-Making

Surrogate decision makers are authorized to reach decisions for doubtfully autonomous or nonautonomous patients. If a patient is not competent to choose or to refuse treatment, a hospital, a physician, or a family member may justifiably exercise a decision-making role or go before a court or other authority to resolve the issues before implementing a decision. Since the Quinlan decision in New Jersey in 1976, courts and legislatures have established many procedures and standards for surrogate decision-making. However, much remains unresolved, particularly with respect to patients who are incompetent and debilitated, yet conscious. Decisions to terminate or continue treatment are made daily for patients in this condition—for example, those suffering from stroke, Alzheimer's disease, Parkinson's disease, chronic depression affecting cognitive function, senility, and psychosis.

Currently, many courts operate on a widely shared view about how treatment decisions should be reached for both formerly competent and never-competent patients. In this account, all patients have a right to decide, and their autonomous choices must be consulted whenever possible as the basis of any decision. Proponents of this position hold that an incompetent person is still a person with the right to choose. We will propose a different account of decision-making standards. In doing so, we will consider three general standards that surrogate decision makers might use: (1) *substituted judgment*, which is often presented as an autonomy-based standard, (2) *pure autonomy*, and (3) *the patient's best interests*. Our objective is to structure and integrate this set of standards for surrogate decision-making. Although we evaluate these standards for law and policy, our underlying argument is a moral argument that extends our earlier discussions of the value of protecting autonomy. Only in Chapter 4 will we consider *who* should be the surrogate decision maker.

The Substituted Judgment Standard

Substituted judgment begins with the premise that decisions about treatment properly belong to the incompetent or nonautonomous patient by virtue of rights of autonomy and privacy. The patient has the right to decide but is incompetent to exercise it, and it would be unfair to deprive an incompetent patient of decision-making rights merely because he or she is no longer (or has never been) autonomous.

The standard of substituted judgment is, at best, a weak autonomy standard. It requires the surrogate decision maker to "don the mental mantle of the incompetent," as the *Saikewicz* court put it—that is, to make the decision the incompetent would have made if competent. In this case, the court invoked the standard of substituted judgment to decide that Joseph Saikewicz, a never-competent patient, would not have chosen treatment had he been competent. Asserting that what the majority of reasonable people would choose could differ from what a particular incompetent person would choose, the court said,

[T]he decision in many cases such as this should be that which would be made by the incompetent person, if that person were competent, but taking into account the present and future incompetency of the individual as one of the factors which would necessarily enter into the decision-making process of the competent person.[88]

As understood in this and other courts, the basic premise of the substituted judgment standard rests on a fiction. An incompetent person cannot literally be said to have the right to make medical decisions if that right can only be exercised by other competent persons. We believe that the standard of substituted judgment should be used for once-competent patients only if reason exists to believe that a decision can be made as the patient would have made it. In such cases, the surrogate's acquaintance with the patient should be sufficiently deep and relevant that a judgment will reflect the patient's views and values. Accordingly, if the surrogate can reliably answer the question, "What would *the patient* want in this circumstance?" substituted judgment is an appropriate standard. But if the surrogate can only answer the question, "What do *you* want for the patient?" then this standard is inappropriate, because all connection to the patient's former autonomy has vanished. Similarly, we should reject the standard of substituted judgment for never-competent patients. No basis exists for a judgment of autonomous choice if a person has never been autonomous.

The standard of substituted judgment helps us understand what we should do for once-competent patients whose relevant prior preferences can be discerned; but, so interpreted, it collapses into a pure autonomy standard that respects previous autonomous choices. We conclude that we should abandon substituted judgment altogether in law and in ethics and substitute a pure autonomy standard whenever explicit prior autonomous judgments are identifiable.

The Pure Autonomy Standard

The second standard eliminates the ghostly autonomy found in substituted judgment. It applies exclusively to formerly autonomous, now-incompetent patients who expressed a relevant autonomous preference. This standard specifies the general commitments of the principle of respect for autonomy. Whether or not a formal advance directive exists, prior autonomous judgments should be accepted.

The Claire Conroy case, in which the New Jersey Supreme Court grappled with several standards of surrogate decision-making, is instructive.[89] Conroy, an 83-year-old nursing home resident, suffered from irreversible physical and mental impairments, including organic brain syndrome, arteriosclerotic heart disease, hypertension, diabetes, necrotic ulcers on her left foot, and a gangrenous left leg. She was awake enough to track persons with her eyes, but was severely demented, lay in a fetal position, and was unable to speak. She had no discernible cognitive or volitional functioning.

Conroy's nephew (Thomas Whittemore), who was her guardian and only surviving blood relative, sought court permission to remove his aunt's nasogastric tube, an action that would result in her dehydration and death in about a week. He appealed to her general fear of doctors and her refusal to have her gangrenous leg amputated as evidence that his request would conform to her wishes. Conroy's physician opposed Whittemore's petition as a violation of medical ethics. However, the trial court authorized removal of the feeding tube, even though her dying might be painful, on the grounds that her life had become permanently burdensome. A court-appointed guardian ad litem appealed the court's order, which was stayed pending appeal.

Even though Conroy died during the appellate process, two courts issued opinions. A first appellate court reversed the trial court's judgment, on grounds that removal of the feeding tube would cause Conroy's death and thus would constitute an active and impermissible killing from dehydration and starvation. On further appeal, the New Jersey Supreme Court held that any medical treatment, including artificial nutrition and hydration, may be withheld or withdrawn from an incompetent patient under some circumstances. It held that life-sustaining treatment is legitimately withheld or withdrawn from an incompetent patient when it is clear from a "subjective test"—with a demonstrable basis in former autonomous choices—that this particular patient, when autonomous, would have refused under the circumstances. If this subjective or autonomy test is not met, a best interests test then must be satisfied. The court reasoned that the subjective or autonomy-based standard is in principle fulfilled by a written document (such as a living will); an oral directive to family member, friend, or health care provider; a durable power of attorney; the patient's convictions about medical treatment administered to others; religious beliefs and tenets; or the "patient's consistent pattern of conduct with respect to prior decisions about his own medical care." *Conroy* rightly noted that "in the absence of adequate proof of the patient's wishes, it is naive to pretend that the right to self-determination serves as the basis for substituted decision-making."

Although we commend a pure autonomy standard, some problems appear in *Conroy* and similar legal decisions regarding satisfactory evidence for acting under this standard. In the absence of explicit instructions, a surrogate decision maker might, for example, selectively choose from the patient's life history those values that accord with the surrogate's own values, and then use only those selected values in reaching decisions. The surrogate's findings might also be based on values of the patient that are only distantly relevant to the immediate decision, such as the patient's expressed dislike of hospitals. It is reasonable to ask what a decision maker can legitimately infer from Conroy's prior conduct, especially her fear and avoidance of doctors and her earlier refusal to consent to amputation of a gangrenous leg.

A troublesome problem is that surrogates often assume an explicitness in a patient's directive about the future that does not, with sufficient directness, apply to the decision at hand. For example, in *Evans v. Bellevue Hospital*, a formerly competent patient had executed a durable power of attorney authorizing another to make medical decisions in a circumstance of incompetence and had executed a second document refusing life-sustaining treatments if he suffered from "illness, disease or injury or experienced extreme mental deterioration, such that there is no reasonable expectation of recovering or regaining a meaningful quality of life." When the patient became incompetent and suffered from brain lesions due to toxoplasmosis (a form of infection), the designated surrogate refused treatment, allegedly following the executed document's declaration. Both physicians and a court rightly refused to recognize the proxy's decision, because the document did not clearly pertain to this condition, which was in principle treatable and had a chance of restoring the patient's capacity to communicate.[90] We see then that imprecise statements, like the one in Evans's advance directive, provide too little guidance and are sometimes dangerous.

The Best Interests Standard

Under the best interests standard, a surrogate decision maker must determine the highest net benefit among the available options, assigning different weights to interests the patient has in each option and discounting or subtracting inherent risks or costs. The term *best* is used because the surrogate's obligation is to maximize benefit through a comparative assessment that locates the highest net benefit. The best interests standard protects another's well-being by assessing risks and benefits of various treatments and alternatives to treatment, by considering pain and suffering, and by evaluating restoration or loss of functioning. It is, therefore, inescapably a quality-of-life criterion. Those applying the best interests standard should consider the formerly autonomous patient's preferences, values, and perspectives only as far as they affect interpretations of quality of life, direct benefit, and the like.

The best interests standard has been widely used both in and beyond health care. Long before autonomy and privacy were pervasively applied through law to incompetents and minors, parents' responsibility toward their children was legally defined as the responsibility to act in their children's best interests. The law assumed that parents generally do act in their children's best interests and that the state should not interfere, except in extreme circumstances in which the state and the parents disagree about some decision with potentially serious consequences for the child—for example, when Jehovah's Witness parents refuse life-saving blood transfusions for their minor children. If a court rather than the family decides, the court has already made a judgment about the unjustifiability of the family's proposed course of action.

We believe the best interests standard, so understood, can in some circumstances validly override advance directives executed by autonomous patients who have now become incompetent, refusals by minors, and refusals by other incompetent patients. This overriding can occur, for example, in a case in which a person has designated another by a durable power of attorney to make medical decisions on his or her behalf. If the designated surrogate makes a decision that clearly threatens the patient's best interests, the decision should be overridden unless there is a clearly worded, second document executed by the patient that specifically supports the surrogate's decision.

Courts, health care institutions, and religious communities have been too eager to assert that they do not make quality-of-life judgments, but only reach decisions in view of what the patient would have chosen. Courts have viewed quality-of-life judgments as comparative ways of expressing a person's social worth, and they have understandably wanted to avoid comparative ranking of the worth of individual lives. However, "quality-of-life judgments," properly used, do not concern the social worth of individuals, but rather the value of the life for the person who must live it. Best interests judgments are one way to focus attention on this point, rather than on the value the person's life has for other persons.

Unfortunately, the best interests standard has sometimes been interpreted as highly malleable, thereby permitting values that are irrelevant to the patient's benefits or burdens. For example, when parents have sought court permission for a kidney transplant from an incompetent minor child to a sibling, parental judgments about the "donor's" best interests have, on occasion, taken into account projected psychological trauma from the death of the sibling and the psychological benefits of the unselfish act of "donation."[91] While we would not exclude such considerations altogether, we should greet them with skepticism and with additional procedural protections, such as committee review.

Questions also arise about whether we should limit the burdens considered under the best interests standard to physical pain and suffering, as judicial language often suggests. If pain and suffering were the only relevant burdens, it would be difficult to justify withholding or withdrawing life-sustaining treatment from a permanently comatose patient. We will examine this range of concerns about the best interests standard in Chapters 4 and 5, where we discuss benefits and harms more comprehensively.

In summary, it is presently popular in biomedical ethics to hold that an ordered set of standards for surrogate decision-making runs from (1) autonomously executed advance directives to (2) substituted judgment to (3) best interests, with (1) having priority over (2) and (1) and (2) having priority over (3) in a circumstance of conflict. We have argued that previously competent patients who autonomously expressed their preferences in an oral or written advance directive should be treated under the pure autonomy standard, and we have suggested an *economy of standards*. That is, we have collapsed (1) and (2), as essentially identical. The principle of respect for autonomy provides their only foundation, and it applies if and only if either a prior autonomous judgment itself constitutes an authorization or such a judgment supports a reasonable basis of inference for a surrogate. Where the previously competent person left no reliable traces of his or her wishes, surrogate decision makers should adhere only to (3).

Conclusion

The intimate connection between autonomy and decision-making in health care and research, especially in various kinds of consent and refusal, unifies this chapter's several sections. Although we have justified the obligation to solicit decisions from patients and potential research subjects by the principle of respect for autonomy, we have acknowledged that the principle's precise demands remain unsettled and open to interpretation and specification. We have also maintained that construing respect for autonomy as a principle with priority over all other moral principles, rather than one principle in a framework of prima facie principles, gives it too much weight. The human moral community, indeed morality itself, is rooted no less deeply in the three clusters of principles to be discussed in the next three chapters.

Notes

1. The core idea of autonomy has been helpfully treated by Isaiah Berlin, "Two Concepts of Liberty," in *Four Essays on Liberty* (Oxford: Oxford University Press, 1969), pp. 118–72; Joel Feinberg, *Harm to Self*, vol. III in *The Moral Limits of Criminal Law*, (New York: Oxford University Press, 1986), chs. 18–19; and Thomas E. Hill, Jr., *Autonomy and Self-Respect* (Cambridge: Cambridge University Press, 1991), chs. 1–4.

2. Gerald Dworkin, *The Theory and Practice of Autonomy* (New York: Cambridge University Press, 1988), chs. 1–4; Harry G. Frankfurt, "Freedom of the Will and the Concept of a Person," *Journal of Philosophy* 68 (1971): 5–20.

3. For practical implications and empirical studies, see Priscilla Alderson, "Consent to Children's Surgery and Intensive Medical Treatment," *Journal of Law and Society* 17 (1990): 52–65; and Barbara Stanley, et al., "The Functional Competency of Elderly at Risk," *The Gerontologist* 28, Suppl. (1988): 53–58.

4. See Robert Paul Wolff, in *Defense of Anarchism* (New York: Harper and Row, 1970), pp. 4–6, 13f; and Arthur Kuflik, "The Inalienability of Autonomy," *Philosophy and Public Affairs* 13 (1984): 271–98. See also Joseph Raz, "Authority and Justification," *Philosophy and Public Affairs* 14 (1985): 3–29; and Christopher McMahon, "Autonomy and Authority," *Philosophy and Public Affairs* 16 (1987): 303–28.

5. Susan Sherwin, *No Longer Patient: Feminist Ethics and Health Care* (Philadelphia: Temple University Press, 1992), p. 138. However, she does not reject the relevance of moral considerations of autonomy. For a view that "feminists have reason to regard institutions and practices that undermine autonomy as especially detrimental to women," see Diana T. Meyers, *Self, Society, and Personal Choice* (New York: Columbia University Press, 1989). For discussions and evaluations of feminist critiques of autonomy, see Marilyn Friedman, "Autonomy and Social relationships: Rethinking the Feminist Critique," in *Feminists Rethink the Self*, ed. Diana Tietjens Meyers (Boulder, CO: Westview, 1997), pp. 40–61; John Christman, "Feminism and Autonomy," in *Nagging Questions: Feminist Ethics in Everyday Life*, ed., Dana Bushnell (Lanham, MD: Rowman & Littlefield, 1995); and several essays in *Relational Autonomy: Feminist Perspectives on Autonomy, Agency, and the Social Self*, ed. Catriona Mackenzie and Natalie Stoljar (New York: Oxford University Press, 2000).

6. See Catriona Mackenzie and Natalie Stoljar, "Introduction: Autonomy Refigured," in *Relational Autonomy*, ed. Mackenzie and Stoljar, pp. 3–31. Other essays in this volume develop aspects of "relational autonomy." For its implications for health care, see the chapters by Susan Dodds, Anne Donchin, and Carolyn McLeod and Susan Sherwin. See also Susan Sherwin, "A Relational Approach to Autonomy in Health-

care," in *The Politics of Women's Health: Exploring Agency and Autonomy*, The Feminist Health Care Ethics Research Network (Philadelphia: Temple University Press, 1998); and Anne Donchin, "Understanding Autonomy Relationally," *Journal of Medicine and Philosophy* 23, No. 4 (1998).

7. See Carl E. Schneider, *The Practice of Autonomy: Patients, Doctors, and Medical Decisions* (New York: Oxford University Press, 1998), p. xi. See, similarly, Paul Root Wolpe, "The Triumph of Autonomy in American Bioethics: A Sociological View," in *Bioethics and Society: Constructing the Ethical Enterprise*, ed. Raymond DeVries and Janardan Subedi (Upper Saddle River, NJ, 1998), pp. 38–59; the essays in *The Right to Know and the Right Not to Know*, ed. Ruth Chadwick (Brookfield, VT: Avebury, 1997); Max Charlesworth, *Bioethics in a Liberal Society* (New York: Cambridge University Press, 1993); Daniel Callahan, "Autonomy: A Moral Good, Not a Moral Obsession," *Hastings Center Report* 14 (October 1984): 40–42; Robert M. Veatch, "Autonomy's Temporary Triumph," *Hastings Center Report* 14 (October 1984): 38–40; and James F. Childress, "The Place of Autonomy in Bioethics," *Hastings Center Report* 20 (January/February 1990): 12–16.

8. Some of the writings of Robert Veatch and Haavi Morreim, for example, seem to suggest such an ideal or duty. See also Schneider's analysis in his *Practice of Autonomy*.

9. For the distinction between an option right and a mandatory right, see Joel Feinberg, "Voluntary Euthanasia and the Inalienable Right to Life," *Philosophy and Public Affairs* 7 (1978): 93–123.

10. Leslie J. Blackhall, Sheila T. Murphy, Gelya Frank, et al., "Ethnicity and Attitudes toward Patient Autonomy," *Journal of the American Medical Association* 274 (September 13, 1995): 820–25.

11. Ibid.

12. Joseph A. Carrese and Lorna A. Rhodes, "Western Bioethics on the Navajo Reservation: Benefit or Harm?" *Journal of the American Medical Association* 274 (September 13, 1995): 826–29.

13. I. Kant, *Foundations of the Metaphysics of Morals*, trans. Lewis White Beck (Indianapolis, IN: Bobbs-Merrill Company, 1959); *The Doctrine of Virtue*, part II of the *Metaphysics of Morals*, trans. Mary Gregor (Philadelphia: University of Pennsylvania Press, 1964), esp. p. 127. J. B. Schneewind has argued that "Kant invented the conception of morality as autonomy," in part in support of conceptions of morality as self-governance that had developed in competition with conceptions of morality as obedience. See Schneewind, *The Invention of Autonomy: A History of Modern Moral Philosophy* (Cambridge: Cambridge University Press, 1998), p. 3.

14. J. S. Mill, *On Liberty,* in *Collected Works of John Stuart Mill*, vol. 18 (Toronto: University of Toronto Press, 1977), chs. I, III.

15. See Barbara Herman, "Mutual Aid and Respect for Persons," *Ethics* 94 (July 1984): 577–602, esp. 600–02; Onora O'Neill, "Universal Laws and Ends-in-Themselves," *Monist* 72 (1989): 341–61.

16. See Bernard Lo, et al., "Voluntary Screening for Human Immunodeficiency Virus (HIV) Infection: Weighing the Benefits and Harms," *Annals of Internal Medicine* 110 (May 1989): 727–33; and Martha S. Swartz, "AIDS Testing and Informed Consent," *Journal of Health Politics, Policy, and Law* 13 (Winter 1988): 607–21.

17. See *Report and Recommendations of the National Bioethics Advisory Commission, Research Involving Human Biological Materials: Ethical Issues and Policy Guidance*, Vol. I (Rockville, MD: National Bioethics Advisory Commission, August 1999).

18. This case was prepared by Gail Povar, M.D.

19. Dax Cowart, "Patient Autonomy: One Man's Story [Interview]," *Journal of the Arkansas Medical Society* 85 (1988): 165–69; "Dax Cowart Speaks," *Health Decisions* 2 (1993); Eric A. Rosenberg and Demetrios A. Karides, "An Interview with Dax Cowart," *Journal of the American Medical Association* 277 (September 7, 1994): 744–45; Dax Cowart and Robert Burt, "Controlling Death: Who Chooses, Who Controls? A Dialogue Between Dax Cowart and Robert Burt," *Hastings Center Report* 28 (Jan./Feb. 1998): 14–24; Denis G. Arnold and Paul T. Menzel, "When Comes 'The End of the Day?' A Comment on the Dialogue Between Dax Cowart and Robert Burt," *Hastings Center Report* 28 (Jan./Feb. 1998): 25–27.

20. See Alison Wickman and Alan L. Sandler, "Research involving Critically Ill Subjects in Emergency Circumstances: New Regulations, New Challenges," *Neurology* 48 (1997): 1151–77. See also Robert J. Levine, "Research in Emergency Situations: The Role of Deferred Consent [editorial]," *Journal of the American Medical Association* 273 (April 26,1995): 1300–02; Robert J. Levine, Norman S. Abramson, and Peter Safar, "Deferred Consent [commentary and response]," *Controlled Clinical Trials* 12 (1991): 546–50 and discussion 551–52; Norman S. Abramson, et al., "Deferred Consent: Use in Clinical Resuscitation," *Annals of Emergency Medicine* 19 (1990): 781–84.

21. See Rebecca Dresser and John Robertson, "Quality of Life and Non-Treatment Decisions for Incompetent Patients: A *Critique* of the Orthodox Approach," *Law, Medicine, and Health Care* 17 (1989): 234–44; Jeffrey Blustein, "Choosing for Others as Continuing a Life Story: The Problem of Personal Identity Revisited," *Journal of Law, Medicine and Ethics* 27 (1999 Spring): 20–31; Helga Kuhse, "Some Reflections or the Problem of Advance Directives, Personhood and Personal Identity." *Kennedy Institute of Ethics Journal* 9 (1999 December): 347–64.

22. Thomas Grisso and Paul S. Appelbaum, *Assessing Competence to Consent to Treatment: A Guide for Physicians and Other Health Professionals* (New York: Oxford University Press, 1998), p. 11.

23. Ibid., e.g., p. 128.

24. The analysis in this section has profited from discussions with Ruth R. Faden, Nancy M. P. King, and Dan Brock.

25. See the analysis of the core meaning in Charles M. Culver and Bernard Gert, *Philosophy in Medicine* (New York: Oxford University Press, 1982), pp. 123–26.

26. See *Lake v. Cameron*, 267 F. Supp. 155 (D.D.C. 1967).

27. *Pratt v. Davis*, 118 Ill. App. 161 (1905), aff'd, 224 Ill. 300, 79 N.E. 562 (1906).

28. See Daniel Wikler, "Paternalism and the Mildly Retarded," *Philosophy and Public Affairs* 8 (Summer 1979): 377–92.

29. Subtleties and needed qualifications in this analysis are discussed by Kenneth F. Schaffner, "Competency: A Triaxial Concept," in *Competency*, ed. M. A. G. Cutter and E. E. Shelp (Dordrecht, the Netherlands: Kluwer Academic Publisher, 1991), pp. 253–81.

30. This case was prepared by P. Browning Hoffman, M.D., for presentation in the series of "Medicine and Society" conferences at the University of Virginia.

31. This schema is indebted to Paul S. Appelbaum, Charles W. Lidz, and Alan Meisel, *Informed Consent: Legal Theory and Clinical Practice* (New York: Oxford University Press, 1987), ch. 5; Ruth Macklin, "Some Problems in Gaining Informed Consent from Psychiatric Patients," *Emory Law Journal* 31 (Spring 1982): 345–74; Paul S. Appelbaum and Thomas Grisso, "Assessing Patients' Capacities to Consent to Treatment," *New England Journal of Medicine* 319 (December 22, 1988): 1635–38.

32. Grisso and Appelbaum focus on four functional abilities in assessments of competence to consent to treatment: (1) ability to express a choice, (2) ability to understand information relevant to treatment decision-making, (3) ability to appreciate the significance of that information for one's own situation, and (4) ability to reason logically using relevant information. Grisso and Appelbaum, *Assessing Competence to Consent to Treatment*, Chapter 3. See also their "Comparison of Standards for Assessing Patients' Capacities to Make Treatment Decisions," *American Journal of Psychiatry* 152 (1995): 1033–37. Our list above does not include "appreciation," which we treat below as part of understanding.

33. For additional ways in which values are incorporated, see Loretta M. Kopelman, "On the Evaluative Nature of Competency and Capacity Judgments," *International Journal of Law and Psychiatry* 13 (1990): 309–29. For conceptual and epistemic problems in available tests, see E. Haavi Morreim, "Competence: At the Intersection of Law, Medicine, and Philosophy," in *Competency*, pp. 93–125, esp., pp., 105–08.

34. *Report and Recommendations of the National Bioethics Advisory Commission, Research Involving Persons with Mental Disorders That May Affect Decision Making Capacity*, Vol. I (Rockville, MD: National Bioethics Advisory Commission, December 1998), pp. 58–59.

35. Grisso and Appelbaum, *Assessing Competence to Consent to Treatment*, p. 139.

36. See Willard Gaylin, "The Competence of Children: No Longer All or None," *Hastings Center Report* 12 (April 1982): 33–38, esp. 35; Allen Buchanan and Dan Brock, *Deciding for Others* (Cambridge: Cambridge University Press, 1989), pp. 51–70; and Brock, "Children's Competence for Health Care Decision Making," in *Children and Health Care*, ed. Loretta Kopelman and John Moskop (Boston: Kluwer Academic Publishers, 1989), pp. 181–212.

37. We also need to distinguish two senses of *standard of competence*. In one sense, *criteria* of competence are at stake—that is, the conditions under which a person is competent. In a second sense, *standard of competence* refers to the *pragmatic guidelines* we use to determine competence. For example, a mature teenager could be competent to decide about a kidney transplant (satisfying criteria of competence) but could also be legally incompetent by virtue of age (failing pragmatic guidelines). To avoid this problem of a dual meaning of *standard of competence,* we will use the term only to mean a criterion for determining competence.

38. Buchanan and Brock, *Deciding for Others*, pp. 52–55. For elaboration and defense, see Brock, "Decisionmaking Competence and Risk," *Bioethics* 5 (1991): 105–12.

39. Related problems in the Buchanan-Brock analysis are discussed in Mark R. Wicclair, "Patient Decision-Making Capacity and Risk," *Bioethics* 5 (1991): 91–104, esp. p. 98 (and see p. 120 for an additional "Response"). See also Wicclair, "The Continuing Debate Over Risk-Related Standards of Competence," *Bioethics* 13 (1999): 149–53; Giia S. Cale, "Risk-Related Standards of Competence: Continuing the Debate over Risk-Related Standards of Competence," *Bioethics* 13 (1999): 131–48.

40. *Report and Recommendations of the National Bioethics Advisory Commission, Research Involving Persons with Mental Disorders That May Affect Decision Making Capacity*, p. 58.

41. For doubts about a justification of informed consent based on considerations of autonomy, see Martin Gunderson, "Justifying a Principle of Informed Consent: A Case Study in Autonomy-Based Ethics," *Public Affairs Quarterly* 4 (1990): 249–65, esp. 250, 255.

42. See Jay Katz, *The Silent World of Doctor and Patient* (New York: The Free Press,

1984), pp. 86–87; and President's Commission for the Study of Ethical Problems in Medicine and Biomedical and Behavioral Research, *Making Health Care Decisions* (Washington, DC: U.S. Government Printing Office, 1982), vol. I, p. 15.

43. The analysis in this subsection is based in part on Faden and Beauchamp, *A History and Theory of Informed Consent*, ch. 8.

44. *Mohr v. Williams*, 95 Minn. 261, 265; 104 N.W. 12, 15 (1905).

45. See Jay Katz, "Disclosure and Consent," in *Genetics and the Law II*, ed. A. Milunsky and G. Annas (New York: Plenum Press, 1980), pp. 122, 128; for amplifications, see Katz, "Physician-Patient Encounters 'On a Darkling Plain,'" *Western New England Law Review* 9 (1987): 207–26, and Alan Meisel, "A 'Dignitary Tort' as a Bridge Between the Idea of Informed Consent and the Law of Informed Consent," *Law, Medicine, and Health Care* 16 (1988): 210–18.

46. See, for example, Alan Meisel and Loren Roth, "What We Do and Do Not Know About Informed Consent," *Journal of the American Medical Association* 246 (1981): 2473–77; President's Commission, *Making Health Care Decisions*, vol. II, pp. 317–410, esp. 318, and vol. I, ch. 1, esp. pp. 38–39; National Commission for the Protection of Human Subjects of Biomedical and Behavioral Research, *The Belmont Report* (Washington, DC: DHEW Publication OS 78–0012, 1978), p. 10.

47. See, for example, *Planned Parenthood of Central Missouri v. Danforth*, 428 U.S. 52 at 67 n.8 (1976) (U.S. Supreme Court).

48. Recent studies suggest that many physician–patient encounters in outpatient practice fail to include a *discussion* of these and other factors that are important for informed consent. For instance, one study of what the investigators call "informed decision-making" revealed that in over 3500 clinical decisions, only nine percent met the investigators' definition of completeness for informed decision-making. The authors conclude: "by the most minimal definition consistent with an ethical framework, decision-making in clinical practice may fall short of a basic level of patient involvement in routine decisions." Clarence H. Braddock III, Kelly A. Edwards, Nicole M. Hasenberg, et al., "Informed Decision Making in Outpatient Practice: Time to Get Back to Basics," *Journal of the American Medical Association* 282 (December 22/29, 1999): 2313–20. See also Michael J. Barry, "Involving Patients in Medical Decisions: How Can Physicians Do Better?" *Journal of the American Medical Association* 282 (December 22/29, 1999): 2356–57.

49. *Moore v. Regents of the University of California*, 793 P.2d 479 (Cal. 1990) at 483.

50. See, for example, Clarence H. Braddock, et al., "How Doctors and Patients Discuss Routine Clinical Decisions: Informed Decision Making in the Outpatient Setting," *Journal of General Internal Medicine* 12 (1997): 339–45; John Briguglio, et al., "Development of a Model Angiography Informed Consent Form Based on a Multiinstitutional Survey of Current Forms," *Journal of Vascular and Interventional Radiology* 6 (1995): 971–78; F. J. Dodd, et al., "Consensus in Medical Communication," *Social Science and Medicine* 37 (1993): 565–69; and Charles Keown, Paul Slovic, and Sarah Lichtenstein, "Attitudes of Physicians, Pharmacists, and Laypersons Toward Seriousness and Need for Disclosure of Prescription Drug Side Effects," *Health Psychology* 3 (1984): 1–11.

51. Ruth R. Faden and Tom L. Beauchamp, "Decision-Making and Informed Consent: A Study of the Impact of Disclosed Information," *Social Indicators Research* 7 (1980): 313–36.

52. Carl H. Fellner and John R. Marshall, "Kidney Donors—The Myth of Informed Consent," *American Journal of Psychiatry* 126 (1970): 1245–50, and "Twelve Kidney

Donors," *Journal of the American Medical Association* 206 (1968): 2703–07. See also Roberta G. Simmons, Susan Klein Marine, and Richard L. Simmons, *Gift of Life: The Effect of Organ Transplantation on Individual, Family, and Societal Dynamics* (New Brunswick, NJ: Transaction Books, 1987), esp. ch. 8.

53. See L. A. Siminoff and J. H. Fetting, "Factors Affecting Treatment Decisions for a Life-Threatening Illness: The Case of Medical Treatment of Breast Cancer," *Social Science and Medicine* 32 (1991): 813–18; Jennifer S. Mark and Howard Spiro, "Informed Consent for Colonoscopy: A Prospective Study," *Archives of Internal Medicine* 150 (1990): 777–80; David G. Scherer and N. D. Reppucci, "Adolescents' Capacities to Provide Voluntary Informed Consent," *Law and Human Behavior* 12(1988): 123–41; Christina G. Blanchard, et al., "Information and Decision-Making Preferences of Hospitalized Adult Cancer Patients," *Social Science and Medicine* 27 (1988): 1139–45.

54. L. A. Siminoff, J. H. Fetting, and M. D. Abeloff, "Doctor–Patient Communication about Breast Cancer Adjuvant Therapy," *Journal of Clinical Oncology* 7 (1989): 1192–1200; and J. H. Fetting, et al., "Effect of Patients' Expectations of Benefit with Standard Breast Cancer Adjuvant Chemotherapy on Participation in Randomized Clinical Trial," *Journal of Clinical Oncology* 8 (1990) 1476–82.

55. The Oklahoma Supreme Court has supported this standard. See *Scott v. Bradford*, 606 P.2d 554 (Okla. 1979) at 559 (together with *Masquat v. Maguire*, 638 P.2d 1105, Okla. 1981).

56. *Canterbury v. Spence*, 464 F.2d 772 (1977), at 785–89. For studies of levels of anxiety and stress produced by informed consent disclosures, see Jeffrey Goldberger, et al., "Effect of Informed Consent on Anxiety in Patients Undergoing Diagnostic Electrophysiology Studies," *American Heart Journal* 134 (1997): 119–26; Kenneth D. Hopper, et al., "The Effect of Informed Consent on the Level of Anxiety in Patients Given IV Contrast Material," *American Journal of Roentgenology* 162 (1994): 531–35; and S. Inglis and D. Farnill, "The Effects of Providing Preoperative Statistical Anaesthetic-Risk Information," *Anaesthesia and Intensive Care* 21 (1993): 799–805.

57. *Thornburgh v. American College of Obstetricians*, 106 S.Ct. 2169, at 2199–2200 (1986) (White, J., dissenting).

58. See Howard Brody, *Placebos and the Philosophy of Medicine: Clinical, Conceptual, and Ethical Issues* (Chicago: University of Chicago Press, 1980), pp. 10–11; and Herbert Benson and Mark Epstein, "The Placebo Effect: A Neglected Aspect in the Care of Patients," *Journal of the American Medical Association* 232 (1975): 1225.

59. Brody, *Placebos and the Philosophy of Medicine*, pp. 110, 113, et *passim*; Katz, *The Silent World*, pp. 189–95. For a defense of placebos, see Howard Spiro, *Doctors, Patients, and Placebos* (New Haven, CT: Yale University Press, 1986).

60. Philip Levendusky and Loren Pankratz, "Self-Control Techniques as an Alternative to Pain Medication," *Journal of Abnormal Psychology* 84 (1975): 165–68.

61. Sally E. McNagy and Ruth M. Parker, "High Prevalence of Recent Cocaine Use and the Unreliability of Patient Self-report in an Inner-city Walk-in Clinic," *Journal of the American Medical Association* 267 (February 26, 1992): 1106–08.

62. Sissela Bok, "Informed Consent in Tests of Patient Reliability," *Journal of the American Medical Association* 267 (February 26, 1992): 1118–19.

63. For a study of the nuances of the problem in one patient population, see Barbara A. Bernhardt, et al., "Educating Patients about Cystic Fibrosis Carrier Screening in a Primary Care Setting," *Archives of Family Medicine* 5 (1996): 336–40.

64. *Bang v. Charles T. Miller Hospital*, 251 Minn. 427, 88 N.W. 2d 186 (1958).

65. C. K. Dougherty, et al., "Perceptions of Cancer Patients and their Physicians Involved in Phase I Clinical Trials," *Journal of Clinical Oncology* 13 (1995): 1062–72; Paul R. Benson, et al., "Information Disclosure, Subject Understanding, and Informed Consent in Psychiatric Research," *Law and Human Behavior* 12 (1988): 455–75.

66. See further Edmund G. Howe, "Approaches (and Possible Contraindications) to Enhancing Patients' Autonomy," *Journal of Clinical Ethics* 5 (1994): 179–88.

67. See, for instance, Cheryl Miller, H. Russell Searight, Deborah Grable, et al., "Comprehension and Recall of the Informational Content of the Informed Consent Document: An Evaluation of 168 Patients in a Controlled Clinical Trial," *Journal of Clinical Research and Drug Development* 8, No. 4 (1994): 237–48; Angela Estey, Georgeann Wilkin, and John Dossetor, "Are Research Subjects Able to Retain the Information They Are Given During the Consent Process?" *Health Law Review* 3 (1994): 37–41; Daniel P. Sulmasy, Lisa S. Lehmann, David M. Levine, et al., "Patients' Perceptions of the Quality of Informed Consent for Common Medical Procedures," *Journal of Clinical Ethics* 5 (1994): 189–94; H. D. Swan and D. C. Borshoff, "Informed Consent—Recall of Risk Information Following Epidural Analgesia in Labour," *Anaesthesia and Intensive Care* 22 (1994): 139–41; Robert J. Hekkenberg, Jonathan C. Irish, Lorne E. Rotstein, et al., "Informed Consent in Head and Neck Surgery: How Much Do Patients Actually Remember?" *Journal of Otolaryngology* 26 (1997): 155–59. For a useful guide to empirical research on informed consent, including studies of understanding, see Jeremy Sugarman, Douglas C. McCrory, Donald Powell, et al., "Empirical Research on Informed Consent: An Annotated Bibliography," Special Supplement, *Hastings Center Report* 29 (January–February 1999): S1–S42.

68. For instance, six months after consenting to total joint replacement, 36 consecutive patients were able to recall few of the risks and benefits of the procedure even though they had understood them at the time of their consent. They remembered the surgery's potential benefits more than the risks. See Lellinda M. Hutson and J. David Blaha, "Patients' Recall of Preoperative Instruction for Informed Consent for an Operation," *Journal of Bone and Joint Surgery* 73 (1991): 160–62.

69. Terence C. Wade, "Patients May Not Recall Disclosure of Risk of Death: Implications for Informed Consent," *Medicine, Science and the Law* 30 (1990): 259–62.

70. See Niels Lynoe, Mikael Sandlund, Gisela Dahlqvist, et al., "Informed Consent: Study of Quality of Information Given to Participants in a Clinical Trial," *British Medical Journal* 303 (1991): 610–13; Irwin Kleinman, Debbie Schacter, Joel Jeffries, et al., "Informed Consent and Tardive Dyskinesia: Long-Term Follow-Up," *Journal of Nervous and Mental Disease* 184 (1996): 517–22.

71. The pioneering work was done by Amos Tversky and Daniel Kahneman. See "Choices, Values and Frames," *American Psychologist* 39 (1984): 341–50; and "The Framing of Decisions and the Psychology of Choice," *Science* 211 (1981): 453–58. On informed consent specifically, see Dennis J. Mazur and Jon F. Merz, "How Age, Outcome Severity, and Scale Influence General Medicine Clinic Patients' Interpretations of Verbal Probability Terms," *Journal of General Internal Medicine* 9 (1994): 268–71; and H. J. Sutherland, et al., "Communicating Probabilistic Information to Cancer Patients: Is There 'Noise' on the Line?" *Social Science and Medicine* 32 (1991): 725–31.

72. S. E. Eraker and H. C. Sox, "Assessment of Patients' Preferences for Therapeutic Outcome," *Medical Decision Making* 1 (1981): 29–39; Barbara McNeil, et al., "On the Elicitation of Preferences for Alternative Therapies," *New England Journal of Medicine* 306 (May 27, 1982): 1259–62.

73. Ruth Faden and Alan Faden, "False Belief and the Refusal of Medical Treatment," *Journal of Medical Ethics* 3 (1977): 133–36.

74. *Cobbs v. Grant*, 502 P.2d 1, 12 (1972).

75. Baruch Brody, *Life and Death Decision Making* (New York: Oxford University Press, 1988), p. 22.

76. See Ralph J. Alfidi, "Controversy, Alternatives, and Decisions in Complying with the Legal Doctrine of Informed Consent," *Radiology* 114 (January 1975): 231–34; "Informed Consent: A Study of Patient Reaction," *Journal of the American Medical Association* 216 (1971): 1325–29.

77. See Joel Feinberg, *Social Philosophy* (Englewood Cliffs, NJ: Prentice-Hall, 1973), p. 48; *Harm to Self*, pp. 112–18.

78. Our formulation is indebted to Robert Nozick, "Coercion," in *Philosophy, Science and Method: Essays in Honor of Ernest Nagel*, ed. Sidney Morgenbesser, Patrick Suppes, and Morton White (New York: St. Martin's Press, 1969), pp. 440–72; and Bernard Gert, "Coercion and Freedom," in *Coercion: Nomos XIV*, ed. J. Roland Pennock and John W. Chapman (Chicago: Aldine, Atherton Inc. 1972), pp. 36–37.

79. Paul S. Appelbaum and Loren H. Roth, "Treatment Refusal in Medical Hospitals," in President's Commission, *Making Health Care Decisions*, vol. II, p. 443; see also pp. 452, 462, 466.

80. See Charles W. Lidz and Alan Meisel, "Informed Consent and the Structure of Medical Care," in President's Commission, *Making Health Care Decisions*, Vol. II, pp. 317–410.

81. See James H. Jones, *Bad Blood*, 2nd ed. (New York: The Free Press 1993); David J. Rothman, "Were Tuskegee & Willowbrook 'Studies in Nature'?" *Hastings Center Report* 12 (April 1982): 5–7.

82. See Sarah E. Hewlett, "Is Consent to Participate in Research Voluntary," *Arthritis Care and Research* 9 (1996): 400–04; and Nancy E. Kass, et al., "Trust: The Fragile Foundation of Contemporary Biomedical Research," *Hastings Center Report* 25 (September–October 1996): 25–29.

83. Henry K. Beecher, *Research and the Individual: Human Studies* (Boston: Little, Brown, and Co., 1970), p. 6.

84. See Charles W. Lidz, et al., *Informed Consent: A Study of Decision Making in Psychiatry* (New York: Guilford Press, 1984), ch. 7, esp. pp. 110–11, 117–23.

85. For the distinction between decisional autonomy and executional autonomy, see Bart J. Collopy, "Autonomy in Long Term Care," *The Gerontologist* 28, Suppl. (June 1988): 10–17. On failures to appreciate both capacity and incapacity to consent in nursing homes, see C. Dennis Barton, et al., "Clinicians' Judgement of Capacity of Nursing Home Patients to Give Informed Consent," *Psychiatric Services* 47 (1996): 956–60; and Meghan B. Gerety, et al., "Medical Treatment Preferences of Nursing Home Residents," *Journal of the American Geriatrics Society* 41 (1993): 953–60.

86. For this case, see "If You Let Them, They'd Stay in Bed All Morning: The Tyranny of Regulation in Nursing Home Life," in *Everyday Ethics: Resolving Dilemmas in Nursing Home Life*, ed. R. A. Kane and A. L. Caplan (New York: Springer Publishing Co., 1990), ch. 7. For autonomy in long-term care, see other chapters in *Everyday Ethics* and a special journal issue devoted to this subject: *The Gerontologist* 28 (June 1988).

87. For a defense of negotiated consent, see Harry R. Moody, *Ethics in an Aging Society* (Baltimore, MD: The Johns Hopkins University Press, 1992), ch. 8.

88. *Superintendent of Belchertown State School v. Saikewicz*, Mass. 370 N.E. 2d 417 (1977). For developments in related court opinions, see Sean M. Dunphy and John H. Cross, "Medical Decision Making for Incompetent Persons: The Massachusetts Substituted Judgment Model," *Western New England Law Review* 9 (1987): 153–67.
89. In re *Conroy*, 486 A.2d 1209 (N.J. 1985). All quotations below are from this source.
90. *In the Matter of the Application of John Evans against Bellevue Hospital*, Supreme Court of the State of New York, Index No. 16536/87 (1987).
91. The classic case is *Strunk v. Strunk*, 445 S.W.2d 145 (Ky 1969), which considered these benefits in terms of a standard of substituted judgment.

4

Nonmaleficence

The principle of nonmaleficence asserts an obligation not to inflict harm on others. In medical ethics it has been closely associated with the maxim *Primum non nocere*: "Above all [or first] do no harm." Health care professionals frequently invoke this maxim, yet its origins are obscure and its implications unclear. Often proclaimed the fundamental principle in the Hippocratic tradition of medical ethics, it does not appear in the Hippocratic corpus, and a venerable statement sometimes confused with it—"at least, do no harm"—is a strained translation of a single Hippocratic passage.[1] Nonetheless, the Hippocratic oath clearly expresses an obligation of nonmaleficence and an obligation of beneficence: "I will use treatment to help the sick according to my ability and judgment, but I will never use it to injure or wrong them."

In this chapter, we examine the principle of nonmaleficence and its implications for biomedical ethics. In particular, we critically examine distinctions between killing and letting die, intending and foreseeing harmful outcomes, withholding and withdrawing life-sustaining treatments, and extraordinary and ordinary treatments. Many of these issues center on the terminally ill and the seriously ill and injured. We therefore need a framework for decision-making about life-sustaining procedures and assistance in dying. The framework we defend here would considerably alter current medical practice and guidelines for both competent and incompetent patients. Central to this framework is an interpretation of the principle of nonmaleficence that sanctions rather than suppresses quality-of-life judgments.

The Concept of Nonmaleficence

The Distinction between Nonmaleficence and Beneficence

Many types of ethical theory, including both utilitarian[2] and nonutilitarian theories, recognize a principle of nonmaleficence.[3] Some philosophers combine nonmaleficence with beneficence in a single principle. William Frankena, for instance, divides the principle of beneficence into four general obligations, the first of which we identify as the obligation of nonmaleficence and the other three of which we refer to as obligations of beneficence:

1. One ought not to inflict evil or harm (what is bad).
2. One ought to prevent evil or harm.
3. One ought to remove evil or harm.
4. One ought to do or promote good.[4]

Frankena arranges these elements serially so that—other things being equal in a circumstance of conflict—the first takes precedence over the second, the second over the third, and the third over the fourth. He acknowledges that the fourth element requires defense as a statement of *obligation* (a problem we address in Chapter 5).

If we bring the ideas of benefiting others and not injuring them under a single principle, we will be forced to distinguish, as does Frankena, the several distinct obligations embedded in this general principle. In our view, conflating nonmaleficence and beneficence into a single principle obscures relevant distinctions. Obligations not to harm others (e.g., those prohibiting theft, disablement, and killing) are distinct from obligations to help others (e.g., those prescribing the provision of benefits, protection of interests, and promotion of welfare).

Obligations not to harm others are sometimes more stringent than obligations to help them, but obligations of beneficence are also sometimes more stringent than obligations of nonmaleficence. For example, although the obligation not to injure others intuitively seems more stringent than the obligation to rescue them (that is, obligations of nonmaleficence seem to take precedence over obligations of beneficence), the obligation not to risk injury to research subjects through low-risk procedures is typically not as stringent as the obligation to rescue an injured research subject who underwent the procedures (here an obligation of beneficence takes precedence over an obligation of nonmaleficence). In general, if in a particular case the injury inflicted is very minor (swelling from a needlestick, say), but the benefit provided by rescue is major (such as a life-saving intervention), then we tend to think that the obligation of beneficence takes priority over the obligation of nonmaleficence.[5]

We might try to reformulate the idea of nonmaleficence's increased stringency as follows: Generally, obligations of nonmaleficence are more stringent than obligations of beneficence; and, in some cases, nonmaleficence overrides beneficence, even if the best utilitarian outcome would be obtained by acting beneficently. For example, if a surgeon could save two innocent lives by killing a prisoner on death row to retrieve his heart and liver for transplantation, this outcome would have the highest net utility (in the circumstances), but it is not morally defensible. This formulation of the stringency of nonmaleficence has an initial ring of plausibility, especially if the act of benefiting involves committing a moral wrong. But again we should be extremely cautious about axioms of priority. A beneficial action does not necessarily take second place to an act of not causing harm. In cases of conflict, nonmaleficence is typically overriding, but the weights of these moral principles—like all moral principles—vary in different circumstances. In our view, no rule in ethics favors avoiding harm over providing benefit in all circumstances. The claim that an absolute order of priority exists among elements 1 through 4 in Frankena's scheme above is therefore unsustainable.

Rather than attempting any form of hierarchical ordering, we group the principles of nonmaleficence and beneficence in an arrangement of four norms:

Nonmaleficence
1. One ought not to inflict evil or harm.

Beneficence
2. One ought to prevent evil or harm.
3. One ought to remove evil or harm.
4. One ought to do or promote good.

Each of the three forms of beneficence requires taking action by helping—preventing harm, removing harm, and promoting good—whereas nonmaleficence only requires *intentionally refraining* from actions that cause harm. Rules of nonmaleficence, therefore, take the form "Do not do X." Some philosophers accept only principles or rules that take this proscriptive form. They even limit rules of respect for autonomy to rules of the form, "Do not interfere with a person's autonomous choices." These philosophers reject all principles or rules that require helping, assisting, or rescuing other persons (although they recognize these norms as legitimate *moral ideals*). However, the mainstream of moral philosophy does not accept such a *sharp* distinction between obligations of harming and helping, preferring instead to recognize and preserve the distinction in other ways. We will take this same path, and in Chapter 5 we will explain further the nature of the distinction and why conditions other than some form of *priority* for nonmaleficence can appropriately account for the distinction (see pp. 168–176).

Legitimate disagreements arise about how to classify actions under categories 1 through 4, as well as about the nature and stringency of the obligations that are involved in various circumstances. Consider, for example, the following case.

Robert McFall was dying of aplastic anemia, and his physicians recommended a bone marrow transplant from a genetically compatible donor to increase his chances of living one additional year from 25% to a range of 40–60%. The patient's cousin, David Shimp, agreed to undergo tests to determine his suitability to be a donor. After completing the test for tissue compatibility, he refused to undergo the test for genetic compatibility. He had changed his mind about donation. Robert McFall's lawyer asked a court to require that Shimp undergo the second test and donate his bone marrow if the test indicated a good match.[6]

Public discussion focused on whether Shimp had an obligation of beneficence toward McFall in the form of an obligation to prevent harm, to remove harm, or to promote McFall's welfare. McFall's lawyer contended (unsuccessfully) that even if Shimp did not have a legal obligation of beneficence to rescue his cousin, he had a legal obligation of nonmaleficence, which required that he not make McFall's situation worse. The lawyer argued that when Shimp agreed to undergo the first test and then backed out, he caused a "delay of critical proportions" and thus violated the obligation of nonmaleficence. The judge ruled that Shimp did not violate any legal obligations but held that his actions were "morally indefensible."[7]

This case illustrates certain difficulties of identifying specific obligations under the principles of beneficence and nonmaleficence. Again, we see the importance of specifying these principles to handle circumstances, such as donating organs or tissues, withholding life-sustaining treatments, and hastening the death of a dying patient.

The Concept of Harm

The concept of nonmaleficence has been explicated by use of the terms *harm* and *injury*, but we will confine our analysis to harm. This term has both a normative and a nonnormative use. "X harmed Y" sometimes means that X wronged Y or treated Y unjustly, but it sometimes means only that X caused an adverse effect on Y's interests. As we use these notions, *wronging* involves violating someone's rights, but *harming* need not involve such a violation, or a wrong, or an injustice. To see this distinction, consider that people are harmed without being wronged in circumstances of attack by disease, acts of God, bad luck, and acts by others to which the harmed person has consented.[8] (People can also be wronged without, on balance, being harmed. For example, if an insurance company improperly refuses to pay a patient's hospital bill and the hospital shoulders the full bill, the patient has been wronged by the insurance company, without beig harmed.)

In order to avoid prejudging cases, we construe harm exclusively in the second and nonnormative sense of thwarting, defeating, or setting back some party's interests. Therefore, a *harmful* action by one party may not be wrong or unjus-

tified *on balance, although acts of harming in general are prima facie wrong.*
The reason for their prima facie wrongness is precisely that they do set back the
interests of the persons affected. Harmful actions that involve *justifiable* setbacks
to another's interests are, of course, not wrong. They include cases of justified
criminal punishment, justified demotion of an employee for poor performance in
a job, and discipline in schools.

Some definitions of harm are so broad that they include setbacks to interests
in reputation, property, privacy, and liberty. So broad is the term *harm* in some
writings that it seems to embrace almost every condition that might restrict autonomous action, such as causing discomfort, humiliation, offense, and annoy-
ance. Such a broad conception distinguishes trivial harms from serious harms by
the magnitude of the interests affected. Other accounts with a narrower focus
view harms exclusively as setbacks to physical and psychological interests, such
as those in health and survival.

Whether a broad or a narrow construal is preferable is not critical for our discussion here. Though *harm* is a contested concept, everyone agrees that significant bodily harms and other setbacks to significant interests are paradigm
instances of harm. We will concentrate on physical harms, especially pain, disability, and death, without denying the importance of mental harms and setbacks
to other interests. In particular, we will concentrate on intending, causing, and
permitting death or the risk of death.

Rules Supported by the Principle of Nonmaleficence

The principle of nonmaleficence supports many more specific moral rules (though
principles other than nonmaleficence help justify these rules in some instances).[9]
Typical examples include:[10]

1. Do not kill.
2. Do not cause pain or suffering.
3. Do not incapacitate.
4. Do not cause offense.
5. Do not deprive others of the goods of life.

Both the principle and its specifications in these moral rules are prima facie,
not absolute.

Negligence and the Standard of Due Care

Obligations of nonmaleficence are not only obligations of not inflicting harms but
also include obligations of not imposing *risks* of harm. A person can harm or place
another person at risk without malicious or harmful intent, and the agent of harm
may or may not be morally or legally responsible for the harms. In some cases,
agents are causally responsible for a harm when they do not intend or are unaware

of the harm caused. For example, if cancer rates are elevated at a chemical plant as the result of exposure to a chemical not previously suspected as a carcinogen, workers have been placed at risk by their employer's actions or decisions, even while the employer did not intentionally or knowingly cause the harm.

In cases of risk imposition, law and morality recognize a standard of due care that determine whether the agent who is causally responsible for the risk is legally or morally responsible as well. We can appropriately view this standard as a specification of the principle of nonmaleficence. Due care is taking sufficient and appropriate care to avoid causing harm, as the circumstances demand of a reasonable and prudent person. This standard requires that the goals pursued justify the risks that must be imposed to achieve those goals. Grave risks require commensurately momentous goals for their justification, and emergencies justify risks that nonemergency situations do not justify. For example, attempting to save lives after a major automobile accident justifies the dangers created by speeding emergency vehicles. A person who takes due care in this sense does not violate moral or legal rules even in imposing great risk on another party.

Negligence is the absence of due care. In the professions, it involves a departure from the professional standards that determine due care in a given set of circumstances. The term *negligence* covers two types of situations: (1) intentionally imposing risks of harm that are unreasonable (advertent negligence or recklessness) and (2) unintentionally, but carelessly, imposing risks of harm (inadvertent negligence). In the first type, an agent knowingly imposes an unwarranted risk. For example, a nurse knowingly fails to change a bandage as scheduled, creating an increased risk of infection. In the second type, an agent unknowingly performs a harmful act that he or she should have known and avoided. For example, a physician acts negligently if he or she forgets that a patient does not want to receive certain types of information and discloses that information, causing fear and shame in the patient. Both types of negligence are generally regarded as blameworthy, though some conditions mitigate the blameworthiness. Subtle forms of such judgments pervade morality and medical ethics, as well as criminal and civil law.[11]

In treating negligence, we will concentrate on conduct that falls below a standard of due care that law or morality establishes to protect others from the careless or unreasonable imposition of risks. Courts often must determine responsibility and liability for harm because a patient, client, or customer seeks compensation for setbacks to interests or punishment of a responsible party, or both. We will not consider legal liability here, but the legal model of responsibility for harmful action suggests a general framework that we can adapt to express moral responsibility for harm caused by health care professionals. The following are essential elements in a professional model of due care:

1. The professional must have a duty to the affected party
2. The professional must breach that duty

3. The affected party must experience a harm
4. The harm must be caused by the breach of duty.

Professional malpractice is an instance of negligence that involves not following professional standards of care.[12] These standards require proper training, skills, and diligence. By entering into the profession of medicine, physicians accept the responsibility to observe the standards specific to their profession. If their conduct falls below these standards, they act negligently. Conversely, even if the therapeutic relationship proves to be harmful or unhelpful, malpractice occurs if and only if professional standards of care are not met. For example, in *Adkins v. Ropp*, the Supreme Court of Indiana considered a patient's claim that a physician had been negligent in removing foreign matter from the patient's eye:

When a physician and surgeon assumes to treat and care for a patient, in the absence of a special agreement, he is held in law to have impliedly contracted that he possesses the reasonable and ordinary qualifications of his profession and that he will exercise at least reasonable skill, care and diligence in his treatment of him. This implied contract on the part of the physician does not include a promise to effect a cure and negligence cannot be imputed because a cure is not effected, but he does impliedly promise that he will use due diligence and ordinary skill in his treatment of the patient so that a cure may follow such care and skill, and this degree of care and skill is required of him, not only in performing an operation or administering first treatments, but he is held to the like degree of care and skill in the necessary subsequent treatments unless he is excused from further service by the patient himself, or the physician or surgeon upon due notice refuses to further treat the case.[13]

The line between due care and care that falls below or exceeds what is due is often difficult to draw. Health risks can sometimes be reduced (in industry, say) by increased safety measures, by investing in epidemiological and toxicological studies, by educational or health promotional programs, by training programs, and the like. But a substantial question remains about the lengths to which physicians, employers, and others must go to avoid or lower risks. We will see that this problem presents difficulties for determining the scope of obligations of nonmaleficence.

Distinctions and Rules Governing Nontreatment

Several guidelines have been developed in religious traditions, philosophical discourse, professional codes, and the law to specify requirements of nonmaleficence in health care, particularly with regard to treatment and nontreatment decisions. Some of these guidelines are thorough and helpful, but others need to be revised or replaced. Many of them draw heavily on at least one of the following distinctions:

1. Withholding and withdrawing life-sustaining treatment
2. Extraordinary (or heroic) and ordinary treatment
3. Artificial feeding and life-sustaining medical technologies
4. Intended effects and merely foreseen effects.

Though enormously influential in medicine and law, these distinctions are all untenable. The venerable position that these traditional distinctions occupy in professional codes, institutional policies, and writings in biomedical ethics provides no warrant whatever for retaining them. Indeed, as we shall now see, some of these distinctions can be morally dangerous.

Withholding vs. Withdrawing Treatments

Much debate about the principle of nonmaleficence and forgoing life-sustaining treatments has centered on the omission–commission distinction, especially the distinction between withholding (not starting) and withdrawing (stopping) treatments. Many professionals and family members feel justified in withholding treatments they never started, but not in withdrawing treatments already initiated. They sense that decisions to stop treatments are more momentous and consequential than decisions not to start them. Stopping a respirator, for example, seems to cause a person's death, whereas not starting the respirator does not seem to have this direct causal role.

Consider the following case: An elderly man suffered from several major medical problems, including cancer, with no reasonable chance of recovery. Comatose and unable to communicate, he was being kept alive by antibiotics to fight infection and by an intravenous (IV) line to provide nutrition and hydration. No evidence indicated that he had expressed his wishes about life-sustaining treatments while competent, and he had no family members to serve as the surrogate decision-maker. The staff quickly agreed on a "no code" or "do not resuscitate" (DNR) order, a signed order not to attempt cardiopulmonary resuscitation if a cardiac or respiratory arrest occurred. In the event of such an arrest, the patient would be allowed to die. The staff was comfortable with this decision because of the patient's overall condition and prognosis and because not resuscitating the patient could be viewed as withholding rather than withdrawing treatment.

Questions arose about whether to continue the interventions in place. Some members of the health care team thought that all medical treatments, including artificial nutrition and hydration, as well as antibiotics, should be stopped, because they were "extraordinary" or "heroic measures." Others, perhaps a majority, thought it was wrong to stop these treatments once they had been started. A disagreement erupted about whether it would be permissible not to insert the IV line again if it became infiltrated—that is, if it broke through the blood vessel and began leaking fluid into surrounding tissue. Some who had opposed stopping treatments felt comfortable about not inserting the IV line again because they viewed the action as withholding rather than withdrawing. They emphatically opposed reinsertion if it required a cutdown (an incision to gain access to the deep large blood vessels) or a central line into the heart. Others viewed the provision of artificial nutrition and hydration as a single process and felt that inserting the IV line again was simply restarting or continuing what had been interrupted. For them, not restarting was equivalent to withdrawing, and thus (unlike withholding) morally wrong.[14]

In many cases approximating this one, caregivers' discomfort about withdrawing life-sustaining treatments appears to reflect the view that such actions render them causally responsible for, and therefore culpable for, a patient's death—whereas they are not responsible if they never initiate a life-sustaining treatment. Another source of caregiver discomfort is the conviction that starting a treatment often creates valid claims or expectations that it will be continued; only if the claim is waived does it seem legitimate to many caregivers to stop treatment. Thus, stopping treatment appears to breach expectations, promises, or contractual obligations to the patient, family, or surrogate decision-maker. Patients for whom treatments have not been initiated seem to have no parallel claim.[15]

Feelings of reluctance about withdrawing treatments are understandable, but the distinction between withdrawing and withholding treatments is both irrelevant and dangerous. The distinction is unclear, inasmuch as withdrawing can happen through an omission (withholding), such as not recharging batteries that power respirators or not putting the infusion into a feeding tube. In multistaged treatments, decisions not to start the next stage of a treatment plan can be tantamount to stopping treatment, even if the early phases of the treatment continue.

Even if the distinction were clear, not starting and stopping can both be justified, depending on the circumstances. Both not starting and stopping can cause a patient's death, and both can be instances of allowing to die. Both can even be instances of killing. Courts recognize that individuals can commit a crime by omission if they have an obligation to act, just as physicians can commit a wrong by omission in medical practice. Such a judgment will depend on whether a physician has an obligation either not to withhold or not to withdraw treatment. If a physician has a duty to treat, then omission of treatment breaches the duty whether withholding or withdrawing is involved; but if a physician does not have a duty to treat or a duty not to treat, then omission of either type involves no moral violation. Indeed, if the physician has a duty not to treat, it would be a moral violation not to withdraw the treatment if it has already begun.

In the *Spring* case (case 5), the court raised a legal problem about continuing kidney dialysis as follows: "The question presented by . . . modern technology is, once undertaken, at what point does it cease to perform its intended function?" This court held that "a physician has no duty to continue treatment, once it has proven to be ineffective." The court emphasized the need to balance benefits and burdens to determine overall effectiveness.[16] Although legal responsibility cannot be equated with moral responsibility in such cases, this conclusion is consistent with the moral conclusions about justified withdrawal for which we are presently arguing.

Giving a priority to withholding over withdrawing treatment also can lead to overtreatment in some cases—that is, to continue a treatment that is no longer beneficial or desirable for the patient. Less obviously, the distinction can lead to undertreatment. Patients and families worry about being trapped by biomedical technology that, once begun, cannot be stopped. To circumvent this problem, they become reluctant to authorize the technology, even when it could be beneficial. Health care professionals often come to exhibit the same reluctance. In one case, a seriously ill newborn died after several months of treatment. Much of the treatment was against the parents' wishes because a physician was unwilling to stop the respirator once it had been connected. Later this physician was reportedly "less eager to attach babies to respirators now."[17]

This example illustrates that the moral burden of proof often should be heavier when the decision is to withhold than when it is to withdraw treatments. Only after starting treatments will it be possible, in many cases, to make a proper diagnosis and prognosis, as well as to balance prospective benefits and burdens. Such a trial period can reduce uncertainty about outcomes. Patients and surrogates often feel less stress and more in control if they can reverse or otherwise change a decision to treat after the treatment has started. Accordingly, responsible health care may require proposing a trial with periodic reevaluation.[18] Caregivers then have time to judge the effectiveness of the treatment, and the patient or surrogate has time to evaluate its benefits and burdens. Not to propose or allow the test at all is morally worse than not trying. Hence, withholding might be worse than withdrawing in such cases.

We conclude that the distinction between withholding and withdrawing is morally untenable and can be morally dangerous. Decisions about beginning or ending treatment should be based on considerations of the patient's rights and welfare, and, therefore, on the benefits and burdens of the treatment, as judged by a patient or authorized surrogate. Moreover, if a caregiver makes decisions about treatment using this irrelevant distinction, or allows a surrogate (without efforts at dissuasion) to make such a decision, the caregiver is morally blameworthy for negative outcomes.

The felt importance of the distinction between not starting and stopping undoubtedly accounts for, although it does not justify, the ease with which hospitals and health care professionals have accepted no code or DNR orders. Hospital policies regarding cardiopulmonary resuscitation (CPR), a variety of interventions aimed at restoring function when a cardiac or respiratory arrest occurs, are particularly consequential, because cardiac arrest inevitably occurs in the dying process regardless of the underlying cause of death.

Policies regarding CPR are often independent of other policies regarding life-sustaining technologies, such as respirators, in part because many health care professionals view not providing CPR as withholding rather than withdrawing treatment. Their decisions to provide or not provide CPR are especially problematic when made without advance consultation with patients or their families.[19] Of course, DNR orders are often appropriate, and physicians should provide the option of such orders to patients or surrogates in a variety of circumstances, including terminal illness, irreversible loss of consciousness, and likely imminent and irreversible cardiac or respiratory arrest. However, hospital staffs, as well as patients or their families, are often unclear about what, if anything, DNR orders imply about other levels of care and other technologies. For example, some patients with DNR orders still receive chemotherapy, surgery, and admission to the intensive care unit, whereas others do not.

It is not justifiable to view decisions about CPR as different from decisions about other life-sustaining technologies. Neither the distinction between withholding and withdrawing treatments nor the distinction between ordinary and extraordinary means of treatment, as we will now argue, provides such a justification.

Ordinary vs. Extraordinary Treatments

The distinction between ordinary and extraordinary treatments was once widely invoked, both to justify and to condemn decisions to use or forgo life-sustaining treatments. The traditional rule is that extraordinary treatments can legitimately be forgone, whereas ordinary treatments cannot legitimately be forgone. The distinction has a prominent history in medical practice, judicial decisions, and Roman Catholic casuistry. It has also been used to determine whether an act that results in death counts as killing. As developed by Roman Catholic theologians to deal with problems of surgery (prior to the development of antisepsis and anesthesia), this distinction was used to determine whether a patient's refusal of treatment should be classified as suicide. More specifically, refusal of ordinary means of life-sustaining treatment was long-considered suicide, but refusal of extraordinary means was not. Likewise, families and physicians did not commit homicide if they withheld or withdrew extraordinary means of treatment from patients.

Unfortunately, neither a long history nor precedent guarantees clarity or acceptability, and the distinction between ordinary and extraordinary means of treatment is unacceptably vague and morally misleading. Throughout its history, the distinction has acquired a confusing array of meanings and functions. Interpretors have often taken *ordinary* to mean "usual" or "customary" and *extraordinary* to mean "unusual" or "uncustomary"—under either the professional practice standard discussed in Chapter 3 or the due care standard discussed earlier in this chapter. According to this interpretation, treatments are extraordinary if they are unusual or uncustomary for physicians to use in the relevant contexts. Over time, the terms thus became attached to particular technologies and alterable standards of practice.

The customary or usual in medical practice can be relevant to a moral judgment, but is not by itself sufficient or decisive. Even if it is customary medical practice to treat a disease by a specific means, whether this treatment should be repeated for a particular patient depends on the patient's wishes and condition as a whole, not solely on what is customary. For example, treating pneumonia with antibiotics is usual, but this treatment may be morally optional for a patient who is irreversibly and imminently dying from cancer or AIDS.

Criteria other than usual and unusual medical practice have also been proposed for so-called extraordinary procedures. These criteria include whether the treatment is simple or complex, natural or artificial, noninvasive or highly invasive, inexpensive or expensive, and routine or heroic. These substitutions, which are rarely analyzed with care, generally offer no improvement over *usual* and *unusual*. A treatment that is simple, natural, noninvasive, inexpensive, or routine, is more likely to be viewed as ordinary (and thus obligatory) than a treatment that is complex, artificial, invasive, expensive, or heroic (and thus optional). But these criteria are relevant only if some deeper moral considerations make them relevant. For instance, it is difficult to see why morally we should distinguish a complex treatment that is available and in accordance with the patient's wishes and interests from a simple treatment that is also available and in accordance with the patient's wishes and interests.

More consequential than these conceptual problems is whether such distinctions give sound moral guidance for treatment and nontreatment decisions. The principal consideration is whether a treatment is beneficial or burdensome, not what its classification is. All of these distinctions appear irrelevant except insofar as they point to a quality-of-life criterion that requires balancing benefits against burdens. The need to balance benefits and burdens of treatments stands out in the following once influential exposition of the ordinary–extraordinary distinction:

Ordinary means are all medicines, treatments, and operations which offer a reasonable hope of benefit and which can be obtained and used without excessive expense, pain, or other inconvenience. Extraordinary means are all medicines, treatments, and operations, which cannot be obtained or used without excessive expense, pain, or other inconvenience, or which, if used, would not offer a reasonable hope of benefit.[20]

If we determine excessiveness by the probability and magnitude of the benefit, as weighed against the likely burdens, then using this distinction is functionally equivalent to balancing burdens and benefits. If no reasonable hope of benefit exists, then any expense, pain, or other inconvenience is excessive, and it is probably obligatory not to treat (because it would cause harm without compensating benefit). If a reasonable hope of benefit exists, along with significant burdensomeness, the treatment is optional. Competent patients have a right to make decisions about treatment in light of their own assessment of burdens and benefits, and even for incompetent patients a treatment is not obligatory if it is greatly burdensome. The ordinary–extraordinary distinction thus rests entirely on the balance between benefits and burdens, including immediate detriment, inconvenience, risk of harm, and other costs.

We conclude that the distinction between ordinary and extraordinary treatment is morally irrelevant and should be replaced by the distinction between optional and obligatory treatment, as determined by the balance of benefits and burdens to the patient.

Sustenance Technologies vs. Medical Treatments

Widespread debate has occurred about whether we can legitimately use the distinction between *medical* technologies and *sustenance* technologies that supply nutrition and hydration using needles, tubes, catheters, and the like to distinguish justified and unjustified forgoing of life-sustaining treatments. Some argue that technologies of caregiving for dispensing sustenance, such as artificially administered nutrition and hydration, are *nonmedical* means of maintaining life that are unlike optional forms of medical life-sustaining technologies, such as respirators and dialysis machines. To determine whether this distinction is more acceptable than the previous distinctions, we begin with three cases.

First, consider the case of a 79-year-old widow who had been a resident of a nursing home for several years. In the past, she had experienced repeated transient ischemic attacks, caused by reductions or stoppages of blood flow to the brain. Because of progressive organic brain syndrome, she had lost most of her mental abilities and had become disoriented. She also had thrombophlebitis (inflammation of a vein associated with clotting) and congestive heart failure. Her daughter and grandchildren visited her frequently and loved her deeply. One day, she suffered a massive stroke. She made no recovery and remained nonverbal, but she continued to manifest a withdrawal reaction to painful stimuli and exhibited some purposeful behaviors. She strongly resisted a nasogastric tube being placed into her stomach to introduce nutritional formulas and water. At each attempt, she thrashed about violently and pushed the tube away. When the tube was finally placed, she managed to remove it. After several days, the staff could not find new sites for inserting IV lines and debated whether to take further "extraordinary" measures to maintain fluid and nutritional intake for this elderly patient who had failed to improve and was largely unaware and unresponsive. After lengthy discussions with nurses on the floor and with the patient's family, the physicians in charge reached the conclusion that they should not provide further IVs, cutdowns, or tube feeding. The patient had minimal oral intake and died quietly the following week.[21]

Second, in a ground-breaking case in 1976 the New Jersey Supreme Court held that it was permissible for a guardian to disconnect Karen Ann Quinlan's respirator and allow her to die.[22] After the respirator was removed, she lived for almost ten years, protected by antibiotics and sustained by nutrition and hydration provided through a nasogastric tube. Unable to communicate, she lay comatose in a fetal position, with increasing respiratory problems, bedsores, and weight loss (from 115 to 70 pounds). A moral issue developed over the course of those ten years. If it is permissible to remove the respirator, is it permissible, for the same reasons, to remove the feeding tube? Several Roman Catholic moral theologians advised the parents that they were not morally required to continue medically administered nutrition and hydration (MN&H) or antibiotics to fight infections. Nevertheless, the Quinlans continued MN&H because they believed that the feeding tube did not cause pain, whereas the respirator did.

Third, while Karen Quinlan lingered, the same state supreme court faced another case involving artificial nutrition and hydration in which a guardian requested withdrawal of MN&H for an 84-year-old nursing home resident. The Court held that the provision of nutrition and hydration through nasogastric tubes and other medical means is not always legally required.[23] A Massachusetts court soon reached a similar decision in the Brophy case, involving a 49-year-old man who had been in a persistent, vegetative state for more than three years.[24] Courts have since increasingly maintained that no relevant difference distinguishes MN&H from other life-support measures. They have viewed MN&H as a medical procedure subject to the same evaluative standards as other medical procedures and thus sometimes unjustifiably burdensome.[25] A similar discussion about MN&H has surfaced in treatment decisions about newborns who are seriously ill or severely disabled.

In the above three cases, the same moral question is present: Should MN&H be construed as obligatory or as optional, and, if so, under which circumstances?[26] We maintain that MN&H may justifiably be forgone in some circumstances for every age group, as is true of other life-sustaining technologies. Our chief reasons are that (1) no morally relevant difference exists between the various life-sustaining technologies and (2) the right to refuse medical treatment for oneself or others is not contingent on the type of treatment. We find no reason to believe that MN&H is always an essential part of palliative care or that it necessarily constitutes, on balance, a beneficial medical treatment.

Although our view is consistent with many recent court decisions, professional codes, and philosophical arguments, it remains controversial. Philosopher G. E. M. Anscombe contends that, "For wilful starvation there can be no excuse. The same can't be said quite without qualification about failing to operate or to adopt some course of treatment."[27] C. Everett Koop, former Surgeon General of the United States, denounces practices of allowing newborns to die by omitting MN&H as infanticide occasioned by "starving a child to death";[28] he condemns similar practices for adults as intentional acts of killing that amount to active euthanasia because they cause a preventable death.[29] From this perspective, although caregivers may legitimately omit some forms of treatment, they cannot justifiably omit MN&H.

Defenders of this position have advanced three main arguments, each of which directly challenges our position. The first argument holds that MN&H are required because they are necessary for the patient's comfort and dignity. This view underlies the controversial rule once proposed by the U.S. Department of Health and Human Services for treatment of disabled newborns: "The basic provision of nourishment, fluids, and routine nursing care is a fundamental matter of human dignity, not an option for medical judgment."[30] A similar conviction about patient comfort and dignity underlies the exclusionary clause in several natural death acts that disallow advance directives for artificial nutrition and hydration, while permitting advance directives for nonsustenance procedures that prolong life.[31]

A second argument that MN&H are never optional focuses on symbolic significance. Medical professionals generally find it intuitively devastating to "starve" someone. Provision of nutrition and hydration symbolizes the essence of care and compassion. As Daniel Callahan puts it, feeding the hungry and nursing by nourishing are "the rudimentary healing gesture" and "the perfect symbol of the fact that human life is inescapably social and communal."[32]

The third argument is a version of the wedge or slippery slope argument considered later in this chapter. The controlling idea is that policies of not providing MN&H will lead to adverse consequences because society will not be able to limit decisions about MN&H to legitimate cases, especially under pressures for cost containment in health care. Whereas "death with dignity" first emerged as a compassionate response to the threat of overtreatment, patients now face the threat of undertreatment because of pressures to contain the escalating costs of health care. Such concerns about psychological and social barriers focus on a slide from acting in the patient's interests to acting in the society's interests, from considering the patient's quality of life to considering the patient's value for society, from decisions about terminally ill patients to decisions about nondying patients, from letting die to killing, and from cessation of artificial feeding to cessation of natural feeding. One fear is that the "right to die" will be transformed into the "obligation to die," perhaps against the patient's wishes and interests.[33]

These arguments merit serious consideration, but in the end they are not persuasive. Procedures of MN&H themselves sometimes involve risks of harm, discomfort, and indignity, such as pain from a central IV and physical restraints that prevent patients from removing the lines or tubes. Evidence also indicates that patients who are allowed to die without artificial hydration sometimes die more comfortably than patients who receive such hydration. It is misleading to project the common experience of hunger and thirst on a dying patient who is malnourished and dehydrated. Malnutrition is not identical with hunger; dehydration is not identical with thirst; and starvation is very different from acute dehydration in a medical setting. Caregivers can also alleviate feelings of hunger, thirst, dryness of the mouth, and related problems by other means, such as ice on the lips, without introducing MN&H.[34]

For some competent patients, the burdens of MN&H outweigh their benefits, and no one should deprive these patients of their right to refuse treatment. The obligation to care for patients entails provision of treatments that are in accordance with their preferences and interests (within the limits set by just allocation policies), not the provision of treatments because of what they symbolize in the larger society. In an approach that represents a compromise for physicians who want to engage in symbolically significant actions, while also acting in accord with the patient's wishes and interests, some physicians start and continue IV lines at a rate that will result in dehydration over time.[35] This approach is both risky and deceptive. These physicians fail to acknowledge their final objective, which is that the patient will become dehydrated and malnourished, and die as a result.

The fears underlying the third argument about the slippery slope are more troubling because of uncertainties about whether lines can be drawn and maintained in order to prevent abuses. In 1997, it was determined that 75% of the over two million people who died that year in the United States died in nursing homes (19%) or hospitals (56%) under the care of strangers, often at considerable cost to their families and to society.[36] These and other patients in long-term care are vulnerable, and when making treatment decisions on their behalf, we should be concerned about the potential loss of broad moral commitments that form the cement of our social universe. However, no evidence exists that protecting these patients requires providing MN&H in all circumstances or that the emotions underlying the symbol of providing nutrition and hydration are either necessary or sufficient to avert social disaster.

We conclude that it is sometimes legitimate not to provide MN&H and that the presumption in favor of MN&H for incompetent patients is rebuttable under one of the following conditions: (1) The procedures are highly unlikely to improve nutritional and fluid levels. (2) The procedures will improve nutritional and fluid levels, but the patient will not benefit (e.g., in cases of anencephaly or permanent vegetative state). (3) The procedures will improve nutritional and fluid levels and the patient will benefit, but the burdens of MN&H will outweigh its benefits. For example, when MN&H can be provided only with essential physical restraints that cause fear and discomfort for a severely demented patient. Of course, a competent patient may refuse the procedures without regard to these conditions.

Intended Effects vs. Merely Foreseen Effects

Another venerable attempt to specify the principle of nonmaleficence appears in the rule of double effect (RDE), often called the principle or doctrine of double effect. This rule incorporates a pivotal distinction between intended effects and merely foreseen effects (where effects are consequences of actions).

Functions and conditions of the RDE. The RDE is invoked to justify claims that a single act having two foreseen effects, one good and one harmful (such as death), is not always morally prohibited.[37] As an example of the use of the RDE, consider a patient experiencing terrible pain and suffering who asks a physician for help in ending his life. If the physician directly kills the patient to end the patient's pain and suffering, he or she intentionally causes the patient's death as a means to end pain and suffering. But suppose the physician could provide medication to relieve the patient's pain and suffering at a substantial risk that the patient would die earlier as a result of the medication. If the physician refuses to administer a toxic analgesia, the patient will endure continuing pain and suffering; if the physician provides the medication, it may hasten the patient's death. If the physician's provision of medication were intended to relieve grave pain and suffering and not to cause or hasten death and the physician does not intend the lethal effect, the act of hastening death is not wrong, according to the rule of double effect.

Classic formulations of the RDE identify four conditions or elements that must be satisfied for an act with a double effect to be justified. Each is a necessary condition, and together they form sufficient conditions of morally permissible action:[38]

1. *The nature of the act.* The act must be good, or at least morally neutral (independent of its consequences).
2. *The agent's intention.* The agent intends only the good effect. The bad effect can be foreseen, tolerated, and permitted, but it must not be intended.
3. *The distinction between means and effects.* The bad effect must not be a means to the good effect. If the good effect were the direct causal result of the bad effect, the agent would intend the bad effect in pursuit of the good effect.
4. *Proportionality between the good effect and the bad effect.* The good effect must outweigh the bad effect. That is, the bad effect is permissible only if a proportionate reason compensates for permitting the foreseen bad effect.

We begin to investigate the cogency of the RDE by considering four cases of what many call therapeutic abortion (limited to protecting maternal life in these examples): (A) A pregnant woman has cancer of the cervix; a hysterectomy is needed to save her life, but it will result in the death of the fetus. (B) A pregnant woman has an ectopic pregnancy—the nonviable fetus is in the fallopian tube—and removal of the tube, which will result in the death of the fetus, is medically indicated to prevent hemorrhage. (C) A pregnant woman has a serious heart disease that will probably result in her death if she attempts to carry the pregnancy to term. (D) A pregnant woman in difficult labor will die unless the physician performs a craniotomy (crushing the head of the unborn fetus). Official Roman Catholic teaching and many moral theologians and philosophers hold that actions that produce fetal deaths in cases A and B sometimes satisfy the four conditions of the RDE and, therefore, are morally acceptable, whereas the actions that produce fetal deaths in cases C and D never meet the conditions of the RDE and, therefore, are morally unacceptable.[39]

In the first two cases, according to the RDE, a physician undertakes a legitimate medical procedure aimed at saving the pregnant woman's life with the foreseen, but unintended, result of fetal death. Viewed as side effects that are not intended (rather than as ends or means), these fetal deaths are said to be justified by a proportionately grave reason (saving the pregnant woman). In both cases C and D, the action of killing the fetus is a means to save the pregnant woman's life. As such, it requires intending the fetus's death (even if the death is not desired). Therefore, in those cases criteria 2 and 3 are violated and the act cannot be justified by proportionality (4).

Critics of the RDE contend that it is difficult and perhaps impossible to establish a morally relevant difference between cases such as A (hysterectomy) and D (craniotomy) in terms of the very abstract conditions that comprise the RDE. In neither case does the agent want or desire the death of the fetus, and the descriptions of the acts in these cases do not indicate morally relevant differences between intending, on the one hand, and foreseeing but not intending, on the other. More specifically, it is not clear why craniotomy is killing the fetus rather than crushing the skull of the fetus with the unintended result that the fetus dies. It is also not clear why, in the hysterectomy case, the fetus' death is foreseen but not intended. Proponents of the RDE must have a practicable way to distinguish the intended from the merely foreseen, but they face major difficulties in developing accounts of intention to draw defensible moral lines between the hysterectomy and craniotomy cases. Some modern reformulations of the RDE (especially those emphasizing the fourth condition) even permit craniotomies to save the pregnant woman because of the proportional value of her life.

Additional problems with the RDE. Adherents of the RDE need an account of intentional actions and intended effects of action that properly distinguishes them from nonintentional actions and unintended effects. The literature on intentional action is itself controversial and focuses on diverse conditions, such as volition, deliberation, willing, reasoning, and planning. One of the few widely shared views in this literature is that intentional actions require that an agent have a plan—a blueprint, map, or representation of the means and ends proposed for the execution of an action.[40] For an action to be intentional, then, it must correspond to the agent's plan for its performance.

Alvin Goldman uses the following example in an attempt to prove that merely foreseen effects are unintentional.[41] Imagine that Mr. G is taking a driver's test to prove competence. He comes to an intersection that requires a right turn and extends his arm to signal for a turn, although he knows it is raining and his hand will become wet. According to Goldman, Mr. G's signaling for a turn is an intentional act. By contrast, his getting a wet hand is an unintended effect or "incidental by-product" of his hand-signaling. The defender of the RDE elects a similarly narrow conception of what is intended in order to avoid the conclusion that an agent intentionally brings about all the consequences of an action that the agent foresees. The defender distinguishes between acts and effects, and then between (1) effects that are desired or wanted and (2) effects that are foreseen but not desired or wanted. The RDE views the latter effects as foreseen, but not intended.

However, it is more suitable in these contexts to discard the language of desiring and wanting altogether, and to say that effects that are foreseen but not desired are "tolerated."[42] These effects are not so undesirable that the actor would choose not to perform the act that results in them, and they are a part of the plan of an intentional action. To account for this point, let us use a model of intentionality based on what is *willed* rather than what is *wanted*. On this model, intentional actions and intentional effects include any action and any effect specifically willed in accordance with a plan, including tolerated as well as wanted effects.[43] On this conception, a physician can desire not to do what he intends to do, in the same way that we can be willing to do something but, at the same time, reluctant to do it or even detest doing it.

Under this conception of intentional acts and intended effects, the distinction between what is intended and what is merely foreseen in a planned action is not viable.[44] For example, if a man enters a room and flips a switch that he knows turns on both a light and a fan, but desires only to activate the light, he cannot say that he activates the fan unintentionally. Even if the fan were to make an obnoxious whirring that he knows about and desires to avoid, it would be mistaken to say that he unintentionally brought about the obnoxious sound by flipping the switch. More generally, a person who knowingly and voluntarily acts to bring about an effect brings about that effect intentionally. The effect is intended, although the person did not desire it, did not will it for its own sake, and did not intend it as the goal of the action.

Finally, we must consider the moral relevance of the RDE and its distinctions. Is it plausible to distinguish morally between intentionally causing the death of a fetus by craniotomy and intentionally removing a cancerous uterus that causes the death of a fetus? In both actions, the intention is to save the woman's life with knowledge that the fetus will die. No agent in either scenario desires the bad result (the fetus's death) for its own sake, and none would have tolerated the bad result if its avoidance were morally preferable to the alternative outcome. Each party accepts the bad effect only because it cannot be eliminated without sacrificing the good effect. Accordingly, the agents in our various examples above do not appear to want, will, or intend in ways that make a moral difference.

In the standard interpretation of the RDE, the fetus's death is a *means* to saving a woman's life in the unacceptable case, but it is merely a *side effect* in the acceptable case. That is, an agent intends a means, but need not intend a side effect. However, this approach seems to allow almost anything to be foreseen as a side effect rather than intended as a means (although it does not follow that we can create or direct intentions as we please). For example, in the craniotomy case, the surgeon might not intend the death of the fetus but only intend to remove it from the birth canal. The fetus will die, but is this outcome more than an unwanted and (in double effect theory) unintended consequence?[45]

Defenders of the RDE may eventually find a way out of these puzzles, but they have not found it thus far. One constructive effort to retain an emphasis on intention without entirely abandoning or neglecting the point of the RDE focuses on the way actions display a person's motives and character. From this perspective, as we saw in Chapter 2, the core issue is whether a person's conduct flows from a proper motivational structure and a good character. Often in evaluating persons we are more concerned with their *motivation* to perform an action (why they performed the action) than with their *intention* in performing the action (what they planned to do). The intention to kill another person may be less relevant morally than the motive or doing so—for example, to defend ourself, to defend an innocent third party, or to meet the request of a dying patient.

In the case of performing a craniotomy to save a pregnant woman's life, a physician may not *want* or *desire* the death of the fetus and may regret performing a craniotomy, just as much as in the case of removing a cancerous uterus. Such facts about the physician's motivation and character can make a decisive difference to a moral assessment of the action and the agent. But the RDE is unable to reach this conclusion on its own. In effect, our proposal to focus on motivation transforms the RDE into the moral framework of character judgments that we established in Chapter 2.

Even if one accepts the RDE, it will be irrelevant in many pressing problems about harm and killing that are currently under discussion in biomedical ethics, including the issues surrounding assisted suicide and euthanasia, which we consider later in this chapter. The RDE is fashioned exclusively for cases with both a bad and a good effect, but often the central matter in dispute is whether an effect such as death is bad or good for a person. Nothing in the RDE decides this issue. For example, the RDE does not determine whether voluntary, active euthanasia produces a bad effect or a good effect. Rather, its goodness or badness must be defended or rejected on independent grounds.

Some parts of the RDE are perfectly acceptable—for example, that we justifiably allow a harmful effect only if we will probably bring about a proportionately weighty good one. But, as we will now see, biomedical ethics can put this same general requirement to many uses beyond those permitted by the conditions of the RDE.

Optional Treatments and Obligatory Treatments

We have now rejected several leading distinctions and rules about forgoing life-sustaining treatment that are sanctioned by various traditions of medical ethics. In their place, we propose a distinction between obligatory and optional treatments. We will rely heavily on an analysis of quality of life that is generally incompatible with the distinctions and rules that we have rejected above. The following categories are basic to our arguments:

I. Obligatory to Treat (Wrong Not to Treat)
II. Obligatory Not to Treat (Wrong to Treat)
III. Optional Whether to Treat (Neither Required nor Prohibited)

Under category II, the question is whether it is ever wrong to treat (or obligatory not to treat). A treatment is optional, under III, if it is morally neutral whether a physician provides it, a surrogate authorizes or refuses it, and the like.

The principles of nonmaleficence and beneficence have often been specified to establish a presumption in favor of providing life-sustaining treatments for sick and injured patients. However, use of life-sustaining treatments occasionally violates patients' interests. For example, pain can be so severe and physical restraints so burdensome that these factors outweigh anticipated benefits, such as brief prolongation of life. In these circumstances, providing the treatment is sometimes inhumane or cruel. Even for the incompetent patient, the burdens can so outweigh the benefits that the treatment is wrong rather than optional, just as it would be in the case of a competent patient who refuses treatment.

Conditions for Overriding the Prima Facie Obligation to Treat

Several conditions justify decisions by patients, surrogates, or health care professionals to withhold or withdraw treatment. We introduce these conditions (other than valid refusal of treatment) in this section.

Futile or pointless treatment. Treatment is not obligatory when it offers no benefit to the patient because it is pointless or futile. Several treatments fit this description. For example, if a patient is dead, although still on a respirator, he or she can no longer be harmed by cessation of treatment. However, in some religious and personal belief systems, a patient is not considered dead according to the criteria recognized in health care institutions. For example, if heart and lung function can be maintained, some religious traditions hold that the person is not dead, and the treatment is therefore not futile, even if health care professionals deem it futile. This is the tip of an iceberg of controversies that surround the notion of futility.

Typically, we think of the term *futile* as referring to a situation in which patients who are irreversibly dying have reached a point at which further treatment provides no physiological benefit or is hopeless and becomes optional. (Palliative interventions may, of course, still be continued.) This model, however, covers only a narrow range of treatments that have been labeled futile in the literature on the subject. All of the following have been referred to as futile: Whatever cannot be performed, whatever is highly unlikely to be efficacious (i.e., statistically, the odds of success are exceedingly small), whatever will probably produce only a low-grade, insignificant outcome (i.e., qualitatively, the results are expected to be exceedingly poor), whatever is highly likely to be more burdensome than beneficial, and whatever is completely speculative because it is an untried "treatment." Thus, the term *futility* is now used to cover many situations of predicted improbable outcomes, improbable success, and unacceptable benefit–burden ratios.[46] This situation of competing conceptions and great ambiguity suggests that we should generally avoid the term *futility* in favor of more precise language.

Ideally, objective medical factors will be central in decisions involving either those who are dead or those who are irreversibly dying. Realistically, though, this ideal is difficult to satisfy. Disagreement often exists among health professionals, and conflicts may arise from a family's belief in a possible miracle, a religious tradition's insistence on doing everything in such circumstances, and so forth. It is sometimes difficult to know whether a judgment of futility is based on a probabilistic prediction of failure or on something closer to medical certainty. If an elderly patient has a one percent chance of surviving an arduous and painful regimen, one physician may call the procedure futile while another may view survival as an unlikely outcome but still a possibility that should be considered. We here encounter a value judgment about what is worth the effort, as well as a judgment based on scientific knowledge. Indeed, "futility" typically is used to express a combined value judgment and scientific judgment.

Writings in biomedical ethics that discuss futility often focus on the patient's or surrogate's right to refuse futile treatment. However, compelling medical circumstances and new legislation have raised the question whether the physician may or even must refuse to provide some treatment. The fact that a treatment is futile is often said to change the physician's moral relationship to patients or surrogates. The physician is not morally required to provide the treatment (and in some cases may be required not to provide the treatment) and may not even be required to discuss the treatment.[47] These circumstances often involve incompetent persons, especially patients in a persistent vegetative state (PVS), where physicians or hospital policies impose decisions to forgo life-support on patients against surrogates' wishes. Increasingly, hospitals are adopting policies aimed at denying therapies that physicians judge to be futile, especially after trying them for a reasonable period of time.

The possibility of judgmental error by physicians should lead to caution in formulating these policies, but, at the same time, unreasonable demands by patients and families should not preclude reasonable policies by health care institutions.

Here, as well as elsewhere, respect for the autonomy of patients or authorized surrogates is not a trump that allows them alone to determine whether a treatment is required or is futile. In one case, for instance, Mr. C., who was irreversibly deteriorating from emphysema, insisted on having his life prolonged as long as possible by all available means. He demanded aggressive treatment, although the staff considered the treatment futile. When he became unconscious, his family and the staff had to decide whether to respect their earlier agreement with him or let him die. Without a prior statement of Mr. C.'s wishes, the caregivers would have faced no moral difficulty in terminating treatment that was only prolonging his dying. But even with the prior agreement, following Mr. C.'s previous wishes might not be justified because of the combination of futility and limited health care resources.[48] For instance, if other patients who were not imminently dying could not otherwise gain access to the ventilator and space in the intensive care unit, we would not be obligated to continue treatment.

The upshot is that a pointless or futile treatment, in the sense of a treatment that has no chance of being efficacious, is morally optional, but some putatively futile treatments must be handled differently.[49]

Burdens of treatment outweigh benefits. A mistaken assumption about law and ethics sometimes found in medical codes and institutional policies is that physicians may terminate life-sustaining treatments for persons not able to consent or refuse the treatments only if the patient is terminally ill. However, even if the patient is not terminally ill, life-sustaining medical treatment is still not obligatory if its burdens outweigh its benefits to the patient (or if the competent patient has other good reasons for refusing the treatment). Medical treatment for those not terminally ill is sometimes optional, even if it could prolong life for an indefinite period and the patient is incompetent and has left no advance directive. The principle of nonmaleficence does not imply the maintenance of biological life, nor does it require the initiation or continuation of treatment without regard to the patient's pain, suffering, and discomfort.

In Case 5, for example, 78-year-old Earle Spring developed numerous medical problems, including chronic organic brain syndrome and kidney failure. Hemodialysis controlled the latter problem. Although several aspects of this case are in dispute—such as whether Spring was aware of his surroundings and able to express his wishes—a plausible argument exists that the family and health care professionals were not morally obligated to continue hemodialysis, because of the balance of benefits and burdens to a patient whose compromised mental condition and kidney function would gradually worsen no matter what was done. However, this case, like many others, is complicated by the family's conflict of interest because of their obligations, both to pay mounting and burdensome health care costs and to make judgments in the patient's best interests.

Few decisions are more momentous than those to withhold or withdraw a medical procedure that sustains life. But, in some cases, it is unjustified for surrogates and clinicians to begin or to continue therapy knowing that it will produce a greater balance of pain and suffering for a patient incapable of choosing for or against such therapy.

The Centrality of Quality-of-Life Judgments

Controversies about quality-of-life judgments. Our arguments thus far give considerable weight to quality-of-life judgments in determining whether treatments are optional or obligatory. We have relied on the premise that, when quality of life is sufficiently low that an intervention produces more harm than benefit for the patient, it is justifiable to withhold or to withdraw treatment. Such judgments require defensible criteria of benefits and burdens in order not to reduce quality of life to arbitrary judgments of personal preference and the patient's social worth.

In a landmark case involving quality-of-life judgments, 68-year-old Joseph Saikewicz, who had an IQ of 10 and a mental age of approximately two years and eight months, suffered from acute myeloblastic monocytic leukemia. Chemotherapy would have produced extensive suffering and possibly serious side effects. Remission under chemotherapy occurs in only 30 to 50% of such cases and typically only for between two and 13 months. Without chemotherapy, Saikewicz could be expected to live for several weeks or perhaps several months, during which he would not experience severe pain or suffering. In not ordering treatment, the lower court considered "the quality of life available to him [Saikewicz] even if the treatment does bring about remission." The supreme judicial court of Massachusetts, however, rejected a construal of the lower court's judgment that equated the value of life with a measure of the quality of life—in particular, with Saikewicz's lower quality of life because of mental retardation. Instead, the court interpreted "the vague, and perhaps ill-chosen, term 'quality of life' . . . as a reference to the continuing state of pain and disorientation precipitated by the chemotherapy treatment."[50] It thus balanced prospective benefit against pain and suffering, finally determining that the patient's interests supported a decision not to provide chemotherapy. From a moral standpoint, we agree with the reasoning and the conclusion reached in this legal opinion.

Nonetheless, "quality of life" needs analysis. Some writers have argued that we should reject *moral* judgments about quality of life and rely exclusively on *medical* indications for treatment decisions. Paul Ramsey, for example, argues that, for incompetent patients, we need only determine which treatment is medically indicated to know which treatment is obligatory and which is optional. For imminently dying patients, responsibilities are not fixed by obligations to provide treatments that serve only to extend the dying process, but rather by obligations to provide appropriate care in dying. The choices are thus between further palliative treatments and no treatments. Ramsey worries that, unless we use these guidelines, we will gradually move toward a policy of active, involuntary euthanasia for unconscious or incompetent, nondying patients, based on loose quality-of-life judgments.[51]

However, putatively objective medical factors—such as general criteria used to determine medical indications for treatment—cannot provide what Ramsey envisions. Indeed, these criteria tend to undermine his fundamental distinction between the medical and the moral. It is impossible to determine what will benefit a patient without presupposing some quality-of-life standard and some conception of the life the patient will live after a medical intervention. Accurate medical diagnosis and prognosis are indispensable, but a judgment about whether to use life-prolonging measures rests unavoidably on the anticipated quality of life, not merely on a standard of what is medically indicated.[52]

Ramsey objects that a quality-of-life approach wrongly shifts the focus from whether treatments are beneficial to patients to whether patients' lives are beneficial to them—a shift that opens the door to active, involuntary euthanasia.[53] But the real issue is whether we can state criteria of quality of life with sufficient precision and cogency to avoid such dangers. We think we can, though the vagueness surrounding terms such as *dignity* and *meaningful life* is a cause for concern, and cases in which seriously ill or disabled newborn infants have been "allowed to die" under questionable justifications provide a reason for caution.

We should exclude several conditions of patients from consideration altogether. For example, mental retardation is irrelevant in determining whether treatment is in the patient's best interest. Proxies should not confuse quality of life for the patient with the value of that patient's life for others, and they should not refuse treatment that would be in the incompetent patient's interests in order to avoid burdens to the family or costs to society. Instead, the incompetent patient's best interests, defined in terms of his or her personal welfare, generally should be the decisive criterion for a proxy, even if the patient's interests conflict with familial or societal interests.

This position contrasts with that of the President's Commission for the Study of Ethical Problems in Medicine and Biomedical and Behavioral Research. It recognized a broader conception of best interests that includes the welfare of the family: "The impact of a decision on an incapacitated patient's loved ones may be taken into account in determining someone's best interests, for most people do have an important interest in the well-being of their families or close associates."[54] It is true that a patient often has an interest in his or her family's welfare, but it is a long step from this premise to a conclusion about whose interests should be overriding. When the incompetent patient has never been competent or never expressed his or her wishes while competent, it is not proper to impute altruism or any other motive to that patient against his or her medical best interests.

Children with serious illnesses or disabilities. Some of the most difficult questions about quality of life and treatment omission involve endangered near-term fetuses, seriously ill newborns, and young children. Prenatal obstetric management and neonatal intensive care can now salvage the lives of many anomalous fetuses and disabled newborns with physical conditions that would have been fatal three decades ago. However, the resultant quality of life is sometimes so low that it raises questions about whether the aggressive obstetric management or intensive care has produced more harm than benefit for the patient. Some commentators argue that avoidance of harm (including iatrogenic harm) is the best guide to decisions on behalf of near-term fetuses and infants in neonatal nurseries,[55] whereas others argue that aggressive intervention violates the obligation of nonmaleficence if any one of three conditions is present: "inability to survive infancy, inability to live without severe pain, and inability to participate, at least minimally, in human experience."[56]

We accept the conclusion that managing high-risk pregnancies nonaggressively and allowing seriously disabled newborns to die are, under some conditions, morally permissible actions that do not violate obligations of nonmaleficence. When quality of life is so low that aggressive intervention or intensive care produces more harm than benefit for the patient, it is justifiable to withhold or to withdraw treatment from near-term fetuses, newborns, or infants—just as it is with persons of other ages. The conditions that would lead to a sufficiently poor quality of life include a number of antenatal conditions that commonly eventuate in stillbirth, severe brain damage caused by birth asphyxia, Tay-Sachs disease (which involves increasing spasticity and dementia and usually results in death by age three or four), and Lesch-Nyhan disease (which involves uncontrollable spasms, mental retardation, compulsive self-mutilation, and early death). Severe cases of neural tube defects in which newborns lack all or most of the brain and death is inevitable would also occasion a justifiable decision not to treat.

The debate about treatment or nontreatment of seriously ill and disabled newborns was stimulated in the United States by an article in which Raymond S. Duff and A. G. M. Campbell reported that 43 of 299 consecutive deaths in the intensive care nursery at the Yale–New Haven Hospital had occurred following a decision for nontreatment based on the infants' extremely poor prognosis for meaningful life.[57] This and similar reports led to a public debate that went unaccompanied by government intervention for almost a decade. Vigorous government action then occurred in response to the Infant Doe case, in which Infant Doe died six days after he was born with Down syndrome and respiratory and digestive complications requiring major surgery, which his parents refused to authorize. Subsequently, Congress passed amendments to the Child Abuse and Treatment Act that defined as child abuse the "withholding of medically indicated treatment" from children.[58] This law and subsequent regulations define "medically indicated treatment" as all treatment that is likely to ameliorate life-threatening conditions, including nutrition and hydration. However, Congress also recognized three exceptions, each of which was sufficient to render life-sustaining treatment optional.

1. The infant is chronically and irreversibly comatose.
2. Provision of such treatment would merely prolong dying or not be effective in ameliorating or correcting the infant's life-threatening conditions.
3. Provision of such treatment would be futile and the treatment would be inhumane.

Some government officials interpreted this approach as involving reasonable *medical* judgments, rather than *quality-of-life* judgments. Such a strategy attempts to keep these judgments in line with sound professional practice, but it is problematic. We have already argued that "medically indicated treatments" themselves presuppose values and, often, standards of quality of life. Conditions 1 through 3, therefore, cannot be reduced to nonevaluative, medically indicated exceptive conditions to otherwise medically indicated treatments. Rather, these conditions express Congress's view of ethically indicated exceptions, and they incorporate quality-of-life judgments about which lives should be saved.

Consistent with our arguments at the end of Chapter 3, the most appropriate standard in cases of never-competent patients, including seriously ill newborns, is that of best interests, as judged by the best obtainable estimate of what reasonable persons would consider the highest net benefit among the available options. As noted above, we need to restrict such quality-of-life judgments by justifiable criteria of benefits and burdens in order not to reduce quality of life to arbitrary and partial judgments of personal preference or of social worth. For example, Down syndrome is not by itself a sufficient reason to allow a newborn to die, and usually it is not sufficient even when the newborn suffers from other life-threatening conditions that require treatment.

We conclude that competent patients and authorized surrogates can use controlled quality-of-life considerations with medical input to legitimately determine whether treatments are optional or obligatory. These categories of optional and obligatory should replace the traditional distinctions and rules examined earlier in this chapter. However, we must now consider the most difficult of all the distinctions that have been used to determine acceptable decisions about treatment and acceptable forms of professional conduct with seriously ill or injured patients, namely that between killing and letting die.

Killing and Letting Die

A persistent body of distinctions and rules about life-sustaining treatments derives from the distinction between killing and letting die (or allowing to die), which in turn draws on the act–omission and active–passive distinctions.[59] The killing–letting die distinction often underlies distinctions (1) between suicide and forgoing treatment and (2) between homicide and natural death. These distinctions are unsatisfactory for many of the purposes to which they have been put and need significant reformulation, both in biomedical ethics and in public policy, if we are to retain them.

This section will address three areas of concern. (1) *A conceptual question:* "What conceptually is the difference between killing and letting die?" (2) *A moral question:* "Is killing in itself morally wrong, whereas allowing to die is not in itself morally wrong?" (3) *A conceptual and causal question:* "Is forgoing life-sustaining treatment sometimes a form of killing, and, if so, is it sometimes suicide and sometimes homicide?"

Conceptual Questions About the Nature of Killing and Letting Die

Can we define *killing* and *letting die* so that they are conceptually distinct and do not overlap? The following two cases suggest that we cannot: (1) A newborn with Down syndrome needed an operation to correct a tracheoesophageal fistula (a congenital deformity in which a connection exists between the trachea and the esophagus, thereby allowing food or milk to get into the lungs). The parents and physicians maintained that survival was not in this infant's best interests and decided to let the infant die rather than perform the operation. However, a public outcry occurred over the case, and critics charged that the parents and physicians had killed the child by negligently allowing the child to die.[60] (2) Dr. Gregory Messenger, a dermatologist, was charged with manslaughter after he unilaterally terminated his premature (25 weeks gestation, 750 g) son's life-support system in a Lansing, Michigan, neonatal intensive care unit. He thought he had merely acted compassionately in letting his son die after a neonatologist had failed to fulfil a promise not to resuscitate the infant.[61]

In such cases, can we legitimately describe actions that involve intentionally not treating a patient as "allowing to die" or "letting die," rather than "killing"? Do at least some of these actions involve both killing and allowing to die? Is "allowing to die" a euphemism in some cases for "acceptable killing" or "acceptable taking of life"? These conceptual questions have moral implications. Unfortunately, both ordinary discourse and legal concepts are vague and equivocal. In ordinary language, *killing* is causal action that brings about death, whereas *letting die* is the intentional avoidance of causal intervention so that disease, system failure, or injury causes death. Killing extends to animal and plant life. Neither in ordinary language nor in law does the word "killing" entail a wrongful act or a crime. Neither source of this language requires an intentional action for killing; for example, we can say properly that, in automobile accidents, one driver killed another even when no awareness, intent, or negligence was present.

Conventional definitions are unsatisfactory for drawing any sharp distinction between killing and letting die. They allow many acts of letting die to count as killing, thereby defeating the very point of the distinction. For example, under these definitions, health professionals kill patients when they intentionally let them die in circumstances in which a duty exists to keep the patients alive. It is unclear in literature on the subject how to distinguish killing from letting die so as to avoid even such simple cases that satisfy the conditions of both killing and letting die. We will confine the terms *killing* and *letting die* to circumstances in which a human being intentionally brings about the death of a human being (oneself or another). Killing and letting die do not occur by accident, chance, mishap, and the like. Killing and letting die also are not mutually exclusive concepts. One person can kill another by intentionally allowing the other to die so that killing can occur by omission as well as by commission. However, this usage does not change the fact that the meaning of "killing" and "letting die" are vague and inherently contestable. Attempts to refine their meanings are likely to produce controversy without closure. We use these terms only because they are so prominent in the literature on the issues we will discuss.

Connecting Right and Wrong to Killing and Letting Die

"Letting die" is (prima facie) acceptable in medicine under one of two justifying conditions: (1) a medical technology is *useless* (medically futile), or (2) patients (or their authorized surrogates) have *validly refused* a medical technology. That is, letting a patient die is acceptable if and only if it satisfies the condition of futility or the condition of a valid refusal of treatment. (Honoring a valid refusal of a useful treatment is here letting die, not killing.) If these conditions are not satisfied, then letting a patient die involves negligence and may constitute a form of killing.

"Killing," by contrast, has been conceptually and morally connected in medicine to *unacceptable* acts. The conditions of medical practice make this connection understandable, but killing's absolute unacceptability is not assumed outside of medical circles. In general, the term "killing" does not necessarily entail a wrongful act or a crime, and the rule "Do not kill" is not an absolute rule. Standard justifications of killing, such as killing in self-defense, killing to rescue a person endangered by other persons' immoral acts, and killing by misadventure (accidental, nonnegligent killing while engaged in a lawful act) prevent us from prejudging an action as wrong merely because it is a killing. To correctly apply the label "killing" or the label "letting die" to a set of events will therefore (outside of traditional assumptions in medicine) fail to determine whether an action is acceptable or unacceptable.[62]

Killing may, of course, generally be wrong and letting die only rarely wrong, but, if so, this conclusion is contingent on the features of particular cases. The general wrongness of killing and general rightness of letting die are not surprising features of the moral world inasmuch as killings are *rarely authorized* by appropriate parties (excepting contexts of warfare and capital punishment) and cases of letting die generally are *validly authorized*. Be that as it may, the *frequency* with which one kind of act is justified, by contrast to the other kind of act, is not relevant to the moral (or legal) justification of either kind of act. Forgoing treatment to allow patients to die can be both as intentional and as immoral as actions that in some more direct manner take their lives (and both can be forms of killing).

Correctly labeling an act as "killing" or as "letting die," therefore, does not determine that one form of action is better or worse, or more or less justified, than the other. Some particular instance of killing (a brutal murder, say) may be worse than some particular instance of allowing someone to die (e.g., forgoing treatment for a patient who is in a persistent vegetative state); but some particular instance of letting die (not resuscitating a patient who could be saved, say) also may be worse than some particular instance of killing (such as mercy killing at the patient's request). Nothing about either killing or allowing to die entails judgments about actual wrongness or rightness, or about the beneficence or nonmaleficence of the action. Rightness and wrongness depend on the merit of the justification underlying the action, not on the type of action it is. Neither killing nor letting die, therefore, is wrongful per se; and in this regard, they are distinguished from murder, which is wrongful per se.

Accordingly, a judgment that an act of either killing or letting die is justified or unjustified entails that we know something else about the act besides these characteristics. We may need to know about the actor's motive (whether it is benevolent or malicious, for example), the patient's or surrogate's request, or the act's consequences. These additional factors will allow us to place the act on a moral map and make a normative judgment about it.

We should, therefore, leave open questions of the justifiability of "killing" and "letting die" when we consider several forms of physician aid-in-dying that we consider later in this chapter. In short, whether letting die is justified and whether killing is unjustified are matters in need of analysis and argument, not matters that medical tradition and legal prohibition have adequately resolved.

Forgoing Life-Sustaining Treatment: Killing or Allowing to Die?

Many writers in medicine, law, and ethics have construed a physician's intentionally forgoing a medical technology as letting die, rather than killing, if and only if an underlying disease or injury causes death. When physicians withhold or withdraw medical technology, according to this doctrine, a natural death occurs, because natural conditions do what they would have done if the technology had never been initiated. By contrast, killings occur when acts of persons rather than natural conditions cause death.[63] From this perspective, one acts nonmaleficently in allowing to die and maleficently in killing.

Though this view is influential in law and medicine, it is seriously flawed. To obtain a satisfactory account, we must add that the forgoing of the medical technology is *validly authorized* and for this reason *justified*. If the physician's forgoing of technology were unjustified and a person died from "natural" causes of injury or disease, the result would be unjustified killing, not justified allowing to die. The validity of the authorization, not some independent assessment of causation, determines the morality of the action.

To bring out this point, consider a thought-experiment: Two patients are in their beds in a semiprivate hospital room, both with the same malady and both respirator-dependent. One has refused the respirator; the other wishes to remain on the respirator. A physician intentionally flips a master switch that turns off both respirators. The two patients die in the same way at the same time of the same physical causes and by the same physical action of the physician. Though they die of the same physical causes, they do not die of the same causes of interest to law and morality, because the proximate cause—that is, the cause responsible for the outcome—is not the same in the two otherwise identically situated patients. The doctor unjustifiably caused the death of and killed one patient (the action caused the death); but the doctor justifiably let the other patient die (a forbearance to treat) and did not cause this patient's death. This argument shows that a valid authorization transforms what would be a maleficent act of killing into a nonmaleficent (and perhaps beneficent) act of allowing to die.

From both a legal and a moral point of view, one reason why physicians do not injure, maltreat, or kill patients when they withhold or withdraw medical technology and thereby physically cause death is that a physician is morally and legally obligated to recognize and act upon a valid refusal. Since a valid refusal of treatment binds the physician, it would be absurd to hold that these legal and moral duties require physicians to cause the deaths of their patients—in the legal and moral sense of "cause"—and thereby to kill them.

Even from a legal perspective, we can provide a better account than, "The preexisting disease caused the death." The better account is that legal liability should not be imposed on physicians and surrogates unless they have an obligation to provide or continue the treatment. If no obligation to treat exists, then questions of causation and liability do not arise. If the categories of obligatory and optional are primary, we have a reason for avoiding discussions about killing and letting die altogether and for focusing instead on health care professionals' obligations and problems of moral and legal responsibility. The value of this reformulation will become clear in the discussion of physician-assisted suicide in the next section.

We conclude for now that the distinction between killing and letting die suffers from vagueness and moral confusion. The language of killing is so thoroughly confusing—causally, legally, and morally—that it can provide little if any help in discussions of assistance in dying.

The Justification of Intentionally Arranged Deaths

We can now address a set of moral questions that builds on the conceptual, causal, and moral conclusions reached in the previous section. We will formulate the issues largely free of the language of "killing." The general question we address is, "Under what conditions, if any, is it permissible for patients and health professionals to arrange for assisted suicide or for voluntary active euthanasia?" (In assisted suicide, the final agent is the one whose death is brought about, and in voluntary active euthanasia, the final agent is another party who has been authorized to act by the one whose death is brought about.)

Many people inside and outside medicine now believe that active physician assistance for a narrow group of seriously ill and dying patients at their request can be morally justified. Many also believe that, under closely monitored supervision, such acts of assistance in dying should be made legally permissible. The literature generally treats these issues under the umbrella of the legal protection of a "right to die,"[64] but underlying the legal issues is a powerful struggle in law, medicine, and ethics over the nature, scope, and foundations of the right to choose the manner of one's death. We will here offer few judgments about legalization, public policy, or institutional policy. Our interest is in moral questions about whether these acts of assistance by health professionals are justified, chiefly, whether autonomy rights justify requests for active forms of aid-in-dying.

We will argue that sufficient moral reasons exist in some cases to justify acts that intentionally hasten death. However, these reasons are not necessarily sufficient to support revisions in either professional codes of ethics or public policies. We begin with the importance of this distinction between acts and policies. We will then work back to more foundational moral issues.

Acts, Practices, and Slippery Slope Problems

To justify an act is distinct from justifying a practice or a policy that permits or even legitimates the act's performance. A rule of practice or a public policy that prohibits various forms of assistance in dying in medicine may be justified, even if it excludes some acts of causing a person's death that in themselves are morally justifiable. For example, a law might not permit physicians to use a drug overdose to cause death for a patient who suffers from terrible pain, who will probably die within three weeks, and who requests a merciful, assisted death. However, this same act might be justified in an individual case.

The problem is that a practice or policy that allows physicians to intervene to cause deaths or help cause deaths runs risks of abuse and, on balance, might cause more harm than benefit. The argument is not that serious abuses will occur immediately, but that they will grow incrementally over time. Society could start by severely restricting the number of patients who qualify for assistance in dying, but might later revise and loosen these restrictions so that cases of unjustified killing began to occur. Unscrupulous persons would learn how to abuse the system, just as they do now with methods of tax evasion that operate on the margins of the system of legitimate tax avoidance. In short, the slope of the trail toward unjustified taking of life will be so slippery and precipitous that, according to some, we ought never to get on it.

Many dismiss these slippery slope or wedge arguments because of a lack of empirical evidence to support their claims as well as their heavily metaphorical character ("the thin edge of the wedge," "the first step on the slippery slope," "the foot in the door," and "the camel's nose under the tent"). However, we should take some arguments of this form with the utmost seriousness.[65] They force us to think carefully about whether unacceptable harm is likely to result from attractive and apparently innocent first steps.

If society removes certain restraints against interventions that cause death, various psychological and social forces would likely make it more difficult to maintain the relevant distinctions in practice. For example, in some settings, it is plausible to argue as follows: (1) To authorize causing patients' deaths for their benefit when they are suffering excruciating pain or have a bleak future risks opening the door to the encouragement of euthanasia in order to relieve burdens on families and financial burdens on society. (2) *Voluntary* active euthanasia (an act of bringing about the death of a person at his or her informed request) invites social changes leading to *nonvoluntary* euthanasia (an act of killing a person who is incapable of making an informed request) and perhaps to *involuntary* euthanasia (an act of killing a person who, while competent, opposes being killed). However plausible these consequences, in assessing the possibilities we should recall that various forms of active assistance in dying can occur by both omission and commission. Withheld or withdrawn treatment (such as hydration and nutrition) can cause death just as a lethal injection can cause death.

This form of slippery slope argument becomes more compelling when we consider the effects of social discrimination based on disability, the increasing number of newborns with disabilities who survive at heavy cost to the public, and the growing number of aging persons with medical problems that require larger and larger proportions of the public's financial resources. If rules permitting voluntary active euthanasia become public policy, the risk increases that persons in these populations will be harmed; for example, the risk increases that families and health professionals may abandon treatments for disabled newborns and severely brain-damaged adults to avoid social and familial burdens. Moreover, if decision-makers can determine that some newborns and adults have overly burdensome conditions or lives with no value, the same logic can be extended to other populations of feeble, debilitated, and seriously ill patients who are financial and emotional burdens on families and society.

Many of these circumstances are relevantly similar to circumstances that already provide the leading justifications for third-party decisions to withhold or withdraw life support. Often the patients did not request these omissions and left no advance directive. For instance, it takes little imagination to suppose that many parents would, if given the opportunity, withhold life-sustaining technologies from their newborns because of disabilities, such as blindness, retardation, and malformed limbs.

Rules in our moral code against passively or actively causing the death of another person are not isolated fragments. They are threads in a fabric of rules that support respect for human life. The more threads we remove, the weaker the fabric may become. If we focus on the modification of *attitudes*, not only on *rules*, shifts in public policy may also erode the general attitude of respect for life. Prohibitions are often both instrumentally and symbolically important, and their removal could weaken a set of attitudes, as well a practices and restraints that we cannot replace.

Rules against bringing about another's death also provide a basis of trust between patients and health care professionals. We expect health care professionals to promote our welfare under all circumstances. We may risk a loss of public trust if physicians become agents of active euthanasia in addition to healers and caregivers. Nonetheless, we may risk a loss of trust if patients and families believe that physicians are abandoning them in their suffering because they lack the courage and will to offer the assistance needed in the darkest hours of their lives.

The ultimate success or failure of slippery slope arguments against assistance in dying depends on speculative predictions of a progressive erosion of moral restraints. If dire consequences will, in fact, flow from the legal legitimation of assisted suicide or voluntary active euthanasia, then these arguments are cogent and such practices are justifiably prohibited. But how good is the evidence that dire consequences will occur? Does the evidence indicate that we cannot maintain firm distinctions in public policies between, for example, patient-requested death and involuntary euthanasia?[66]

Scant evidence supports any of the answers traditionally given to these questions, so far as we can see. Those, including the present authors, who take seriously some versions of the slippery slope argument should simply admit that the argument needs a premise on the order of a precautionary principle, such as "better safe than sorry." The likelihood of the projected moral erosion, then, is not something we can easily assess. Arguments on every side are speculative and analogical, and different assessors of the same evidence reach different conclusions. An intractable controversy also is likely to persist over what counts as good evidence. Although we cannot here resolve these public issues about evidence, social attitudes, and legitimate practices, we can go to the heart of the moral problem, which is whether some acts of assisting another in dying are justified.

Valid Requests for Aid-in-Dying

At least since the passage of legislation in Oregon that allows physician-assisted suicide in limited circumstances,[67] the frontier of the social and legal acceptance of expanded rights to control one's death has shifted in biomedical ethics from *refusal* of treatment to *request* for aid-in-dying.[68] Now that law and morality ensure that competent patients have a right to refuse treatment, and health professionals have an obligation to implement the refusals, many have turned their attention to the question whether patients have a similar right to request the assistance of physicians willing to help them die. Assuming that the principles of respect for autonomy and nonmaleficence justify forgoing treatment, the same form of justification might extend to physicians prescribing barbiturates or providing other forms of help requested by seriously ill patients.

This strategy rests on the premise that reform in professional ethics and law is needed because of the apparent inconsistency between (1) the strong rights of autonomy that allow persons in grim circumstances to refuse treatment so as to bring about their deaths and (2) the apparent denial of a similar autonomy right to arrange for death by mutual agreement between patient and physician under equally grim circumstances. The argument for reform seems particularly compelling when a condition has become overwhelmingly burdensome for a patient, pain management is inadequate, and only a physician can and is willing to bring relief. At present, medicine and law are in the awkward position of having to say to such patients, "If you were on life-sustaining treatment, you would have a right to withdraw the treatment and then we could let you die. But since you are not, we can only allow you to refuse nutrition and hydration or give you palliative care until you can die a natural death, however painful, undignified, and costly." This seems tantamount to condemning the patient to live a life or to suffer an end to life that he or she does not want.

Clearly, the two types of authorization—refusal of treatment and request for aid-in-dying—are not perfectly analogous. A health professional is obligated to honor an autonomous refusal of a life-prolonging technology, but he or she is not (under ordinary circumstances) obligated to honor an autonomous request for aid-in-dying. This difference does not, however, cut to the heart of the problem, because the issue is not about whether physicians are *obligated* to lend assistance. The issue is whether valid requests render it *permissible* for a physician (or some other person) to lend aid-in-dying. Refusals in medical settings have a moral power lacking in requests, but requests do not lack all power to confer on another a right to act in response.

A physician's precise responsibilities to a patient may depend on the nature of the request made and the nature of the pre-established patient–physician relationship. In some cases of physician-compliance with requests, the patient and the physician pursue the patient's best interest under an agreement that the physician will not abandon the patient or resist what they jointly determine to serve the patient's best interests. In some cases, patients in a close relationship with a physician *both* refuse a medical technology *and* request a hastened death in order to lessen pain or suffering. Refusal and request are parts of a single plan. If the physician accepts the plan, assisted suicide (or possibly euthanasia) grows out of the pre-established relationship.

From this perspective, a valid request for aid-in-dying frees a responder of moral culpability for the death, just as a valid refusal precludes culpability. This logic underlies Oregon's law and helps explain why many adamantly opposed it: This law conspicuously subscribes to the principle that valid requests for assistance are licit and that physicians may respond affirmatively to such requests without fear of legal liability.

We can conceive of no moral grounds for restricting the liberty of a competent individual to make such a request for aid-in-dying. The serious moral questions concern whether physicians are obligated not to implement such requests under certain conditions, such as a depressed state of mind that is serious but does not render a patient incompetent. We believe that physicians sometimes have sufficient moral reason to refuse to comply with such a request, but also that they sometimes have sufficient reason to comply.

These arguments suggest that causing a person's death is morally wrong, when it is wrong, because an unauthorized intervention thwarted or set back a person's interests. It is an evil act when it deprives the person who dies of opportunities and goods.[69] However, if a person freely elects and authorizes death and makes an autonomous judgment that the event constitutes a personal benefit rather than a setback to his or her interests, then active aid-in-dying at the person's request involves no harm or moral wrong. To the contrary, not to help such persons in their dying will frustrate their plans and cause them a loss, thereby harming them. It can also bring them indignity and despair. From this perspective, causing death is not always an evil act.

If letting die based on valid refusals does not harm or wrong persons or violate the rights of persons who die earlier than they otherwise would, how can assisted suicide or voluntary active euthanasia harm or wrong persons who make autonomous choices to die earlier than they otherwise would? In each case, persons seek what for them, in their bleak circumstances, is the best means to the end of quitting life. That is, the person in search of assisted suicide, the person who seeks active euthanasia, and the person who forgoes life-sustaining technology to end life may be identically situated in regard to prognosis and suffering. They simply select different means to end their lives.

Assisting an autonomous person at his or her request to bring about death is, from this perspective, a way of showing respect for the person's autonomous choices. Similarly, denying the person access to other individuals who are willing and qualified to comply with the request shows a fundamental disrespect for the person's autonomy. From a *social* and *legal* perspective there may be good grounds for more zealously protecting one type of patient (e.g., those without health insurance or those who speak no English) than another, but it is unclear why we should protect the one more than the other from the *moral* perspective of a right to make an autonomous choice. What basis could give one type of competent patient a right to choose that is weightier than the right of the other type of competent patient?

Unjustified Physician-Assisted Suicide

The fact that the autonomous requests of patient for aid-in-dying should be respected in some circumstances does not entail that *all* cases of physician-assisted death are justifiable. Jack Kevorkian's practices provide an example of the kind of *unjustified* physician-assisted suicide that medical ethics should discourage. In his first case of assisting in suicide, Janet Adkins, an Oregon grandmother with Alzheimer's disease, had reached a decision that she wanted to take her life rather than lose her cognitive capacities, which she was convinced were slowly deteriorating. After Adkins read about Kevorkian's machine in the news media, she communicated with him by phone and then flew from Oregon to Michigan to meet with him. Following brief discussions over a weekend, she and Kevorkian drove to a park in north Oakland County. He inserted a tube in her arm and started saline flow. His machine was constructed so that Adkins could then press a button to inject other drugs, eventuating in potassium chloride, which physically caused her death. She then pressed the button.[70]

This case raises several concerns. Janet Adkins was in the fairly early stages of the crippling effects of Alzheimer's and was not yet debilitated. At 54 years of age, she was still capable of enjoying a full schedule of activities with her husband and playing tennis with her son, and she might have been able to live a meaningful life for several more years. A slight possibility existed that the Alzheimer's diagnosis was incorrect, and she might have been more psychologically depressed than Kevorkian appreciated. She had limited contact with him before they collaborated in her death, and he did not administer examinations to confirm either her diagnosis or her level of competence to commit suicide. He also lacked the professional expertise to evaluate her. The glare of media attention also raises the question whether Kevorkian acted imprudently in order to generate publicity for his social goals and for his forthcoming book.

Lawyers, physicians, and writers in bioethics have almost universally condemned Kevorkian's actions. The case raises all the fears present in the arguments mentioned previously about physicians who assist in dying: abuse, lack of social control, acting without accountability, and unverifiable circumstances of a patient's death. Although Kevorkian's approach to assisted suicide is regrettable, his "patients" raise profoundly distressing questions about the lack of a support system in medicine or another domain for handling their problems. Having thought for over a year about her future, Janet Adkins decided that the suffering of continued existence exceeded its benefits. Judging from her friends' reports, she knew what she wanted and appreciated both the costs and the benefits. Her family supported her decision. She faced a bleak future from the perspective of a person who had lived an unusually vigorous life, both physically and mentally. She believed that her brain would slowly deteriorate, with progressive and devastating cognitive loss and confusion, fading memory, immense frustration, and loss of all capacity to take care of herself. She also believed that the full burden of responsibility for her care would fall on her family. From her perspective, what Kevorkian offered was preferable to what other physicians offered.

Current social institutions, including the medical system, are inadequate to help many patients in a similar condition who have reached a similar conclusion about their fates. Many dying persons face inadequate counseling, emotional support, and pain control. To them, their condition is intolerable, and no avenue of hope exists. They would rather kill themselves or be killed than face what they understand to be a bleak future without relief. To judge Kevorkian harshly is appropriate, but to say that his "patients" act immorally by arranging for death at their own hand or with a physician's assistance is, for the reasons just mentioned, an overly harsh and unwarranted judgment.

Justified Physician-Assisted Suicide

Balancing the errors of the Kevorkian strategy are several prominent cases of *justified* assisted suicide. First, consider the case of Larry McAfee, in which a court as well as physicians faced a dilemma about legitimate forms of assistance. McAfee was a competent adult, paralyzed from the neck down as the result of an automobile accident. He was not terminally ill, but he found his life as a quadriplegic intolerable. A professional engineer, he devised a self-disconnecting, mouth-controlled mechanism that would separate him from his ventilator, thereby causing his death. A Georgia court found that McAfee's right to refuse treatment and disconnect himself outweighed the state's interest in the preservation of life and in preventing suicide. This finding endorsed the right of a competent patient to refuse customary life-sustaining treatment.

But McAfee wanted more, from the courts and from his physicians. He had previously attempted to disconnect himself from the respirator, but had been unable to follow through with the act because the loss of oxygen incapacitated him. He therefore asked for a physician's assistance in administering a sedative to control pain enough so that he could disconnect himself. The court found that no criminal or civil liability would be attached to a physician who helped him by administering the sedative, but this court hinted (agreeing with a trial court) that courts could not order a physician to administer the sedative. Nevertheless, the court found that "McAfee's right to have a sedative (a medication that in no way causes or accelerates death) administered before the ventilator is disconnected is a part of his right to control his medical treatment."[71]

Such confusing and troublesome cases should never reach a court. The right acknowledged is a right that health care facilities should recognize without the patient having to meet repeated refusals of assistance from physicians. We do not propose a right that requires coercion of physicians' consciences, a troubled area of medical ethics. Instead, we recommend that medical professionals themselves confront these issues and acknowledge that it is permissible to assist some patients in their dying. The problem is that law and medicine (and to some extent ethics) have conspired to insist on the maintenance of traditional sanctions against physician-assisted suicide. Larry McAfee is a striking example of how the current system drives patients who need medical attention to physicians like Jack Kevorkian who are willing to take aggressive actions.

Second, consider the case of the physician Timothy Quill, who prescribed the barbiturates desired by a 45-year-old patient who had refused a risky, painful, and often unsuccessful treatment for leukemia. She had been his patient for many years, and members of her family had, as a group, come to this decision with his counsel. The patient was competent, and had discussed and rejected all reasonable alternatives for the relief of suffering. This case satisfied most of the conditions that the present authors consider sufficient for justified assisted suicide. These conditions include:

1. A voluntary request by a competent patient
2. An ongoing patient–physician relationship
3. Mutual and informed decision-making by patient and physician
4. A supportive yet critical and probing environment of decision-making
5. A considered rejection of alternatives
6. Structured consultation with other parties in medicine
7. A patient's expression of a durable preference for death
8. Unacceptable suffering by the patient
9. Use of a means that is as painless and comfortable as possible.

Even though Quill's actions satisfied most of these conditions, some people found his involvement as a physician unsettling and unjustified. Some critics invoked the wedge argument, because so many patients, especially in elderly populations, are potentially affected if acts like Quill's are legalized. Others were troubled by the fact that Quill potentially violated a New York State law against assisted suicide. Furthermore, to reduce the risks of criminal liability, Quill lied to the medical examiner by informing him that a hospice patient had died of acute leukemia.[72]

Despite these problems, we do not oppose Quill's act, his patient's decision, or their relationship. Suffering and loss of cognitive capacity can ravage and dehumanize patients so severely that death is in their best interests. In these tragic situations, physicians like Quill do not act wrongly in assisting competent patients to bring about their deaths. Public policy issues regarding how to avoid abuses and discourage unjustified acts should be part of our discussion about assisted suicide, but these issues do not affect the moral justifiability of the physician's act itself.

In general, we have thus far been able to respect the line between unjustifiable and justifiable passive euthanasia in medical practice, and we should be able to hold the line between justified and unjustified assistance in suicide. We appreciate that this observation conflicts somewhat with our earlier comments on wedge or slippery slope arguments, but we believe that these two points of view can be reconciled—that is, brought into reflective equilibrium.

Protecting Incompetent Patients

In Chapter 3, we treated standards for surrogate decisions for incompetent patients. We will now consult those standards in order to discuss *who* should decide for the incompetent patient. This question largely concerns the best system for protecting such patients from negligence and harm. Most of us think first of families as the proper decision-makers, because they generally have the deepest interest in protecting their incompetent members. However, this focus is sometimes too narrow. We need a system that will shield incompetent individuals whose family members are caught in conflicts of interest, while also protecting residents of nursing homes, psychiatric hospitals, and facilities for the disabled and mentally retarded who rarely, if ever, see a family member. The appropriate roles of families and courts, guardians, conservators, hospital committees, and health professionals all merit consideration.

Advance Directives

In an increasingly popular procedure rooted more in respect for autonomy than in obligations of nonmaleficence, a person, while competent, either writes a directive for health care professionals or selects a surrogate to make decisions about life-sustaining treatments during periods of incompetence.[73] Two types of *advance directive* aim at governing future decision-making: (1) *living wills*, which are substantive directives regarding medical procedures that should be provided or forgone in specific circumstances, and (2) *durable power of attorney* (DPA) for health care, or proxy directives. A DPA is a legal document in which one person assigns another person as authority to perform specified actions on behalf of the signer. The power is "durable" because, unlike the usual power of attorney, it continues in effect if the signer of the document becomes incompetent.

Much of the early legislative action on this topic focused on the agent's decisions through living wills, in the form of advance directives to physicians that specify the treatment a person welcomes or declines in foreseeable circumstances, such as a persistent vegetative state (PVS), irreversible loss of cognitive capacities, and incompetence. However, individuals have difficulty in specifying decisions or guidelines that adequately anticipate the full range of medical situations that might occur. As a result, designating surrogate decision-makers has become more prevalent. Both kinds of advance directive can be combined in some legal jurisdictions in a single document, and both can be used for refusal of life-sustaining treatment.

Living wills and DPAs protect autonomy interests and may reduce stress for families and health professionals who fear making the wrong decision, but they also generate practical and moral problems.[74] First, relatively few persons compose them or leave explicit instructions.[75] Second, a designated decision-maker might be unavailable when needed, might be incompetent to make good decisions for the patient, or might have a conflict of interest (for example, because of a prospective inheritance or an improved position in a family-owned business). Third, some patients who change their preferences about treatment fail to change their directives, and a few when legally incompetent, protest a surrogate's decision. Fourth, state laws often severely restrict the use of advance directives. For example, advance directive have legal effect in some states if and only if the patient is terminally ill and death is imminent. But decisions must be made in some cases when death is not imminent or the medical condition cannot appropriately be described as a terminal illness. Fifth, living wills provide no basis for health professionals to overturn instructions that turn out not to be in the patient's best medical interest, although the patient could not have reasonably anticipated this circumstance while competent. Surrogate decision-makers too make decisions with which physicians sharply disagree, in some cases asking the physician to act against his or her conscience. Sixth, some patients do not have an adequate understanding of the range of decisions a health professional or a surrogate might be called upon to make and, even with an adequate understanding, cannot foresee clinical situations and possible future experiences.

Vague language is found in many living wills. For example, The Pennsylvania Advance Directive for Health Care "declares" as follows: "I direct my attending physician to withhold or withdraw life-sustaining treatment that serves only to prolong the process of my dying, if I should be in a terminal condition or in a state of permanent unconsciousness."[76] Additional questions often must be answered, such as "Is this condition terminal?" "Is NG-feeding (nasogastric feeding) extraordinary means?" "Is CPR heroic?" and "Is death imminent?" Answering such questions requires inference and discretion.

The following case illustrates the need for resourceful interpretation: Mrs. Z., a 55-year-old teacher of foreign languages, developed aspiration pneumonia, which required admission to the intensive care unit. Her condition was probably caused by a diminished gag reflex, the result of 20 years of multiple sclerosis. To prevent future occurrence, the staff discussed oversewing the patient's epiglottis (part of the larynx), which would require a permanent tracheostomy and entail loss of laryngeal speech capability. Because of her multiple sclerosis,

Mrs. Z. was confined to bed at home. Her only interaction with friends involved speech, and she tutored students at home. Without the medical procedure, a future episode of aspiration pneumonia would probably be fatal. Mrs. Z. stated that she would rather die than be unable to speak, but she was not clearly competent at the time, in part because of what was believed to be a mild organic brain syndrome. Mrs. Z.'s prior living will was then submitted by her sister. The document contained Mrs. Z.'s directive not to be kept alive artificially if she could not lead a "useful life." The sister—in effect serving as a proxy, as if there were a DPA—interpreted Mrs. Z.'s use of the phrase "useful life" to include the ability to relate to others meaningfully by verbal communication. The staff felt comfortable in accepting this judgment and in refraining from performing procedures they had been considering.[77]

Despite the questionable interpretation of "useful life" in this case, and despite the six problems cited previously, the advance directive is a promising and valid way for competent persons to exercise their autonomy.[78] From the perspective of biomedical ethics, the problems are primarily practical, and we can overcome some of them by adequate methods of implementation that follow the outlines of procedures for informed consent discussed in Chapter 3.

Surrogate Decision-making Without Advance Directives

When an incompetent patient has not left an advance directive, who should make the decision, and with whom should the decision-maker consult?

Qualifications of surrogate decision-makers. We propose the following list of qualifications for decision-makers for incompetent patients (including newborns):

1. Ability to make reasoned judgments (competence)
2. Adequate knowledge and information
3. Emotional stability
4. A commitment to the incompetent patient's interests that is free of conflicts of interest and free of controlling influence by those who might not act in the patient's best interests.

The first three conditions are familiar from discussion of informed consent in Chapter 3. The only potentially controversial condition is the fourth. Here we endorse a criterion of *partiality*—that is, acting as an advocate in the incompetent patient's best interests—rather than *impartiality*, which requires neutrality in the consideration of the interests of the various affected parties.

Four classes of decision-makers have been proposed and used in cases of withholding and terminating treatment for incompetent patients: families, physicians and other health care professionals, institutional committees, and courts. If a court-appointed guardian exists, that person will be the primary responsible party.

Absent the intervention of a court, we need a defeasible structure of decision-making authority that places the family as the presumptive authority when the patient cannot make the decision and has not previously designated a decision-maker.

The role of the family. Wide agreement exists that the patient's closest family member is the first choice as a surrogate. The family's role should be presumptively primary because of its presumed identification with the patient's interests, depth of concern about the patient, and intimate knowledge of his or her wishes, as well as its traditional role in society. However, the patient's closest family member(s) are demonstrably unsatisfactory in some cases, and the authority of the family is not final or ultimate.[79] Circumstances occur in which physicians rightly feel compelled to reject a family's decision or to require its review by an ethics committee or the courts. Even the closest family member can have a conflict of interest, can be poorly informed, or can be too distant personally—and even estranged from the patient.[80]

Unfortunately, the term *family* is imprecise, especially if it includes the extended family. Our reasons for assigning presumptive priority to the patient's closest family member also support assigning relative priority to other family members, as most state statutes now require. The ranking varies in these statutes, but an example we find acceptable is the ordering in the Virginia Natural Death Act. If the patient is incompetent and has not specified standards through an advance directive, a decision to withhold or withdraw life-prolonging treatment must involve consultation and agreement between the attending physician and "any of the following individuals in the following order of priority if no individual in a prior class is reasonably available, willing and competent to act:" judicially appointed guardian (if necessary in the circumstances), patient-designated decision-maker, spouse, adult child or a majority of the adult children reasonably available, parents of the patient, and nearest living relative of the patient.[81]

This suggested ranking is not absolute, and health care professionals sometimes should seek to disqualify potential decision-makers because of their incompetence, ignorance, bad faith, or conflict of interest. Serious conflicts of interest in the family may be more common than either physicians or the courts have generally appreciated.

The role of health care professionals. Physicians and other health care professionals can help the family become adequate decision-makers and can safeguard the patient's interests and preferences (where known) by monitoring the quality of surrogate decision-making. Physicians can sometimes discharge their obligations by withdrawing from the case or transferring the patient, but typically they have obligations to help patients and to ensure that surrogates do not violate their own obligations. If physicians contest a surrogate's decision and disagreements persist, they will need an independent source of review, such as a hospital ethics committee or the judicial system. In the event that a surrogate, a member of the health care team, or an independent reviewer asks a caregiver to perform an act that the caregiver regards as futile or unconscionable, the caregiver is not obligated to perform the act, but may still be obligated to help the surrogate or patient make other arrangements for care.

In examining the role of physicians and other health care professionals, we need more empirical evidence about their willingness to override surrogate decisions and their reasons for doing so. Much of the available evidence is derived from decisions about particular classes of patients and may not be accurate beyond these classes. This evidence indicates that physicians not infrequently displace surrogates as decision-makers or act without surrogate permission for a wide variety of reasons, such as poor prognoses, medical futility, and protecting parents of infants.[82] Such actions usually involve nondisclosure or manipulation of information rather than coercion. For example, physicians sometimes do not adequately inform surrogates on grounds that the information would overburden them, upset them, or make them feel guilty. Such actions may be justified, but alternatives such as counseling also may alleviate the problems.

Institutional ethics committees. Surrogate decision-makers sometimes refuse treatments that are in the interests of those they should protect, and physicians sometimes too readily acquiesce. In other cases, these decision-makers may need help in reaching difficult decisions. In such circumstances, a mechanism or procedure is needed to help make a decision or to break a closed, private circle of refusal and acquiescence. A similar need exists for assistance in decisions regarding residents of nursing homes and hospices, psychiatric hospitals, and many residential facilities in which families often play no significant role. One promising, but loosely structured, mechanism is the institutional ethics committee. Some state laws now mandate or legally empower these committees.

Institutional committees were first established to allocate time on kidney machines and for research involving human subjects. Their use for decision-making about treatment or nontreatment for incompetent patients is more recent and more controversial. These committees differ widely in their composition and function. Many create or recommend explicit policies to govern actions, such as withholding and withdrawing treatment, and many serve educational functions in the hospital. Controversy centers on additional functions, such as whether, apart from evidence of abuse of incompetent patients, committees should make, facilitate, or monitor decisions about patients in particular cases.

The decisions of committees on occasion need to be reviewed or criticized, perhaps by an auditor or impartial party. This procedural check is similar to the legal use of "neutral factfinders" appointed to monitor medical decisions made by parents for children who reject parental judgments. These committees do not have formal procedures of evidence or legal representation, and checks help protect confidentiality, ensure fair representation, and provide for equal consideration.[83]

Nonetheless, the benefits of good committee review generally outweigh its risks. These committees help resolve disagreements, generate reasoned options, and help the parties conform to institutional guidelines and federal regulations. A major justification for committee review is that open discussion and debate foster better thinking than can be expected of parties with a narrower perspective. These committees have a particularly robust role to play in circumstances in which physicians acquiesce too readily to parental, familial, or guardian wishes when they are contrary to the best interests these surrogates are meant to promote. Until we better understand the extent to which families or guardians and physicians act or fail to act to pursue the best interests of infants, minors, or incompetent individuals, it is prudent and morally appropriate to require internal committee review whenever parents, families, or guardians decide that life-sustaining therapy should be forgone (whether or not the physician concurs with the surrogate's decision).

The judicial system. Courts have sometimes been unduly intrusive as final decision-makers, but in many cases they are the last and the fairest recourse. In a widely discussed declaration, for example, the supreme judicial court of Massachusetts held in *Saikewicz* that questions of life and death require the "process of detached but passionate investigation and decision that forms the ideal on which the judicial branch of government was created."[84]

The courts should be invoked when there are good reasons to seek to disqualify the family or health care professionals in order to protect an incompetent patient's interests or to adjudicate conflicts over those interests. The courts also sometimes need to intervene in nontreatment decisions for salvageable incompetent patients in mental institutions, nursing homes, and the like. If no family members are available or willing to be involved, and if the patient is confined to a state mental institution or is in a nursing home, it may be appropriate to establish safeguards beyond the health care team and the institutional ethics committee. For example, the New Jersey Supreme Court in *Conroy* recommended the involvement of the state ombudsman, created several years earlier as an established administrative office for the surveillance of nursing homes.[85]

Conclusion

We have concentrated in this chapter on specifying the principle of nonmaleficence. From the premise that we can and should protect persons against some types and levels of harm, as well as avoid causing harm to them, it is a short step to the conclusion that a positive obligation exists to provide benefits such as health care. The step may be shorter still because of the conceptual and moral uncertainty that surrounds the distinctions between the obligation to avoid harm to others, the obligation to benefit them, and the obligation to treat them justly. We engage these topics in Chapters 5 and 6.

Notes

1. W. H. S. Jones, *Hippocrates*, vol. I (Cambridge, MA: Harvard University Press, 1923), p. 165. See also Albert R. Jonsen, "Do No Harm: Axiom of Medical Ethics," in *Philosophical and Medical Ethics: Its Nature and Significance*, ed. Stuart F. Spicker and H. Tristram Engelhardt, Jr. (Dordrecht, the Netherlands: D. Reidel, 1977), pp. 27–41. On the connection of "Do No Harm" to nonmaleficence and beneficence, see Virginia A. Sharpe, "Why 'Do No Harm'?" *Theoretical Medicine* 18 (1997): 197–215.

2. See H. L. A. Hart, *The Concept of Law* (Oxford: Clarendon Press, 1961), p. 190.

3. See, for example, W. D. Ross, *The Right and the Good* (Oxford: Clarendon Press, 1930), pp. 21–26; and John Rawls, *A Theory of Justice* (Cambridge, MA: Harvard University Press, 1971; revised edition, 1999), p. 114 (1999: p. 98).

4. William Frankena, *Ethics*, 2nd ed. (Englewood Cliffs, NJ: Prentice-Hall, 1973), p. 47.

5. On the priority of avoiding harm, see criticisms by N. Ann Davis, "The Priority of Avoiding Harm," in *Killing and Letting Die*, 2nd ed., ed. Bonnie Steinbock and Alastair Norcross (New York: Fordham University Press, 1994), pp. 298–354.

6. *McFall v. Shimp*, no. 78-1771 in Equity (C. P. Allegheny County, Pa., July 26, 1978). See Barbara J. Culliton, "Court Upholds Refusal to Be Medical Good Samaritan," *Science* 201 (August 18, 1978): 596–97; "Judge Upholds Transplant Denial," *New York Times*, July 27, 1978, p. A10; Mark F. Anderson, "Encouraging Bone Marrow Transplants from Unrelated Donors," *University of Pittsburgh Law Review* 54 (1993): 477ff.

7. Alan Meisel and Loren H. Roth, "Must a Man Be His Cousin's Keeper?" *Hastings Center Report* 8 (October 1978): 5–6.

8. See Joel Feinberg, *Harm to Others*, vol. I of *The Moral Limits of the Criminal Law* (New York: Oxford University Press, 1984), esp. pp. 32–36.

9. On the roles of harm and nonmaleficence in bioethics, see Bettina Schöne-Seifert, "Harm," in Warren Reich, ed. *Encyclopedia of Bioethics*, rev. ed. (New York: Simon & Schuster Macmillan, 1995): 1021–1026.

10. For a useful arrangement of rules of nonmaleficence, see Bernard Gert, *Morality: A New Justification of Morality* (New York: Oxford University Press, 1988), ch. 6–7.

11. See H. L. A. Hart, *Punishment and Responsibility* (Oxford: Clarendon Press, 1968), esp. pp. 136–57; Joel Feinberg, *Doing and Deserving* (Princeton, NJ: Princeton University Press, 1970), esp. pp. 187–221; Holly Smith, "Culpable Ignorance," *Philosophical Review* 92 (1983): 543–71; and Eric D'Arcy, *Human Acts: An Essay in their Moral Evaluation* (Oxford: Clarendon Press, 1963), esp. p. 121.

12. On medical negligence, physician-caused harm, and their connection to medical ethics, see Virginia A. Sharpe and Alan I. Faden, *Medical Harm: Historical, Conceptual, and Ethical Dimensions of Iatrogenic Illness* (New York: Cambridge University Press, 1998). On the legal model, see "Physician's Duty to Inform of Risks," *American Law Reports*, 3d, 88 (1986): 1010–25; and Martin Curd and Larry May, *Professional Responsibility for Harmful Actions* (Dubuque, IA: Kendall/Hunt, 1984).

13. Quoted in Angela Roddy Holder, *Medical Malpractice Law* (New York: John Wiley & Sons, 1975), p. 42.

14. This case was presented to one of the authors during a consultation. On some of the intuitions at work in this and similar cases, see Anna Maria Cugliari and Tracy E. Miller, "Moral and Religious Objections by Hospitals to Withholding and Withdrawing Life-Sustaining Treatment," *Journal of Community Health* 19 (1994): 87–100.

15. For defenses of the distinction along these or similar lines, see Daniel P. Sulmasy and Jeremy Sugarman, "Are Withholding and Withdrawing Therapy Always Morally Equivalent?" *Journal of Medical Ethics* 20 (1994): 218–22 (commented on by John Harris, pp. 223–24); and Kenneth V. Iserson, "Withholding and Withdrawing Medical Treatment: An Emergency Medicine Perspective," *Annals of Emergency Medicine* 28 (1996): 51–54.

16. *In the matter of Spring*, Mass. 405 N.E. 2d 115 (1980), at 488–89.

17. Robert Stinson and Peggy Stinson, *The Long Dying of Baby Andrew* (Boston: Little, Brown and Co., 1983), p. 355.

18. On responsible and compassionate management generally, see Howard Brody, et al., "Withdrawing Intensive Life-Sustaining Treatment—Recommendations for Compassionate Clinical Management," *New England Journal of Medicine* 336 (Feb. 27, 1997): 652–57.

19. Susanna E. Bedell and Thomas L. Delbanco, "Choices about Cardiopulmonary Resuscitation in the Hospital: When Do Physicians Talk with Patients?," *New England Journal of Medicine* 310 (April 26, 1984): 1089–93. See also Marcia Angell, "Respecting the Autonomy of Competent Patients," *New England Journal of Medicine* 310 (April 26, 1984): 1115–16.

20. Gerald Kelly, S.J., "The Duty to Preserve Life," *Theological Studies* 12 (December 1951): 550.

21. This case has been adapted with permission from a case presented by Dr. Martin P. Albert of Charlottesville, Virginia. On continuing debates and problems in nursing homes, see Alan Meisel, "Barriers to Forgoing Nutrition and Hydration in Nursing Homes," *American Journal of Law and Medicine* 21 (1995): 335–82; Elizabeth H. Bradley, Vasum Peiris, and Terrie Wetle, "Discussions About End-of-Life Care in Nursing Homes," *Journal of the American Geriatrics Society* 46 (1998): 1235–41.

22. In the matter of Quinlan, 70 N.J. 10, 355 A.2d 647, *cert. denied*, 429 U.S. 922 (1976). The New Jersey Supreme Court ruled that the Quinlans could disconnect the mechanical ventilator so that the patient could "die with dignity."

23. In re *Conroy*, 98 NJ 321, 486 A2d 1209 (N.J. 1985).

24. *Brophy v. New England Sinai Hospital, Inc.*, 398 Mass. 417, 497 N.E. 2d 626 (1986).

25. These issues were first raised in 1982, in *Barber v. Superior Court*, 147 Cal. App. 3d 1006, 195 Cal. Rptr. 484 (1983). By 1988, many courts accepted this trend as determinative. For a review of the massive court literature during this formative period, see Alan Meisel, *The Right to Die*, 2nd ed. (New York: John Wiley & Sons, 1995). In *Cruzan v. Director, Missouri Department of Health*, 110 S.Ct. 2841 (1990), the U.S. Supreme Court focused on procedural requirements for termination of life-sustaining treatment for incompetent patients. The court assumed that a competent person has a constitutionally protected right to refuse lifesaving hydration and nutrition. Its dicta reflected no distinction between medical and sustenance treatments.

26. See Joann Lynn and James F. Childress, "Must Patients Always Be Given Food and Water?" *Hastings Center Report* 13 (October 1983): 17–21. See also the essays in Joanne Lynn, ed., *By No Extraordinary Means* (Bloomington, IN: Indiana University Press, 1986).

27. G. E. M. Anscombe, "Ethical Problems in the Management of Some Severely Handicapped Children: Commentary," *Journal of Medical Ethics* 7 (1981): 122.

28. C. Everett Koop, "Ethical and Surgical Considerations in the Care of the Newborn with Congenital Abnormalities," in *Infanticide and the Handicapped Newborn*, ed. Dennis J. Horan and Melinda Delahoyde (Provo, UT: Brigham Young University Press, 1982), pp. 89–106, esp. 105; Koop, "Life and Death and the Handicapped Newborn," *Ethics and Medicine: A Christian Perspective* 3 (1987): 39–44.

29. C. Everett Koop and Edward R. Grant, "The 'Small Beginnings' of Euthanasia," *Notre Dame Journal of Law, Ethics & Public Policy* 2 (1986): 607–32; C. Everett Koop, "The Challenge of Definition," *Hastings Center Report* 19 (1989): S2–S3.

30. *Federal Register* 48, No. 129, July 5, 1983.

31. See Alan Meisel, "Legal Issues in Decision Making for Incompetent Patients: Advance Directives and Surrogate Decision Making," *Advance Directives and Surrogate Decision Making in Health Care: United States, Germany and Japan*, eds. Hans-Martin Sass, Robert M. Veatch, and Rihito Kimura (Baltimore, MD: The Johns Hopkins University Press, 1998), 38–65, esp. 41–44.

32. Daniel Callahan, "On Feeding the Dying," *Hastings Center Report* 13 (October 1983): 22; Paolo Cattorini and Massimo Reichlin, "Persistent Vegetative State: A Presumption to Treat," *Theoretical Medicine* 18 (1997): 263–81; and see Ronald A. Carson, "The Symbolic Significance of Giving to Eat and Drink," in Lynn, ed., *By No Extraordinary Means*, pp. 85, 87.

33. See Mark Siegler and Alan J. Weisbard, "Against the Emerging Stream: Should Fluids and Nutritional Support Be Discontinued?" *Archives of Internal Medicine* 145 (January 1985): 129–32; and Patrick Derr, "Why Food and Fluids Can Never Be Denied," *Hastings Center Report* 16 (February 1986): 28–30; Gillian M. Craig, "On Withholding Nutrition and Hydration in the Terminally Ill: Has Palliative Medicine Gone Too Far?", *Journal of Medical Ethics* 20 (1994): 139–43.

34. Robert M. McCann, William J. Hall, and Ann Marie Groth-Juncker, "Comfort Care for Terminally Ill Patients: The Appropriate Use of Nutrition and Hydration," *Journal of the American Medical Association* 272 (Oct. 26, 1994): 1263–66; Robin L. Fainsinger, et al., "Nutrition and Hydration for the Terminally Ill" [Letters and Response], *Journal of the American Medical Association* 273 (June 15, 1995): 1736–37; Ronald Cranford, "Neurologic Syndromes and Prolonged Survival: When Can Artificial Nutrition and Hydration be Foregone?" *Law, Medicine, and Health Care* 19 (1991): 13–22, esp. 18–19.

35. Kenneth C. Micetich, Patricia H. Steinecker, and David C. Thomasma, "Are Intravenous Fluids Morally Required for Dying Patients?" *Archives of Internal Medicine* 143 (May, 1983): 975–78.

36. Centers for Disease Control (CDC), National Center for Health Statistics, "New Study of Patterns of Death in the United States" (February 23, 1998), http://www.cdc.gov/nchs/releases/98facts/98sheets/93nmfs.htm. See earlier, President's Commission, *Deciding to Forego Life-Sustaining Treatment*, pp. 17–18.

37. The rule of double effect has rough precedents that predate the writings of St. Thomas Aquinas (e.g., in Augustine and Abelard). However, the history primarily flows from Aquinas. See Anthony Kenny, "The History of Intention in Ethics," *Anatomy of the Soul* (Oxford: Basil Blackwell, 1973), Appendix; and Joseph T. Mangan, S.J., "An Historical Analysis of the Principle of Double Effect," *Theological Studies* 10 (1949): 41–61. For reservations about attributing the doctrine to St. Thomas, see Gareth Matthews, "Saint Thomas and the Principle of Double Effect," in *Aquinas's Moral Theory*, ed. Scott MacDonald (Ithaca, NY: Cornell University Press, 1998); and Thomas A. Cavanaugh, "Aquinas's Account of Double Effect," *Thomist* 61 (1997): 107–21.

38. Joseph Boyle reduces the RDE to two conditions: intention and proportionality. "Who Is Entitled to Double Effect?" *Journal of Medicine and Philosophy* 16 (1991): 475–94, and "Toward Understanding the Principle of Double Effect," *Ethics* 90 (1980): 527–38. For an emphasis on intention, see Charles Fried, *Right and Wrong* (Cambridge, MA: Harvard University Press, 1978); and Thomas Nagel, *The View from Nowhere* (New York: Oxford University Press, 1986). For criticisms of intention-weighted views, see Sophie Botros, "An Error about the Doctrine of Double Effect," *Philosophy* 74 (1999): 71–83; and Timothy E. Quill, Rebecca Dresser, and Dan Brock, "The Rule of Double Effect–A Critique of Its Role in End-of-Life Decision Making," *New England Journal of Medicine* 337 (1997): 1768–71. For an emphasis on proportionality, see Richard McCormick, S.J., *Ambiguity in Moral Choice* (Milwaukee, WI: Marquette University, 1973) and his contribution to Paul Ramsey and Richard A. McCormick, S.J., eds., *Doing Evil to Achieve Good: Moral Choice in Conflict Situations* (Chicago: Loyola University Press, 1978).

39. See David Granfield, *The Abortion Decision* (Garden City, NY: Image Books, 1971), which defends the RDE, and Susan Nicholson, *Abortion and the Roman Catholic Church* (Knoxville, TN: Religious Ethics, Inc., 1978), which criticizes it. See also the criticisms in Donald Marquis, "Four Versions of Double Effect," *Journal of Medicine and Philosophy* 16 (1991): 515–44.

40. See the analysis in Michael Bratman, *Intention, Plans, and Practical Reason* (Cambridge, MA: Harvard University Press, 1987).

41. Alvin I. Goldman, *A Theory of Human Action* (Englewood Cliffs, NJ: Prentice-Hall, 1970), pp. 49–85.

42. See Hector–Neri Castañeda, "Intentionality and Identity in Human Action and Philosophical Method," *Nous* 13 (1979): 235–60, esp. 255.

43. Our analysis here borrows from Ruth R. Faden and Tom L. Beauchamp, *A History and Theory of Informed Consent* (New York: Oxford University Press, 1986), ch. 7.

44. We follow John Searle in thinking that we cannot reliably distinguish in many situations among acts, effects, consequences, and events. Searle, "The Intentionality of Intention and Action," *Cognitive Science* 4 (1980): 65.

45. Such an interpretation of double effect is defended by Boyle, "Who Is Entitled to Double Effect?"

46. For debates about the nature of futility, see Baruch A. Brody and Amir Halevy, "Is Futility a Futile Concept?" *Journal of Medicine and Philosophy* 20 (1995): 123–44; Loretta M. Kopelman, "Conceptual and Moral Disputes about Futile and Useful Treatments," *Journal of Medicine and Philosophy* 20 (1995): 109–21; Steven H. Miles, "Medical Futility," in *Health Care Ethics: Critical Issues*, ed. John F. Monagle and David C. Thomasma (Gaithersburg, MD: Aspen Publishers, 1994): 233–40; Stuart J. Youngner, "Who Defines Futility?" *Journal of the American Medical Association* 260 (October 14, 1988): 2094–95; and Youngner, "Futility in Context," *Journal of the American Medical Association* 264: (September 12, 1990): 1295–96.

47. See Susan B. Rubin, *When Doctors Say No: The Battleground of Medical Futility* (Bloomington: Indiana University Press, 1998); and Lawrence J. Schneiderman, Nancy Jecker, and Albert R. Jonsen, "Medical Futility: Response to Critiques," *Annals of Internal Medicine* 125 (1996): 669–74.

48. This case was recorded by Robert Baker in his project on Moral Methodologies in ICUs.

49. For constructive proposals that take account of legitimate disagreement, see Robert Truog, "Progress in the Futility Debate," *Journal of Clinical Ethics* 6 (1995): 128–32; Rosemarie Tong, "Towards a Just, Courageous, and Honest Resolution of the Futil-

ity Debate," *Journal of Medicine and Philosophy* 20 (1995): 165–89; and Baruch A. Brody and Amir Halevy, "The Houston Process-Based Approach to Medical Futility," *Bioethics Forum* 14 (1998): 10–18.

50. *Superintendent of Belchertown State School v. Saikewicz*, Mass., 370 N.E. 2d 417 (1977), at 428.

51. Ramsey, *Ethics at the Edges of Life* (New Haven: Yale University Press, 1978), p. 155.

52. See President's Commission, *Deciding to Forego Life-Sustaining Treatment*, ch. 5, and the articles on "The Persistent Problem of PVS," *Hastings Center Report* 18 (February/March 1988): 26–47.

53. Ramsey, *Ethics at the Edges of Life*, p. 172.

54. President's Commission, *Deciding to Forego Life-Sustaining Treatment*.

55. See Frank A. Chervenak and Laurence B. McCullough, "Nonaggressive Obstetric Management," *Journal of the American Medical Association* 261 (June 16, 1989): 3439–40; and their "The Fetus as Patient: Implications for Directive versus Nondirective Counseling for Fetal Benefit," *Fetal Diagnosis and Therapy* 6 (1991): 93–100.

56. Albert R. Jonsen and Michael J. Garland, "A Moral Policy for Life/Death Decisions in the Intensive Care Nursery," in *Ethics of Newborn Intensive Care*, ed. Jonsen and Garland (Berkeley: University of California, Institute of Governmental Studies, 1976), p. 148.

57. Raymond S. Duff and A. G. M. Campbell, "Moral and Ethical Dilemmas in the Special-Care Nursery," *New England Journal of Medicine* 289 (October 25, 1973): 890–94.

58. "Child Abuse Prevention and Treatment and Adoption Reform Act Amendments of 1984," Public Law 98–457, 42 U.S.C. 5101ff (1984); "Child Abuse and Neglect Prevention and Treatment Program: Final Rule," *Federal Register* 50 (April 15, 1985): 14878–901. See also the U.S. Supreme Court ruling on June 9, 1986 in *Bowen v. American Hospital Association et al*, No. 84–1529, 54 LW 4579.

59. See Steinbock and Norcross, eds., *Killing and Letting Die*; Tom L. Beauchamp, ed., *Intending Death* (Upper Saddle River, NJ: Prentice Hall, 1996); H. M. Malm, "Killing, Letting Die, and Simple Conflicts," *Philosophy and Public Affairs* 18 (1989): 238–58; and Jeff McMahan, "Killing, Letting Die, and Withdrawing Aid," *Ethics* 103 (1993): 250–79.

60. See Fred Barbash and Christina Russell, "The Demise of 'Infant . . . ': Permitted Death Gives Life to an Old Debate," *Washington Post*, April 17, 1982.

61. Howard Brody, "Messenger Case: Lessons and Reflections," *Ethics-in-Formation* 5 (1995): 8–9; "Man Acquitted in Son's Death," *New York Times*, 4 February 1995, p. 10; John Roberts, "Doctor Charged for Switching Off His Baby's Ventilator," *British Medical Journal* 309 (13 August 1994): 430. In February 1995, a jury in a lower court cleared Dr. Messenger of the manslaughter charges brought in 1994.

62. Cf. James Rachels, "Active and Passive Euthanasia," *New England Journal of Medicine* 292 (January 9, 1975): 78–80; Rachels, "Killing, Letting Die, and the Value of Life," in his *Can Ethics Provide Answers? And Other Essays in Moral Philosophy* (Lanham, MD: Rowman and Littlefield, 1997): 69–79; Roy W. Perrett, "Killing, Letting Die and the Bare Difference Argument," *Bioethics* 10 (1996): 131–39; and Dan W. Brock, "Voluntary Active Euthanasia," *Hastings Center Report* 22, no. 2 (March/April 1992): 10–22.

63. In both *Quinlan* and *Conroy*, for example, the New Jersey Supreme Court held that the respirator was only delaying the patient's inevitable death, which would be a "nat-

ural death" if the life-support apparatus were removed. For moral accounts that rely on this traditional medical and legal model to defend the killing/letting die distinction, see Kevin P. Quinn, "Assisted Suicide and Equal Protection: In defense of the Distinction between Killing and Letting Die," *Issues in Law and Medicine* 13 (1997): 145–71; and Daniel Callahan, *The Troubled Dream of Life* (New York: Simon & Schuster, 1993), ch. 2.

64. See Lawrence O. Gostin, "Deciding Life and Death in the Courtroom: From Quinlan to Cruzan, Glucksberg, and Vacco—A Brief History and Analysis of Constitutional Protection of the 'Right to Die'," *Journal of the American Medical Association* 278 (Nov. 12, 1997): 1523–28.

65. For fuller discussions, see Douglas Walton, *Slippery Slope Arguments* (Oxford: Clarendon Press, 1992); Govert den Hartogh, "The Slippery Slope Argument," in *A Companion to Bioethics*, ed. Helga Kuhse and Peter Singer (Malden, MA: Blackwell, 1998): 280–90; Christopher James Ryan, "Pulling up the Runaway: The Effect of New Evidence on Euthanasia's Slippery Slope," *Journal of Medical Ethics* 24 (1998): 341–44; Frederick Schauer, "Slippery Slopes," *Harvard Law Review* 99 (1985): 361–83; Bernard Williams, "Which Slopes Are Slippery?" in *Moral Dilemmas in Modern Medicine*, ed. Michael Lockwood (Oxford: Oxford University Press, 1985), pp. 126–37; Wibren van der Burg, "The Slippery Slope Arguments," *Ethics* 102 (October 1991): 42–65; and James Rachels, *The End of Life: Euthanasia and Morality* (Oxford: Oxford University Press, 1986), ch. 10.

66. See Franklin G. Miller, Howard Brody, and Timothy E. Quill, "Can Physician-Assisted Suicide Be Regulated Effectively?" *Journal of Law, Medicine and Ethics* 24 (1996): 225–32.

67. Oregon. Legislature. Measure No. 16. *The Oregon Death with Dignity Act* (1994). Voters first approved Measure 16 in a November 8, 1994 referendum. Under its provision, a terminally ill patient must wish to escape unbearable suffering and must three times request a physician's prescription for lethal drugs. The doctor then must wait 15 days after the first request before writing a prescription for the requested lethal drugs. On November 4, 1997, voters rejected Measure 51, which would have repealed Measure 16. For empirical studies of subsequent developments in Oregon, see Linda Ganzini, et al., "Physicians' Experiences with the Oregon Death with Dignity Act," *The New England Journal of Medicine* 342 (Feb. 24, 2000): 557–63; and Amy D. Sullivan, et al., "Legalized Physician-Assisted Suicide in Oregon—The Second Year," *The New England Journal of Medicine* 342 (Feb. 24, 2000): 598–604.

68. On the nature and importance of the distinction, see Bernard Gert, James L. Bernat, and R. Peter Mogielnicki, "Distinguishing Between Patients' Refusals and Requests," *Hastings Center Report* 24 (July–Aug. 1994): 13–15; Leigh C. Bishop, et al., "Refusals Involving Requests" [Letters and Responses], *Hastings Center Report* 25 (July–Aug. 1995): 4; and Diane E. Meier, et al., "On the Frequency of Requests for Physician Assisted Suicide in American Medicine," *New England Journal of Medicine* 338 (April 23, 1998): 1193–1201.

69. Cf. Allen Buchanan, "Intending Death: The Structure of the Problem and Proposed Solutions," in *Intending Death*, esp. 34–38; Frances M. Kamm, *Morality, Mortality*, vol. I (New York: Oxford University Press, 1993), ch. 1; Kamm, "Physician-Assisted Suicide, the Doctrine of Double Effect, and the Ground of Value," *Ethics* 109 (1999): 586–605; and Matthew Hanser, "Why are Killing and Letting Die Wrong?", *Philosophy and Public Affairs* 24 (1995): 175–201.

70. See *New York Times*, June 6, pp. A1, B6; June 7, 1990, pp. A1, D22; June 9, p. A6;

June 12, p. C3; *Newsweek*, June 18, 1990, p. 46. For Kevorkian's description, see his *Prescription: Medicide* (Buffalo, NY: Prometheus Books, 1991), pp. 221–31.

71. *State of Georgia v. McAfee*, 385 S.E.2d 651 (Ga. 1989).

72. See Timothy E. Quill, "Death and Dignity: A Case of Individualized Decision Making," *New England Journal of Medicine* 324 (March 7, 1991): 691–94, reprinted with additional analysis in Quill, *Death and Dignity* (New York: W. W. Norton & Co., 1993). After Quill wrote the article, a grand jury in Rochester, New York, where the events occurred, declined to indict him, apparently because jurors sympathized with his motives and possibly his action.

73. See Hans-Martin Sass, Robert M. Veatch, and Rihito Kimura, eds., *Advance Directives and Surrogate Decision Making in Health Care: United States, Germany, and Japan*; Nancy M. P. King, *Making Sense of Advance Directives* (Dordrecht, the Netherlands: Kluwer Academic Publishers, 1991; rev. ed. 1996).

74. For balanced accounts of problems and promise in advance directives, see Norman L. Cantor, "Making Advance Directives Meaningful," *Psychology, Public Policy, and Law* 4 (1998): 629–52; and Dan Brock, "Trumping Advance Directives," *Hastings Center Report* 21 (Sept.–Oct. 1991): S5-S6.

75. See E. R. Gamble et al., "Knowledge, Attitudes, and Behavior of Elderly Persons Regarding Living Wills," *Archives of Internal Medicine* 151 (February 1991): 277–80.

76. General Assembly of Pennsylvania, Senate Bill No. 3, Session of 1991, as amended April 6, 1992, as published in *Philadelphia Medicine* 88 (August 1992): 329–33.

77. Stuart J. Eisendrath and Albert R. Jonsen, "The Living Will," *Journal of the American Medical Association* 249 (April 15, 1983): 2054–58.

78. See the empirical study by Donald Patrick, et al., "Validation of Preferences for Life-Sustaining Treatment: Implications for Advance Care Planning," *Annals of Internal Medicine* 127 (1997): 509–17.

79. See Judith Areen, "The Legal Status of Consent Obtained from Families of Adult Patients to Withhold or Withdraw Treatment," *Journal of the American Medical Association* 258 (July 10, 1987): 229–35; and John W. Warren, et al., "Informed Consent by Proxy: An Issue in Research with Elderly Patients," *New England Journal of Medicine* 315 (October, 1986): 1124–28.

80. See Nancy Rhoden, "Litigating Life and Death," *Harvard Law Review* 102 (1988): 437; and Patricia King, "The Authority of Families to Make Medical Decisions for Incompetent Patients after the *Cruzan* Decision," *Law, Medicine & Health Care* 19 (1991): 76–79.

81. Virginia Natural Death Act, Va. Code §§ 54–325.8: 1–13 (1983).

82. See David Asch, John Hansen–Flaschen, and Paul N. Lanken, "Decisions to Limit or Continue Life-Sustaining Treatment by Critical Care Physicians in the United States: Conflicts between Physicians' Practices and Patients' Wishes," *American Journal of Respiratory and Critical Care Medicine* 151 (1995): 288–92; Virginia Tilden, et al., "Decisions about Life-Sustaining Treatment: Impact of Physicians' Behaviors on the Family," *Archives of Internal Medicine* 155 (1995): 633–38; President's Commission, *Deciding to Forego Life-Sustaining Treatment*, pp. 210–11.

83. See Susan M. Wolf, "Ethics Committees and Due Process: Nesting Rights in a Community of Caring," *Maryland Law Review* 50 (1991): 798–858.

84. *Superintendent of Belchertown State School v. Saikewicz*, Mass., 370 N.E. 2d 417 (1977).

85. *In re Conroy*, 486 A.2d 1209 (N.J. 1985), at 1239–42.

5

Beneficence

Morality requires not only that we treat persons autonomously and refrain from harming them, but also that we contribute to their welfare. Such beneficial actions fall under the heading of "beneficence." No sharp breaks exist on the continuum from not inflicting harm to providing benefit, but principles of beneficence potentially demand more than the principle of nonmaleficence because agents must take positive steps to help others, not merely refrain from harmful acts.

This chapter examines two principles of beneficence: positive beneficence and utility. *Positive beneficence* requires agents to provide benefits. *Utility* requires that agents balance benefits and drawbacks to produce the best overall results. We distinguish the virtue of benevolence, various forms of care, and nonobligatory ideals of beneficence from these two principles of beneficence. Building on these distinctions, we discuss the conflicts between beneficence and respect for autonomy that occur in paternalistic refusals to acquiesce in a patient's wishes or choices. The remainder of the chapter focuses on balancing benefits, risks, and costs through analytical methods designed to implement the principle of utility in health policy and clinical care. We conclude that these analytical methods have a useful, although limited, role as aids to decision-making.

The Concept of Beneficence

In ordinary English, the term *beneficence* connotes acts of mercy, kindness, and charity. Forms of beneficence also typically include altruism, love, and humanity. We will understand beneficent action even more broadly, so that it includes all forms of action intended to benefit other persons. *Beneficence* refers to an *action* done to benefit others; *benevolence* refers to the *character trait* or *virtue* of being disposed to act for the benefit of others; and *principle of beneficence* refers to a moral *obligation* to act for the benefit of others. Many acts of beneficence are not obligatory, but a principle of beneficence, in our usage, establishes an obligation to help others further their important and legitimate interests.

Beneficence and benevolence have played central roles in some ethical theories. Utilitarianism, for example, is systematically arranged on a principle of beneficence (the principle of utility), and, during the Scottish Enlightenment, major figures, such as Francis Hutcheson and David Hume, made benevolence the centerpiece of their common-morality theories. In all of these theories, benefitting others is conceived as an aspect of human nature that motivates us to act in the interests of others. These theories closely associate this goal with the goal of morality itself.

We agree that obligations to confer benefits, to prevent and remove harms, and to weigh and balance an action's possible goods against its costs and possible harms are central to biomedical ethics. However, in contrast to some theories, principles of beneficence are not broad enough, in our account, to include all other principles. The principle of utility is itself an extension of the principle of positive beneficence. This extension is necessary because the moral life typically does not provide the opportunity to produce benefits or eliminate harms without creating risks or incurring costs. To be appropriately beneficent generally requires that one determine which actions produce an amount of benefit sufficient to warrant their costs.

This principle of utility is not identical, in our analysis, to the classic utilitarian principle of utility, which is an absolute or preeminent principle. Our principle should be construed neither as the sole principle of ethics nor as one that justifies or overrides all other principles. It is one among a number of prima facie principles. This principle is also limited to balancing probable outcomes of actions—benefits, harms, and costs—in order to achieve the highest net benefit. It does not determine the overall balance of obligations.

Critics often charge that the principle of utility (sometimes called "proportionality") allows society's interests to override individual interests and rights. In biomedical research, for example, the principle of utility suggests that dangerous research on human subjects can be undertaken, and ought to be undertaken, if its likely benefit to society outweighs its danger to the individual subjects. Yet this charge can only be leveled at an *unconstrained* principle of utilitarian balancing. An advantage of our account is that the principle of utility that we defend can be legitimately constrained by the other principles we advance.

Obligatory and Ideal Beneficence

Although philosophers as different as Jeremy Bentham and W. D. Ross have employed the term *beneficence* to identify positive obligations to others, many critics deny that we have these positive obligations. They hold that beneficence is purely a virtuous ideal or an act of charity, and thus that persons are not morally deficient if they fail to act beneficently. These concerns rightly point to a need to clarify and specify beneficence, taking care to note the limits of our obligations and the points at which beneficence is optional rather than obligatory.

One of the most famous examples of beneficence is found in the New Testament parable of the Good Samaritan, which illustrates several problems in interpreting beneficence. In this parable, robbers have beaten and left "half-dead" a man traveling from Jerusalem to Jericho. After two other travelers passed by the injured man without rendering help, a Samaritan who saw him "had compassion, and went to him and bound up his wounds . . . brought him to an inn, and took care of him." In having compassion and showing mercy, the good Samaritan expressed an attitude of caring for the injured man and also took care of him. Both the Samaritan's motives and his actions were beneficent. Common interpretations of the parable suggest that positive beneficence is more an *ideal* than an *obligation*, because the Samaritan's act seems to exceed ordinary morality.

Virtually everyone agrees that the common morality does not contain a principle of beneficence that requires severe sacrifice and extreme altruism in the moral life (e.g., giving both of one's kidneys for transplantation). Only *ideals* of beneficence incorporate such extreme generosity. We are likewise not morally required to benefit persons on all occasions, even if we are in a position to do so. For example, we are not morally required to perform all possible acts of generosity or charity that would benefit others. We can readily grant, then, both that much beneficent conduct is ideal, rather than obligatory, and that the line between an obligation and a moral ideal is often unclear in the case of beneficence.

Nonetheless, the principle of positive beneficence does support an array of more specific moral rules of obligation, including some that we have already noted without referring to them as rules. Examples of these rules of beneficence, in their most general forms, are:

1. Protect and defend the rights of others.
2. Prevent harm from occurring to others.
3. Remove conditions that will cause harm to others.
4. Help persons with disabilities.
5. Rescue persons in danger.

Distinguishing Rules of Beneficence from Rules of Nonmaleficence

Principles and rules of beneficence differ in several ways from those of non-maleficence. As we mentioned in Chapter 4, rules of nonmaleficence (1) are neg-ative prohibitions of action that (2) must be followed impartially, and (3) provide moral reasons for legal prohibitions of certain forms of conduct. By contrast, rules of beneficence (1) present positive requirements of action, (2) need not al-ways be followed impartially, and (3) rarely, if ever, provide reasons for legal punishment when agents fail to abide by the rules.

The second condition, impartial adherence, is especially important and merits additional attention. We are morally prohibited from causing harm to anyone (a perfect obligation). However, we are morally permitted to help or benefit those with whom we have special relationships, and we are very commonly not re-quired to help or benefit those with whom we have no such special relationship. Morality thus allows us to exhibit our beneficence with partiality in regard to those with whom we have special relationships (an imperfect obligation). These distinctions are not arbitrary. It is possible to act nonmaleficently toward all per-sons at all times, but it is generally not possible to act beneficently toward all persons. Accordingly, failing to act nonmaleficently toward a party is (prima facie) immoral, but failing to act beneficently toward a party is very often not immoral. Nonetheless, we are obligated to follow impartially *some* rules of benef-icence, such as those requiring efforts to rescue strangers under conditions of minimal risk. Even some legal punishments for failure to rescue strangers may be justifiable.

Not only do various norms of beneficence establish obligations, but the oblig-ations are sufficiently strong that they sometimes *override obligations of non-maleficence*. For example, obligations of beneficence can require us to meet the demands of the principle of utility: The requirement to benefit may be overrid-ing if we can produce a major benefit by causing a minor harm, or a major ben-efit for many people while causing a minor harm for only a few. For example, many public health programs, such as vaccinations, cause harm to a certain per-centage of the population, while providing a major benefit to other parts of the population. Coercive taxation schemes that fund health care for the indigent jus-tifiably set back the interests of those taxed to benefit the indigent. If there were no obligations of beneficence—only moral ideals of beneficence—such actions would be unjustified. Thus, nonmaleficence does not necessarily override or al-ways take priority over beneficence.

General Beneficence

A distinction between *specific* and *general* beneficence can eliminate some of the confusion that surrounds the distinction between obligatory beneficence and nonobligatory moral ideals. Specific beneficence is directed at specific parties, such as children, friends, and patients; whereas general beneficence is directed beyond these special relationships to all persons. A significant moral dispute underlies these categories. Virtually everyone agrees that all persons are obligated to act in certain circumstances in the interests of their children, friends, and other special parties, but general beneficence is more controversial.

Ross suggests that obligations of general beneficence "rest on the mere fact that there are other beings in the world whose condition we can make better."[1] Such an unqalified form of general beneficence obligates us to benefit persons whom we do not know and with whose views we are not ourselves sympathetic. Obligations of beneficence, so understood, are potentially very demanding. To take an example in contemporary ethical theory, Shelly Kagan argues that we should recognize no limits, in principle, to the sacrifice that morality can demand of us in promoting the overall good.[2]

The thesis that we have the same impartial obligation to persons we do not know as we have to our own families is both overly romantic and impractical. It is also perilous because this unrealistic and alien standard may divert attention from our obligations to those to whom we are close or indebted, and to whom our responsibilities are clear rather than clouded. The more widely we generalize obligations of beneficence, the less likely we will be to meet our primary responsibilities, which many of us already find difficult to meet. For this reason, in part, we believe that the common morality does recognize significant limits to the demands of obligatory beneficence.[3]

Some writers set limits by distinguishing between the removal of harm, the prevention of harm, and the promotion of benefit (see Chapter 4). For instance, in developing "the obligation to assist," Peter Singer distinguishes preventing evil from promoting good, and contends that "if it is in our power to prevent something bad from happening, without thereby sacrificing anything of comparable moral importance, we ought, morally, to do it."[4] Singer's criterion of comparable importance sets a limit on sacrifice: We ought to donate time and resources until we reach a level at which, by giving more, we would cause as much suffering to ourselves as we would relieve through our gift. This argument implies that morality sometimes requires us to make large sacrifices and to reduce our standard of living substantially in the effort to rescue needy persons around the world. However, Singer's proposed obligation of beneficence and his limit on the obligation are too demanding. The requirement that persons must seriously disrupt their life plans in order to benefit those who are sick, undereducated, or starving exceeds the limits built into common-morality obligations. Standards in the common morality assume that the level of cost, risk, or sacrifice that Singer proposes as morally obligatory is actually beyond moral obligation—a commendable moral ideal, but not an obligation.

Michael Slote has argued against Singer that beneficent prevention of evil or harm is not sufficiently strong to require the sacrifice of a "basic life plan." He

formulates the "principle of positive obligation" in this way: "One has an obligation to prevent serious evil or harm when one can do so without seriously interfering with one's life plans or style and without doing any wrongs of
commission."[5] Slote's formulation may contain ambiguities and its own unresolved moral problems,[6] but the common morality (which contrasts with Singer's
utilitarian perspective) surely does not demand much more beneficence than
Slote's statement suggests. Moral standards probably could not demand the beneficence Singer proposes without requiring sacrifice beyond the capability of most
agents. If these standards were to be as demanding as they are in Singer's account, this would put agents in the precarious position of moral disenfranchise-
ment. Whenever moral standards are too high for many persons to achieve, those
persons cannot participate in ways they are "obligated" to participate.

Later Singer attempted to take account of the objection that his principle sets
"too high a standard." He came to the conclusion that his principle requires a
more guarded formulation. To the question, "What level of assistance should we
advocate?," he offered a more realistic answer:

Any figure will be arbitrary, but there may be something to be said for a round percentage of one's income like, say, 10 per cent—more than a token donation, yet not so high
as to be beyond all but saints. . . . No figure should be advocated as a rigid minimum or
maximum; . . . [but by] any reasonable ethical standards this is the minimum we ought
to do, and we do wrong if we do less.[7]

It is difficult to assess a percentage of income as an expression of one's obligation, especially in light of vast differences in income and wealth and also in light
of conditions we identify below. It is even more difficult to assess whether "any
reasonable ethical standard" sets such a figure as ten percent as the minimum.
Nonetheless, Singer's revised thesis rightly attempts to set additional limits on
the scope of the obligation of beneficence—limits that reduce required costs and
impacts on the agent's life plans and that make meeting one's obligations a realistic possibility.

Specific Beneficence and the Obligation to Rescue

Some circumstances eliminate the discretion allowed by general beneficence. In
the stock example of a passerby who observes someone drowning, but stands in
no special moral relationship with the person, the obligation of beneficence is
not strong enough, in our view, to require a passerby, who is a very poor swimmer, to risk his or her life by trying to swim a hundred yards to rescue someone
who is drowning in deep water. There is a critical relationship between the victim and the passerby of a different kind, because the passerby well-placed at that
moment to help the victim. As such, a specific obligation to beneficent action
arises in this circumstance. If the passerby does nothing (e.g., fails to alert a
nearby lifeguard) the failure to help is morally culpable.

Apart from special moral relationships, such as contracts or the ties of family or friendship, a person X has a determinate obligation of beneficence toward person Y if and only if each of the following conditions is satisfied (assuming X is aware of the relevant facts):

1. Y is at risk of significant loss of or damage to life or health or some other major interest.
2. X's action is needed (singly or in concert with others) to prevent this loss or damage.
3. X's action (singly or in concert with others) has a high probability of preventing it.
4. X's action would not present significant risks, costs, or burdens to X.
5. The benefit that Y can be expected to gain outweighs any harms, costs, or burdens that X is likely to incur.[8]

The fourth condition is critical because it enables us to engage the problems that surround formulations of the obligation of beneficence. Although it is difficult to specify "significant risks, costs, or burdens," the implication of the fourth condition is clear: Even if X's action would probably save Y's life and would meet all conditions except the fourth, the action would not be obligatory on grounds of beneficence.

We shall now test these theses about the demands of beneficence with two cases. The first is a borderline case of specific obligatory beneficence, involving rescue, whereas the second presents a clear-cut case of specific obligatory beneficence. In the first case, originally introduced in Chapter 4, Robert McFall was diagnosed as having aplastic anemia, which is usually fatal, but his physician believed that a bone marrow transplant from a genetically compatible donor could increase his chances of surviving. David Shimp, McFall's cousin, was the only relative willing to undergo the first test, which established tissue compatibility. However, Shimp then refused to undergo the second test for genetic compatibility. When McFall sued to force his cousin to undergo the second test and to donate bone marrow if he turned out to be compatible, the judge ruled that the *law* did not allow him to force Shimp to engage in such acts of positive beneficence, but added that Shimp's refusal was "*morally* indefensible."

Conditions (1) and (2) above were met for an obligation of specific beneficence, but condition (3) was not clearly satisfied. McFall's chance of surviving one year would have only increased from 25 to between 40 and 60%. These contingencies make it difficult to determine whether principles of beneficence demanded a particular course of action. Although most medical commentators agreed that the risks to the donor were minimal, Shimp was especially concerned about the fourth condition. Bone marrow transplants require 100 to 150 punctures of the pelvic bone. These punctures can be painlessly performed under anesthesia, and the major risk is a one-in-10,000 chance of death from anesthesia.

Shimp, however, believed that the risks were greater ("What if I become a cripple?," he asked) and that they outweighed the probability and magnitude of benefit to McFall, despite the lack of medical evidence to support his fears. This case, then, is a borderline case of obligatory specific beneficence.

In the *Tarasoff* case (Case 1), upon learning of his patient's intention to kill an identified woman, the therapist notified the police but not the intended victim because of constraints of confidentiality. Suppose we modify the actual circumstances in this case in order to create the following hypothetical situation: A psychiatrist has informed his patient that he does not believe in keeping information confidential. The patient agrees to treatment under these conditions and subsequently reveals a serious intention to kill an identified woman. The psychiatrist may now either remain aloof or make some move to protect the woman (by notifying her or the police). What does morality—and specifically beneficence—demand of the psychiatrist in this case?

Only a remarkably narrow account of moral obligation would assert that the psychiatrist is under no obligation to protect the woman by contacting her or the police. The psychiatrist is not at risk and, moreover, will suffer virtually no inconvenience or interference with his life plan. If morality does not demand this much beneficence, it is hard to see how morality imposes any positive obligations at all. Even if a competing obligation exists, such as protection of confidentiality, requirements of beneficence will sometimes override it. Sometimes, for example, health care professionals have an obligation to warn spouses or lovers of HIV-infected patients who refuse to disclose their status and who refuse to engage in safer sex practices. (See Chapter 7.)

Nevertheless, the limits of obligatory, specific beneficence can explode when we encounter large-scale social problems. The principle that we are obligated to save a human life when we can do so without making major sacrifices will lead us step by step to enormous burdens.[9] The large number of such situations and the large number of recipients who could benefit create the burden. For example, an individual could provide food for a starving person for a small amount of money, but if numerous starving people exist, each of whom could be rescued by a small additional contribution, the burden would quickly surpass an individual's resources.

This conclusion is both practically and theoretically puzzling. It is *practically* puzzling because it makes pinning down and discharging obligations of beneficence extremely difficult. We vacillate between viewing actions as charitable and as obligatory; and we sometimes feel guilty for not doing more, at the same time doubting that we are obligated to do more. The conclusion is *theoretically* puzzling because every time we try to formulate the limits of obligatory specific beneficence through general conditions, the problem of incremental obligations tends to undermine the analysis. For example, a one-dollar gift to a famine relief organization would not make a noticeable dent in our standard of living. But if we gave away everything in our savings and investment accounts by contributing each time a dollar was needed, most of us would regard the personal sacrifice as immense. It is therefore doubtful that ethical theory or practical deliberation can set precise, determinate conditions of beneficence, so that apparently faultless assumptions about obligations of minimal giving do not engulf us in a morass of obligations that exceeds defensible limits.

No doubt more precise limits of obligatory beneficence can be drawn, but it is certain to be a revisionary line in the sense that it will draw a sharper boundary for our obligations than exists in the common morality. Singer's proposed ten percent criterion, for example, represents a revision of our ordinary moral outlook, despite its faint presence in the history of Western morality (primarily in religious obligations of tithing). Any attempt to specify the limits of our obligations of positive beneficence will both sharpen and alter the common morality, which is not sufficiently refined to supply an answer.

Specific Beneficence, Role Obligations, and Other Special Relations

Obligations of specific beneficence usually rest on special moral relations (for example, in families and friendships) or on special commitments, such as explicit promises and roles with attendant responsibilities. These special moral relationships and role relationships may not appear to generate the problems about specifying limits of obligatory beneficent risk-taking and cost-bearing that we have encountered thus far. However, there are limits in these contexts as well. For instance: How far are parents obligated to go in providing expensive care for their severely ill children?[10] Are physicians and other health care professionals obligated to accept extraordinary risks while caring for difficult or contagious patients?

At this stage in the discussion, we note only the implicit assumption of beneficence that exists in medical and health care professions and their institutional contexts: Promoting the welfare of patients—not merely avoiding harm—expresses medicine's goal, rationale, and justification. As the American Nurses' Association puts it, "The nurse's primary commitment is to the health, welfare, and safety of the client."[11] Likewise, in the Hippocratic oath, physicians pledge that they will "come for the benefit of the sick," will apply treatments "for the benefit of the sick according to [their] ability and judgment," and "will keep [patients] from harm and injustice."[12] Preventive medicine and active public health interventions have also long embraced concerted social actions of beneficence, such as vaccination programs and health education as obligatory rather than optional.

A Reciprocity-Based Justification of Obligations of Beneficence

Several justifications have been proposed for obligations of general and specific beneficence. We will defend a reciprocity-based account, since it is particularly well-suited to biomedical ethics. However, we do not believe that reciprocity can account for the full range of obligations of beneficence.

David Hume argued that the obligation to benefit others arises from social interactions: "All our obligations to do good to society seem to imply something reciprocal. I receive the benefits of society, and therefore ought to promote its interests."[13] Reciprocity is the act or practice of making an appropriate (often proportional) return—for example, returning benefit by proportional benefit, harm by proportional criminal sentencing, and friendliness by gratitude. Hume's reciprocity account rightly maintains that we incur obligations to help or benefit others at least in part because we have received or will receive beneficial assistance from them (understood as assistance that they intend in good faith to provide).

As Hume and others recognize, reciprocity functions in circumstances of justice and friendship, as well as in relationships of benefit. Reciprocity is therefore a pervasive feature of social life, although not so pervasive that we can reduce all of the moral life to obligations of reciprocity. We certainly cannot justify all forms of the virtue of benevolence in terms of reciprocity (e.g., the loving care of children). It is even doubtful that all *obligations* of beneficence can be so justified. For example, a physician may have a moral obligation to take care of an indigent stranger at the scene of an automobile accident (even though it is unlikely that the stranger will ever be able to reciprocate). In general, we do not hold that persons who are devoid of reciprocal relationships of benefit thereby escape obligations to act beneficently.

Nonetheless, obligations of beneficence to society (as distinct from those to identified individuals) are typically derived from some form of reciprocity. It is implausible to maintain that we are largely free of or can free ourselves of a broad range of indebtedness to our parents, to researchers in medicine and public health, to educators, and to social institutions such as schools. The claim that we make our way independent of our benefactors is as unrealistic as the idea that we can always act autonomously without affecting others. Accordingly, many obligations of beneficence are appropriately justified by implicit arrangements underlying the necessary give-and-take of social life. Even some obligations of specific beneficence to rescue people in severe need who stand outside special moral relations or institutional relationships can be so justified.[14]

Traditionally, codes of medical ethics have inappropriately viewed physicians as independent, self-sufficient philanthropists whose beneficence is analogous to generous acts of giving. According to the Hippocratic oath, for example, physicians' obligations to patients represent philanthropic service, whereas obligations to their teachers represent debts incurred in the course of becoming physicians. However, many physicians and health care professionals are today deeply indebted to society (e.g., for education and privileges) and to patients, past and present (e.g., for research and "practice"). Because of this indebtedness, the medical profession's role of beneficent care of patients is misconstrued if modeled primarily on philanthropy, altruism, and personal commitment. Rather, this care is rooted in what William May has called the "reciprocity of giving and receiving."[15] Such reciprocity creates an obligation of general beneficence both to patients and to society, although the precise terms of the obligation are rarely specified (and are very difficult to specify).

Obligations of specific beneficence, by contrast, typically derive from special moral relationships with persons, frequently through institutional roles and contractual arrangements. These obligations arise from implicit and explicit commitments, such as promises and roles, as well as from the acceptance of specific benefits. Both our "station and its duties" and our promises impose obligations. For example, a lifeguard on duty is obligated to try to rescue a drowning swimmer, despite personal risk, just as a physician is obligated to meet the needs of his or her patients, despite potential health risks. The claims that we make on each other as parents, spouses, and friends stem not only from interpersonal encounters, but from settled rules, roles, and relations that constitute the matrix of social obligations and role-derived obligations.

When a patient contracts with a physician for services, the latter assumes a role-specific obligation of beneficent treatment that would not be present apart from the relationship. Although physicians in private practice typically have no legal obligation to see patients in emergencies or to help those injured in an automobile accident, moral obligations of beneficence do, on occasion, require such acts. The obligation to render assistance in extraordinary circumstances, such as an automobile accident, is not limited to physicians or to health care professionals. If a lawyer or student, say, had happened on the scene of an accident in the same way, then he or she too would have had an obligation to assist. Anyone who falls under our five-condition analysis of the specific obligation of beneficence has an obligation to provide such assistance, as he or she is able.

Of course, physicians are typically able to lend more assistance in a medical emergency than other citizens, and we can therefore ask whether the physician has a specific obligation of assistance unique to persons with such skills and training. Here we encounter a gray area between a role-specific obligation and a non-role-specific obligation. The physician at the scene of an accident is obligated to do more than the lawyer or student to aid the injured, to the degree there is a need for medical skills. Yet a physician-stranger is not morally required to assume the same level of commitment and risk that a prior contractual relationship with a patient or hospital would morally require.

More generally, controversy exists about the extent to which society should enforce obligations of general and specific beneficence that do not stem from explicit contracts and agreements. So-called Good Samaritan laws are perhaps most effective when they do not require physicians or other health care professionals to provide assistance under threat of a sanction, but rather protect them from civil or criminal liability when they act in good faith and render aid in emergencies.

For example, if a threat of liability exists for rendering medical assistance in an emergency, the professional may view the legal risk of intervening as a valid excuse for not fulfilling a moral obligation to intervene.

Paternalism: Conflicts Between Beneficence and Autonomy

In an inchoate form, the idea that beneficence expresses the primary obligation in health care is ancient. Throughout the history of health care, the professional's obligations and virtues have been interpreted as commitments of beneficence. We find perhaps the most celebrated expression in the Hippocratic work *Epidemics*: "As to disease, make a habit of two things—*to help, or at least to do no harm.*"[16] Traditionally, physicians were able to rely almost exclusively on their own judgments about their patients' needs for treatment, information, and consultation. However, medicine has in recent years increasingly confronted assertions of patients' rights to make independent judgments about their medical fate. As assertions of autonomy rights have increased, the problem of paternalism has loomed larger.

Disputes About the Primacy of Beneficence

Whether respect for the autonomy of patients should have priority over professional beneficence directed at those patients is a central problem in biomedical ethics. Proponents of autonomy rights for patients, the physician's obligations to the patient of disclosure, seeking consent, confidentiality, and privacy are established primarily (and perhaps exclusively) by the principle of respect for autonomy. Others ground such obligations on the professional's obligatory beneficence. For them, the physician's primary obligation is to act for the patient's medical benefit, not to encourage autonomous decision-making.

Confusion has often marked the debate between proponents of the autonomy model and proponents of the beneficence model—as we will refer to these two contrasting paradigms—because of a failure to distinguish two views of principles of beneficence: sometimes beneficence is viewed as *competing* with a principle of respect for autonomy and sometimes beneficence is viewed as *incorporating* the patient's autonomous choices (in the sense that the patient's preferences help to determine what counts as a medical benefit). For example, two exponents of the preeminence of the beneficence model—Edmund Pellegrino and David Thomasma—argue that "the best interests of the patients are intimately linked with their preferences," from which "are derived our primary duties toward them."[17] This formulation of the beneficence model appears to be little more than a restatement of the autonomy model. If the patient's preferences alone determine the content of the physician's obligation to act beneficently, respect for autonomy rather than beneficence has triumphed.[18]

Elsewhere, however, Pellegrino and Thomasma interpret the meaning and authority of beneficence as independent of—and potentially in conflict with—the patient's preferences: "Both autonomy and paternalism are superseded by the obligation to act beneficently. . . . In the real world of clinical medicine, there are no absolute moral principles except the injunction to act in the patient's best interest." They then present several circumstances in which medical beneficence appropriately overrides the patient's autonomy because the patient has made irresponsible choices. For example, "autonomy would be wrongly exercised if [the patient] rejected penicillin treatment for pneumococcal or meningococcal meningitis."[19] The latter infections are life-threatening and can produce serious central nervous system damage. Pellegrino and Thomasma believe that, in this case, refusal of treatment would be irresponsible, and a caring physician, therefore, should override the patient's refusal. Here we find a robust defense of a beneficence model.

We will argue that debate about which principle or model should be overriding in medical practice cannot be solved in this streamlined manner by defending one principle against the other principle, or by making one principle absolute. Neither the patient nor the physician has premier and overriding authority, and no preeminent principle exists in biomedical ethics, not even the obligation to act in the patient's best interest. This position is consistent with our earlier claim that beneficence provides the primary goal and rationale of medicine and health care, whereas respect for autonomy (along with nonmaleficence and justice) sets moral limits on the professional's actions in pursuit of this goal. To demonstrate the consistency between these two theses, we must examine several aspects of the problem of paternalism, beginning with conceptual issues.

The Nature of Paternalism

Philosophical analyses of paternalism are at least as old as Immanuel Kant, who denounced paternalistic government ("imperium paternale," he called it) for benevolently restricting the freedoms of its subjects. Kant was concerned about a government that "cancels freedom." He never considered the possibility that a parental model of benevolence—one that likens the state to a protective parent caring for an incompetent minor—might be considered a form of paternalism. Nor did John Stuart Mill contemplate the possibility that paternalism might encompass interventions with those who have limited or no autonomy.[20]

However, what they never anticipated came to pass. Intervention in the life of a substantially nonautonomous dependent became and remains the most widely accepted model of justified paternalism. That is, the paradigmatic form of justified paternalism starts with incompetent children in need of parental supervision and extends to other incompetents in need of care analogous to beneficent parental guidance.

The *Oxford English Dictionary (O.E.D.)* dates the term *paternalism* from the 1880s (after Kant and Mill), giving its root meaning as "the principle and practice of paternal administration; government as by a father; the claim or attempt to supply the needs or to regulate the life of a nation or community in the same way a father does those of his children." The analogy with the father presupposes two features of the paternal role: that the father acts beneficently (that is, in accordance with his conception of the interests of his children) and that he makes all or at least some of the decisions relating to his children's welfare, rather than letting them make those decisions. In health care relationships, the analogy extends further: A professional has superior training, knowledge, and insight and is thus in an authoritative position to determine the patient's best interests. From this perspective, a health care professional is like a loving parent with dependent and often ignorant and fearful children.

Paternalism always involves some form of interference with or refusal to conform to another person's preferences regarding his or her own good. Paternalistic acts typically involve force or coercion, on the one hand, or deception, lying, manipulation of information, or nondisclosure of information, on the other. According to some definitions in the literature, all paternalistic actions restrict autonomous choice. Although one author of this text prefers this conception,[21] we will not follow it here. Instead, we will follow the current mainstream of the literature on paternalism and accept the broader definition suggested by the *O.E.D.*: intentional nonacquiescence or intervention in another person's preferences, desires, or actions with the intention of either avoiding harm to or benefiting the person. Even if a person's desires, intentional actions, and the like do not derive from a substantially autonomous choice, then overriding them can still be paternalistic under this definition.[22] For example, if a man ignorant of his fragile, life-threatening condition and sick with a raging fever attempts to leave a hospital, it would be paternalistic to detain him, even if his attempt to leave did not derive from a substantially autonomous choice.

Paternalism, then, is *the intentional overriding of one person's known preferences or actions by another person, where the person who overrides justifies the action by the goal of benefiting or avoiding harm to the person whose preferences or actions are overridden.* This definition is normatively neutral, and therefore does not presume that paternalism is either justified or unjustified. Although the definition assumes an act of beneficence analogous to parental beneficence, it does not assume whether the beneficence is justified, misplaced, obligatory, and so forth.

Sometimes an action may appear to be paternalistic under this definition when in fact it is nonpaternalistic. An example appears in biomedical research involving prisoners. In its report on research involving prisoners, the National Commission for the Protection of Human Subjects of Biomedical and Behavioral Research argued that the closed nature of prison environments creates a potential for abuse of authority and therefore invites the exploitation and coercion of prisoners.[23] Although a Commission-authorized study indicated that most prisoners believe that neither coercion nor undue influence compromises their consent to research, the commission argued that prisons' coercive and exploitative possibilities justify regulations prohibiting the use of prisoners in research, even if they wish to participate.

This restriction appears to be paternalistic, but closer analysis shows that it is not. The commission maintained that if a prison environment were not exploitative or coercive (and if a few other conditions were met), then prisoners should be allowed to choose to participate in research. The commission's justifying ground was that we cannot predict or control whether prisoners will be exploited in settings that render them vulnerable, and that society should prohibit even research to which prisoners *might validly consent* because society cannot adequately monitor whether the subjects' consent is, in fact, valid and what the subsequent conditions of participation will be.

Many circumstances in biomedical ethics suggest a need to examine carefully whether classes of persons are being exploited, but special restrictions placed on members of those classes may or may not be paternalistic. For example, healthy, nonrelated organ donors and cancer patients solicited for research, are in this respect sometimes treated like the prisoners just mentioned; but even stringent protective requirements aimed at their welfare may not be paternalistic. In some cases, the justification of an act, policy, or practice of nonacquiescence or intervention in a person's preferences is partially, but not purely, paternalistic because it is intermixed with nonpaternalistic reasons, such as protection of third parties. Such impure or mixed paternalism is common in public policy debates.

Moral Problems of Medical Paternalism

Throughout the history of medical ethics both the principles of nonmaleficence and beneficence have provided a basis for paternalistic actions toward patients. For example, physicians have traditionally taken the view that disclosing certain forms of information can cause harm to patients under their care and that medical ethics obligates them not to cause such harm.

In Case 3, a man brings his father, who is in his late sixties, to his physician because he has a suspicion that his father's problems in interpreting and responding to daily events indicate Alzheimer's disease. The man also makes an "impassioned plea" that the physician not tell his father whether the tests suggest Alzheimer's. Tests subsequently indicate that the father probably does have the disease. The physician now faces a dilemma, because of the conflict between demands of respect for autonomy and demands of beneficence. The physician first considers the now widely recognized obligation to inform patients of a diagnosis of cancer. (See our discussion in Chapter 7.) This obligation typically presupposes accuracy in the diagnosis, a relatively clear course of the disease, and a competent patient—none of which is clearly present in this case. The physician also notes that disclosure of Alzheimer's disease adversely affects patients' coping mechanisms, and thus could harm the patient, particularly by causing further decline, depression, agitation, and paranoia.

Some patients—for example, those who are depressed or addicted to potentially harmful drugs—are unlikely to reach adequately reasoned decisions. Other patients who are competent and deliberative may make poor choices against the courses of action that their physicians recommend. When patients of either type choose harmful courses of action, some health care professionals respect autonomy by not interfering beyond attempts at persuasion, whereas others act beneficently by attempting to protect patients against the potentially harmful consequences of their own choices. Problems of how to specify these principles, which principle to follow under which conditions, and how to intervene in the decisions and affairs of such patients when intervention is warranted are all central to debates about medical paternalism.[24]

In an article published in 1935, L. J. Henderson argued that "the best physicians" use the following as their primary guide: "So far as possible, 'Do No Harm.' You can do harm by the process that is quaintly called telling the truth. You can do harm by lying. . . . But try to do as little harm as possible, not only in treatment with drugs, or with the knife, but also in treatment with words." Henderson insisted that, for the patient's good, physicians should withhold some information or disclose it only to the family. He also argued that physician deference to the patients' autonomy rights is dangerous because it compromises clinical judgment and presents a hazard to the patient's health.[25]

An example of Henderson's strategy in action appears in Case 2, where a physician discovered an inoperable, incurable carcinoma in a 69-year-old man. Because of their long relationship, the physician knew that the patient was fragile in several respects. The patient was neurotic, had a history of psychiatric disease, and had recently suffered a severe depressive reaction, during which he had behaved irrationally and attempted suicide. When he blurted out, "Am I OK?" and, "I don't have cancer, do I?" the physician answered, "You're as good as you were ten years ago," knowing that the response was a paternalistic lie but also believing it was justified. The physician was worried that a truthful disclosure would seriously disrupt the man's life plans—he was undergoing this routine physical examination in preparation for a brief but greatly anticipated trip to Australia—and would possibly cause mental instability or even lead to suicide. The physician planned to disclose the diagnosis to the patient later—after the trip to Australia, when he could also give proper attention to the man's mental condition.

Mill, despite his stringent opposition to paternalism, considered temporary beneficent interventions in a person's actions to be justified on some occasions.

He argued that a person who is ignorant of a significant risk—for example, in starting to cross a dangerous bridge—may justifiably be restrained in order to ensure that he or she is acting intentionally and with adequate knowledge of the consequences of this action. Once warned, the person should be free to choose whatever course he or she desires. Because Mill did not regard this temporary intervention as a "real infringement" of liberty, he did not view it as paternalistic. However, under our definition of paternalism, such a temporary intervention is paternalistic.

If a paternalistic intervention does not override autonomy because no substantial autonomy is present, it is far easier to justify the intervention than it would be if a comparable preference or action were autonomous. However, in contrast to much of the literature on paternalism, we will argue that beneficence does sometimes provide grounds for justifiably restricting autonomous actions as well as nonautonomous ones.

Weak (Soft) and Strong (Hard) Paternalism

We can further clarify paternalism by a distinction Joel Feinberg introduced between strong and weak paternalism, which he later referred to as hard and soft paternalism.[26] In weak paternalism, an agent intervenes on grounds of beneficence or nonmaleficence only to prevent *substantially nonvoluntary* conduct—that is, to protect persons against their own substantially nonautonomous action(s). Substantially nonvoluntary or nonautonomous actions include cases of consent or refusal that is not adequately informed, severe depression that precludes rational deliberation, and addiction that prevents free choice and action.[27] In weak paternalism, then, a person's ability must be compromised in some way.

Strong paternalism, by contrast, involves interventions intended to benefit a person, despite the fact that the person's risky choices and actions are informed, voluntary, and autonomous. A strong paternalist refuses to acquiesce in a person's autonomous wishes, choices, and actions when there is a need to protect that person. The strong paternalist will restrict the information available to the person or will override the person's informed and voluntary choices. These choices need not be *fully* informed or voluntary, but for the interventions to qualify as strong paternalism, the choices must be *substantially* autonomous.

Reasons exist to doubt that weak paternalism qualifies as a form of paternalism that needs a defense. That we should protect persons from harm caused *to* them by conditions *beyond* their control is not a controversial premise. Paternalism is a problem about the conditions under which we can and should protect others against *self*-caused harm. Accordingly, as Feinberg has bluntly argued, it may be "severely misleading to think of [weak paternalism] as any kind of [real] paternalism."[28]

The Justification of Paternalism and Antipaternalism

Three main positions have been defended regarding the justifiability of paternalism: (1) antipaternalism, (2) a justified paternalism that appeals primarily to
some form of the principle of respect for autonomy, and (3) a justified paternalism that appeals primarily to principles of beneficence. All three positions agree
that some acts of weak paternalism are justified, such as preventing a man under the influence of an hallucinogenic drug from killing himself. Even antipaternalists will not object to these interventions because substantially autonomous
actions are not at stake.

Antipaternalism. Antipaternalists oppose (strong) paternalistic intervention because it violates individual rights and unduly restricts free choice. The serious
adverse consequences of giving paternalistic authority to the state or to a class
of individuals, such as physicians, provide one basis for the rejection of (strong)
paternalism, but another and more influential basis is that rightful authority resides in the individual. The argument for this conclusion rests on the analysis of
autonomy rights in Chapter 3: Strong paternalistic interventions display disrespect toward autonomous agents and fail to treat them as moral equals, treating
them instead as less than independent determiners of their own good. If others
impose their conception of the good on us, they deny us the respect they owe us,
even if they in fact provide us with a benefit and have a better conception of our
needs than we do.[29]

Antipaternalists also argue that paternalistic standards are too broad and therefore would authorize and institutionalize too much intervention if made the basis of policy. Using an extreme example, Robert Harris argues that paternalism
would in principle "justify the imposition of a Spartan-like regimen requiring rigorous physical exercise and abstention from smoking, drinking, and hazardous
pastimes,"[30] subject to the threat of criminal sanctions.

Careful defenses of paternalism would disallow these extreme interventions, and
at best these antipaternalist arguments establish only a rebuttable presumption
against paternalistic intervention. Nonetheless, antipaternalists believe that an unacceptable latitude of judgment would remain in contexts involving potential abuses
of power. For example, suppose a woman risks her life for the advancement of
medicine by submitting to a highly risky experiment, an act most would think not
in her best interests. Are we to commend her, ignore her, or coercively restrain her?
Strong paternalism suggests that it would be permissible and perhaps obligatory to
restrain her. If so, antipaternalists argue, the state is permitted, in principle, to coerce its morally heroic citizens if they act in a manner "harmful" to themselves.
More generally, strong paternalism would empower the state to take away persons'
rights to make decisions over their lives when officials view those decisions as excessively risky. Similarly, it would authorize health care institutions, physicians,
and nurses to override patients' plans and preferences in many cases.

The medical example with the most extensive antipaternalistic literature is the involuntary hospitalization of persons who have neither been harmed by others nor actually harmed themselves, but who are thought to be at risk of such harm. These cases involve a double paternalism: A paternalistic justification for both therapy and commitment. Consider, for example, Catherine Lake, who suffered from arteriosclerosis, which caused temporary confusion and mild loss of memory. Her condition was interspersed with periods of mental alertness and rationality. All parties agreed that Lake had never harmed anyone or presented a threat of danger, but she was committed to a mental institution because she often seemed confused and defenseless. At her trial, while apparently rational, she testified that she knew the risks of living outside the hospital and preferred to assume those risks rather than remain in the hospital environment. The court of appeals denied her petition, arguing that she was "mentally ill," a "danger to herself," and "not competent to care for herself." In its legal justification, the court cited a statute that "provides for involuntary hospitalization of a person who is 'mentally ill and, because of that illness is likely to injure himself'."[31] Antipaternalists would argue that since Lake did not harm others and understood the dangers under which she placed herself, her freedom should not have been restricted.

Antipaternalists would view this case differently if Lake had not been substantially autonomous. The antipaternalist would then regard the intervention as justified by the intent to benefit, and would note that, in these cases, beneficence does not conflict with respect for autonomy because no substantial autonomy exists.

Is paternalism justified by consent or by benefit? Some influential supporters of paternalistic intervention hold that a paternalistic action can be justified only if (1) the harms prevented from occurring or the benefits provided to the person outweigh the loss of independence and the sense of invasion the intervention causes, (2) the person's condition seriously limits his or her ability to make an autonomous choice, (3) the intervention is universally justified under relevantly similar circumstances, and (4) the beneficiary of the paternalistic actions has consented, will consent, or would, if rational, consent to those actions on his or her behalf.

The following case presents an example of a paternalistic action that some would hold satisfies these criteria of justified paternalism. An involuntarily committed mental patient wishes to leave the hospital, although his family opposes his release. The patient argues that his mental condition does not justify confinement. However, after one previous release, he had plucked out his right eye, and after another release, he had severed his right hand. The patient functions competently in the state hospital, where he sells news materials to fellow patients and handles limited financial affairs. The source of his "problems" is his religious beliefs. He regards himself as a true prophet of God and believes that "it is far better for one man to believe and accept an appropriate message from God to sacrifice an eye or a hand according to the sacred scriptures rather than for the present course of the world to cause even greater loss of human life." Acting on this belief, he engages in self-mutilation. According to the paternalist, this person functions rationally from day to day, yet at times needs and deserves help. His capacities are too diminished and his dangerousness to himself too severe to allow complete independence without custodial care.[32]

Several prominent theories appeal to *consent* to justify paternalistic interventions in such cases—be it rational consent, subsequent consent, hypothetical consent, or some other type of consent. As Gerald Dworkin puts it, "the basic notion of consent is important and seems to me the only acceptable way to try to delimit an area of justified paternalism." Rosemary Carter agrees, arguing that "consent plays the central role in justifying paternalism, and indeed . . . no other concepts are relevant." Donald VanDeVeer similarly justifies paternalistic interventions for persons "acting in a seriously encumbered manner [where] it is highly probable that they would give valid consent to the intervention if the opportunity were available."[33]

For those who support a consent-based theory, paternalism is a "social insurance policy" to which fully rational persons would subscribe in order to protect themselves.[34] Such persons would know, for example, that they might be tempted at times to make decisions that are far-reaching, potentially dangerous, and irreversible. At other times, they might suffer irresistible psychological or social pressures to take actions that are unjustifiably risky—for example, a challenge to fight might place their honor in question, causing them to accept the challenge. In still other cases, persons might not sufficiently understand the dangers of their actions, such as medical facts about the effects of smoking, although they might believe they have a sufficient understanding. Those who use consent as a justification thus conclude that we would consent to a limited authorization for others to control our actions in situations like these through paternalistic policies and practices.

John Rawls and Gerald Dworkin espouse a form of justified paternalism based on the premise that completely rational agents (those fully aware of their circumstances) would consent to paternalism and would even consent to a system of penalties to motivate them to avoid foolish actions. According to this theory of consent, those whose autonomy is defective are unable to make the prudent decision that they would otherwise make. Rawls and Dworkin do not propose a *predictive* consent theory, according to which a particular individual would give consent if his or her present impairment were removed. Rather, they argue from a Kantian conception of what the rational and autonomous agent would agree to in hypothetical circumstances of consent.[35]

A theory that appeals to rational consent to justify paternalistic interventions has attractive features, particularly its attempt to harmonize principles of beneficence and respect for autonomy so that paternalistic interventions respect autonomy rather than override it. However, this approach does not incorporate an individual's actual *consent*, and, without further specification, it will also likely justify more paternalism than its original defenders anticipated. Almost any risk an agent accepts can form the basis of an intervention on grounds that no rational person would assume the risk.

More importantly, consent in this (or any) form is not necessary to justify paternalistic interventions, and appeals to consent obscure more than they clarify the issues. It is best to keep autonomy-based justifications at arm's length from paternalism. Beneficence alone justifies truly paternalistic actions, just as it justifies parental actions that override children's preferences.[36] We do not control children because we believe that they will subsequently consent to or would rationally approve our interventions. We control them because we believe they will have better (or at least less risky) lives, whether they know it or not. Even if we hope for subsequent consent or approval from our children or our patients, the justification for our intervention rests on their welfare, not on their autonomous choices.

The most plausible justification of paternalistic actions places benefit on a scale with autonomy interests and balances both: As a person's interests in autonomy increase and the benefits for that person decrease, the justification of paternalistic action becomes less cogent; conversely, as the benefits for a person increase and that person's interests in autonomy decrease, the justification of paternalistic action becomes more plausible. Thus, preventing minor harms or providing minor benefits while deeply disrespecting autonomy lacks plausible justification; but actions that prevent major harms or provide major benefits while only trivially disrespecting autonomy have a highly plausible paternalistic rationale. Although many in contemporary biomedical ethics contest this claim, we will now argue that this form of paternalism is warranted.

Justified Strong Paternalism

Although strong paternalism is a dangerous position that is subject to abuse, under some conditions a narrow range of strongly paternalistic acts is justified. In reaching this conclusion, we do not defend public and institutional *policies* of strong paternalism, but only certain *acts* of strong paternalism.

Two cases provide starting points for reflection on the conditions of justified strong paternalism. In the first, a physician obtains the results of a myelogram (a graph of the spinal region) following examination of a patient. Although the test yields inconclusive results and needs to be repeated, it also suggests a serious pathology. When the patient asks about the test results, the physician decides on grounds of beneficence to withhold potentially negative information, knowing that, upon disclosure, the patient would be distressed and anxious. Based on her experience with other patients and her ten-year knowledge of this patient, the physician is confident that the information would not affect the patient's decision to consent to another myelogram. Her sole motivation in withholding the information is to spare the patient the emotional distress of thinking through a painful decision prematurely and perhaps unnecessarily. However, the physician intends to be completely truthful with the patient about the results of the second test and will disclose the information well before the patient will need to decide about surgery. This physician's act of temporary nondisclosure seems to us morally justified, though beneficence has (temporarily) received priority over respect for autonomy. (See also our discussion of the disclosure of "bad news" in Chapter 7.)

A more commonplace example of justified strong paternalism appears in the following case reported by Mary Silva:

> After receiving his preoperative medicine, C, a 23-year-old male athlete scheduled for a hernia repair, states that he does not want the side rails up. C is of clear mind and understands why the rule is required; however, C does not feel the rule should apply to him because he is not the least bit drowsy from the preoperative medication and he has no intention of falling out of bed. After considerable discussion between the nurse and patient, the nurse responsible for C's care puts the side rails up. Her justification is as follows: C is not drowsy because he has just received the preoperative medication, and its effects have not occurred. Furthermore, if he follows the typical pattern of patients receiving this medication in this dosage, he will become drowsy very quickly. A drowsy patient is at risk for a fall. Since there is no family at the hospital to remain with the patient, and since the nurses on the unit are exceptionally busy, no one can constantly stay with C to monitor his level of alertness. Under these circumstances, the patient must be protected from the potential harm of a fall, despite the fact that he does not want this protection. . . . The nurse restricted this autonomous patient's liberty based on . . . protection of the patient from potential harm . . . and *not* as a hedge against liability or for protection from criticism.[37]

Such minor strong paternalistic actions are common in hospitals. If there is no reasonable alternative or if, for example, these actions spare dying patients totally pointless grief and suffering, they are cases of justified strong paternalism.

Normally, strong paternalism is appropriate and justified in health care only if the following conditions are satisfied:

1. A patient is at risk of a significant, preventable harm.
2. The paternalistic action will probably prevent the harm.
3. The projected benefits to the patient of the paternalistic action outweigh its risks to the patient.
4. The least autonomy-restrictive alternative that will secure the benefits and reduce the risks is adopted.

These conditions justify strong paternalism, but the interpretation and limits of each condition need more analysis than we can provide here. (See also our more general interpretation of conditions for overriding prima facie obligations in Chapter 1.)

We are tempted to add a fifth condition requiring that a paternalistic action not *substantially* restrict autonomy. This condition could be satisfied only if vital or substantial autonomy interests are not at stake. This would not be the case if, for example, a Jehovah's Witness refuses a blood transfusion because of a deeply held conviction, because here a vital autonomy interest is at stake. To intervene coercively by providing the transfusion would substantially infringe the patient's autonomy and thus could not be justified under this additional condition. However, some rare cases of justified strong paternalism cross this line of minimal infringement. In general, as the risk to a patient's welfare increases or the likelihood of an irreversible harm increases, the likelihood of a justified paternalistic intervention correspondingly increases.[38]

The following case plausibly supports strong paternalistic intervention, even though it involves more than minimal infringement of respect for autonomy: A psychiatrist is treating a patient similar to the patient discussed above who plucked out his eye and cut off his hand for religious reasons. However, this patient is not insane and acts conscientiously on his unique religious views. He asks the psychiatrist a question about his condition, a question that has a definite answer but which, if answered, would lead him to engage in self-maiming behavior in order to fulfill what he believes to be his religion's demands. Many, including the present authors, would maintain that the doctor acts paternalistically, but justifiably, by concealing information from this patient, even if he is rational and otherwise informed. Because the infringement of the principle of respect for autonomy is *more than minimal* in this case (the religious views being central to the patient's life plan), a fifth condition requiring no substantial infringement of autonomy cannot be a necessary condition for *all* cases of justified strong paternalism.

We may seem to have suggested at various points in this section that a judgment about the justifiability of paternalistic actions depends on assigning overriding status to either respect for autonomy or beneficence. However, framing the issues in this way is overly simplistic and can be seriously misleading. A better strategy is to return to the arguments about specification, balancing, and coherence presented in Chapter 1. Developing a position on paternalism requires appreciating the limits of principles and the need to give them additional content, while attempting to render specifications and particular judgments as coherent with other commitments as possible. The problem of medical paternalism is the problem of rightly specifying and balancing physician beneficence and patient autonomy in the patient–physician relationship. It is a messy and complicated problem, and coherence in our judgments is difficult to achieve. Determining which paternalistic actions are justifiable requires persons with good judgment in the handling of contingent conflicts.

Problems of Suicide Intervention

The state, religious institutions, and health care professionals have all traditionally assumed some jurisdiction to intervene with suicide. Those who intervene do not always attempt to justify their actions on paternalistic grounds, but paternalism, in both weak and strong forms, has been the primary justification.

Approximately 30,000 certified suicides occur in the United States each year, and many other suicides are routinely classified as accidental deaths, in part because too little is known about the decedents' intentions. Several conceptual questions about the term *suicide* also make it difficult to classify acts as suicides.[39] For example, when Barney Clark became the first human to receive an artificial heart, he was given a key that he could use to turn off the compressor if he wanted to die. As Dr. Willem Kolff noted, if the patient "suffers and feels it isn't worth it any more, he has a key that he can apply. . . . I think it is entirely legitimate that this man whose life has been extended should have the right to cut it off if he doesn't want it, if [his] life ceases to be enjoyable."[40] Would Clark's use of the key to turn off the artificial heart have been an act of suicide? If he had refused to accept the artificial heart in the first place, few would have labeled his act a suicide. His overall condition was extremely poor, the artificial heart was experimental, and no suicidal intention was evident. If, on the other hand, Clark had intentionally shot himself with a gun while on the artificial heart, the act would have been classified as suicide. If Clark had used the key to turn off his artificial heart, controversy would have erupted about whether to characterize his act as forgoing life-sustaining treatment, as withdrawing from an experiment, as suicide, or as all of the above.

Pursuing conceptual problems about the vagueness of *suicide* would take us too far from our topic. Our concern is paternalistic intervention in cases that are generally agreed to be acts of suicide or attempted suicide. The primary moral issue is the following: Do individuals have a moral right to decide about the acceptability of suicide for themselves and to act on their convictions without interference? If suicide is a protected moral right, then the state, health professionals, and others have no legitimate grounds for intervention in autonomous suicide attempts. No one seriously doubts that we should intervene to prevent suicide by nonautonomous persons, and few people wish to return to the days when suicide was a criminal act. But if we accept an autonomy right, then we could not legitimately attempt to prevent the imprudent (though autonomous) individual from committing suicide.

A clear and relevant example of attempted suicide appears in the following case, involving John K., a 32-year-old lawyer. Two neurologists independently confirmed that his facial twitching, which had been evident for three months, was an early sign of Huntington's disease, a neurological disorder that progressively worsens, leads to irreversible dementia, and is uniformly fatal in approximately ten years. His mother suffered a horrible death from the same disease, and John K. had often said that he would prefer to die than to suffer the way his mother had suffered. Over several years, he had been anxious, had drunk heavily, and had sought psychiatric help for intermittent depression. Following a confirming diagnosis, he told his psychiatrist about his situation and asked for help in committing suicide. After the psychiatrist refused to help, John K. attempted to take his own life by ingesting his antidepressant medication, leaving a note of explanation to his wife and child.[41]

Several interventions occurred or were possible in this case. First, the psychiatrist refused to assist John K.'s suicide and would have sought involuntary commitment had John K. not insisted that he did not plan to attempt suicide anytime soon. The psychiatrist probably thought that he could provide appropriate psychotherapy over time. Second, John K.'s wife found him unconscious and rushed him to the emergency room. Third, the emergency room staff decided to treat him, despite the suicide note. The question is which, if any, of these possible or actual interventions is justifiable?

One widely accepted account of our obligations relies on John Stuart Mill's strategy of temporary intervention. On this account, intervention is justified to ascertain whether a person is acting autonomously; further intervention is unjustified once it is clear that the person's actions are substantially autonomous. Glanville Williams used this strategy in an influential statement:

If one suddenly comes upon another person attempting suicide, the natural and humane thing to do is to try to stop him, for the purpose of ascertaining the cause of his distress and attempting to remedy it, or else of attempting moral dissuasion if it seems that the act of suicide shows lack of consideration for others, or else again from the purpose of trying to persuade him to accept psychiatric help if this seems to be called for. . . . But nothing longer than a temporary restraint could be defended. I would gravely doubt whether a suicide attempt should be a factor leading to a diagnosis of psychosis or to compulsory admissions to a hospital. Psychiatrists are too ready to assume that an attempt to commit suicide is the act of mentally sick persons.[42]

This antipaternalist stance is vulnerable to criticism on two grounds. First, failure to intervene with strong efforts symbolically communicates to potential suicides a lack of communal concern and diminishes our sense of communal responsibility. Second, many persons who commit suicide are mentally ill, clinically depressed, or destabilized by a crisis and are, therefore, not acting autonomously. From a clinical perspective, many suicidal persons are beset with ambivalence, simply wish to reduce or interrupt anxiety, or are under the influence of drugs, alcohol, or intense pressure. Many mental health professionals believe that suicides almost always result from maladaptive attitudes or illnesses needing therapeutic attention and social support.[43]

In a typical circumstance, the potential suicide plans how to end life while simultaneously holding fantasies about how rescue will occur, not only rescue from death but from the negative circumstances prompting the suicide. If the suicide springs from clinical depression or is a call for help, a failure to intervene seems to show disrespect for the person's deepest autonomous wishes, including his or her hopes for the future. Surface intentions do not always capture deeper desires or inclinations, and, in a matter as serious as suicide, deeper motives should receive a heavy weighting in justifying intervention.

Several public policy problems are connected to these claims. Many people are concerned that changes in suicide laws either to legalize physician-assisted suicide or to discourage suicide intervention will encourage suicides by persons who are not substantially autonomous, especially those who are terminally ill and in need of both care and resources. Some studies indicate that people diagnosed with AIDS commit suicide at a rate significantly greater than the general population, though AIDS may be only one among several conditions leading to suicide.[44] Some patients with AIDS want to commit suicide rather than face the prospect of suffering and dying from their disease, but their medical condition may also cause central nervous system complications, such as delirium or dementia, that may render them unable at some point to make a substantially autonomous choice. While recognizing the case for "rational suicide" by patients with AIDS, one physician contends that "from the clinical point of view, careful evaluations of suicides, even in terminally ill patients, almost invariably reveal evidence that the suicide occurred as a manifestation of a psychiatric disorder rather than as a rational choice."[45]

Another worry is that new suicide laws would foster insensitive attitudes on the part of health care professionals, especially in a medical system organized around cost reduction. Some institutions devoted to caring for the ill and elderly, such as the modern nursing home, already communicate a message of indifference to various forms of suffering that lead patients to end their lives. These institutions contrast sharply with the ethos of a hospice, which provides a supportive community. Hospices are but one of many concrete examples of social institutions that counterbalance an undue emphasis on rights of autonomy, independence, and self-reliance.

However, caution is also needed in calls for communal beneficence, which may express itself paternalistically through forceful interventions or criminal sanctions. Although suicide has been decriminalized, a suicide attempt, irrespective of motive, almost universally provides a legal basis for public officers to intervene, as well as grounds for involuntary hospitalization.[46] Often the burden of proof is more appropriately placed on those who claim that the patient's judgment is imprudent or not autonomous. For example, Ida Rollin, 74 years old, suffered from ovarian cancer, and her physicians told her that she had only a few months to live and that her dying would be very painful and upsetting. Rollin indicated to her daughter that she wanted to commit suicide and requested her assistance. The daughter secured some pills and conveyed a doctor's instructions about how they should be taken. When the daughter expressed reservations about these plans, her husband reminded her that they "weren't driving, she [Ida Rollin] was" and that they were only "navigators."[47]

This metaphor-laden reference to rightful authority is a reminder that those who propose suicide intervention require a moral justification that fits the context. Occasions arise in health care (and elsewhere) when it is appropriate to step aside and allow a suicide, and even to assist in a person's suicide, just as occasions exist when it is appropriate to intervene. (See Chapter 4.)

Denying Requests for Nonbeneficial Procedures

Patients or their surrogates occasionally request medical procedures that the clinician is convinced will not be beneficial. The clinician may believe that the procedure is ineffective or futile or that its harms or risks will prevent a net benefit. Often, though not always, denials of such requests are instances of paternalism.

Passive paternalism. Debates about paternalism typically focus on active paternalistic interventions when the patient prefers nonintervention. A comparatively neglected form of paternalism, what we might call *passive paternalism*, appears in the professional's refusal, for reasons of patient-centered beneficence, to execute a patient's positive preferences for an intervention.[48] The following case illustrates passive paternalism. Elizabeth Stanley, a sexually active 26-year-old intern, requests a tubal ligation, insisting that she has thought about this request for months, dislikes available contraceptives, does not want children, and understands that tubal ligation is irreversible. When the gynecologist suggests that she might someday want to get married and have children, she responds that she would either find a husband who did not want children or adopt children. She thinks that she is not likely to change her mind and wants the tubal ligation to make it impossible for her to reconsider. She has scheduled a vacation in two weeks and wants the surgery then.[49]

If a physician justifies a refusal to perform the tubal ligation on grounds of the patient's benefit, the action is paternalistic. Such passive paternalism is usually easier to justify than active paternalism because physicians generally do not have a moral obligation to carry out their patients' desires when they are incompatible with acceptable standards of medical practice or are against the physicians' conscience. If a physician believes that providing a requested treatment, such as antibiotics for a cold or a worthless drug for cancer, is not in the patient's best interests, he or she is not compelled to violate his or her conscience, even when the patient is substantially autonomous. Of course, setting a professional standard of practice may itself be a paternalistic effort to protect patients' interests, but that is a separate problem.

Medical futility. Passive paternalism has been central to recent debates about medical futility, a topic we introduced in Chapter 4. Consider the case of 85-year-old Helga Wanglie, who was maintained on a respirator in a persistent vegetative state (Case 6 in the appendix). The hospital sought to stop the respirator on grounds that it was "nonbeneficial," in that it could not heal her lungs, palliate her suffering, or enable her to experience the benefits of life. The surrogate decision-makers—her husband, a son, and a daughter—wanted life support continued on grounds that Mrs. Wanglie would not be better off dead, that a miracle could occur, that physicians should not play God, and that efforts to remove her life support indicated "moral decay in our civilization."

If life support for such patients is futile, denying patients' or surrogates' requests for treatment is warranted. Even the restrictive Baby Doe regulations (see pp. 138-139) allowed physicians to withhold treatment that they considered "futile in terms of the survival of the infant" or "virtually futile." A justified claim that a medical procedure is futile removes it from the range of otherwise beneficial acts among which patients or their surrogates may choose. The claim is typically not that an intervention will harm the patient (in violation of the principle of nonmaleficence), but that it will not produce the benefit sought by the patient or the surrogate. A justified claim of futility effectively cancels a professional's obligation to provide a medical procedure. But does the language of futility illuminate these issues, and does futility raise a genuine issue of passive paternalism or only an issue about wasted resources and coercion of health professionals' consciences?

As noted in Chapter 4, "medical futility" has several distinguishable meanings in the literature, including the following: (1) the procedure cannot be performed because of a patient's biological condition, (2) the procedure cannot produce the intended physiological effect, (3) the procedure cannot reasonably be expected to produce the benefit that is sought, and (4) the procedure's burdens, harms, and costs will outweigh its anticipated benefits. In our judgment, only the first three are bona fide instances of "medical futility," because the fourth is an on-balance judgment having nothing to do with futility. Claims of medical futility are often presented as objective and value-free, when in fact they are subjective and value-laden. For example, some clinicians insist that a treatment is futile only if there is no chance it will work, while others label a treatment as futile if it has a thirteen percent or lower chance of success.[50]

Claims of futility involve the prediction and evaluation of outcomes, which are usually probable rather than certain. Even determining a statistical threshold is in part evaluative; that is, a line must be fixed in light of values. Even if we assume consensus among clinicians about the statistical threshold, problems will still appear in clinical estimates of the probability that an intervention will be successful.[51] Some contend that a medical procedure is reasonably judged futile when physicians determine through personal experiences and reported empirical data that "in the last 100 cases, a medical treatment has been useless."[52] However, dissimilarities among otherwise similar patients may call this sweeping conclusion into question.

It is always appropriate to ask for a specification of the objectives with respect to which a procedure is said to be futile. An inquiry may reveal that the benefit the physician doubts can be achieved may not be the same benefit the patient seeks. For example, studies often assume that the legitimate objective of cardiopulmonary resuscitation (CPR) is survival to discharge from the hospital; thus, CPR is deemed futile for patients in the categories that statistically do not survive to discharge.[53] However, short-term survival is the main objective for some patients' families. Hence, medical judgment alone cannot determine whether efforts should be undertaken to gain several days or weeks of additional time, even if survival to discharge cannot be reasonably expected.

Furthermore, some acts, such as providing artificial nutrition and hydration, may have symbolic significance in expressing commitments of care, while accomplishing no other medical benefit for patients. Lantos and colleagues argue that "feeding patients in a persistent, vegetative state may be futile if the goal is to restore cognition, but it may provide emotional and symbolic benefits to the patient's family or to society. These goals may be relevant to futility determinations and should not be automatically excluded."[54] In short, the debate about futility is often at bottom a debate about goals, and disputes about appropriate goals involve conflicts of values.

Returning to the Wanglie case (Case 6), we note that the issue is whether the prolongation of life is a sufficient goal for a patient in PVS in the absence of all other benefits. We can best interpret debates about answers to this question as disputes about the legitimacy of goals, rather than as disputes about futility, in the sense of utter hopelessness. Nothing is gained—and much is obscured—by using the label *futility*. The rhetorical power of claims of medical futility derives from the supposition that these judgments are objective and value-free. However, as we have seen, it is a fiction to describe many judgments of medical futility in this way, and such appeals risk unwarranted paternalism.

Despite these precautions about appeals to " medical futility," it is occasionally a justifiable act of paternalism to withhold procedures *without* the knowledge of patients or their surrogates. Physicians may actually mislead patients and their surrogates and diminish autonomy by providing information about a useless procedure. Consider in-hospital CPR as an example. Hospital policies usually require attempts at CPR, unless a written do-not-resuscitate (DNR) order exists that includes patient or family consent. However, some argue that when resuscitation would provide no medical benefit to the patient, hospitals should not require staff to discuss options with either the patient or the family. Both beneficence and nonmaleficence support a paternalistic policy of not presenting nonbeneficial interventions as an option for decision-making. Clinicians often put families in a difficult emotional position by informing them about CPR and then attempting to convince them that it would produce no medical benefit.[55] In addition, such an approach could reduce rather than enhance autonomous decision-making by implying that a meaningful choice exists when in fact it does not.[56]

Finally, conceptions of medical futility are often presented as independent of considerations of financial costs, even though the need to control the costs of health care has fueled much of the interest in medical futility. We develop a framework for justly allocating health care in Chapter 6, but first we need to examine policies that balance benefits, costs, and risks to determine whether they can play a legitimate role in judgments about acceptable care and the distribution of care.

Balancing Benefits, Costs, and Risks

Thus far, we have concentrated primarily on the role of the principle of beneficence in clinical medicine. We shift now to the practices and institutions that are intended to support public beneficence through health policies. These policies reflect reasoned choices about appropriate benefits relative to costs and risks. Particularly influential and controversial are various forms of analysis that implement the principle of utility in health policies. Within limits the tools we will examine are morally unobjectionable and may even be morally required to illuminate trade-offs and enhance our ability to make reasoned assessments and wise judgments that will maximize beneficent outcomes.

Questions commonly arise about the comparison and relative weights of costs, risks, and benefits. Judgments about the most suitable *medical treatments* are routinely based on probable benefits and harms for patients, and judgments about the ethical acceptability of *research involving human subjects* reflect, in part, judgments about whether the probable overall benefits outweigh the risks to subjects. For example, in submitting a research protocol involving human subjects to an institutional review board (IRB) for approval, an investigator is expected to array the risks to subjects and probable benefits to both subjects and society, and then to explain why the probable benefits outweigh the risks. The IRB then offers its reasoned assessment of the protocol.

When IRBs array risks and benefits, determine their respective weights, and reach decisions on this basis, they typically use *informal* techniques. These strategies include expert judgments based on the most reliable data that can be assembled and analogical reasoning based on precedents. IRBs virtually never use formal techniques that manipulate numbers in order to express the objective probability that a research protocol will produce a net benefit. However, we will focus in this section on techniques that do employ *formal, quantitative* analysis of costs, risks, and benefits, because these methods have been at the center of recent controversies over appropriate health-related public policies and are likely to gain in influence in upcoming years.

The Nature of Costs, Risks, and Benefits

Costs are the resources required to bring about a benefit, as well as the negative effects of pursuing and realizing that benefit. They represent, in effect, sacrifices made in the attempt to reach some important objective. We will concentrate on costs expressed in monetary terms—the primary (but not exclusive) interpretation of costs in cost–benefit and cost–effectiveness analysis. The term *risk*, by contrast, refers to a possible future harm, where harm is defined as a setback to interests, particularly in life, health, and welfare. Expressions such as *minimal risk, reasonable risk,* and *high risk* usually refer to the chance of experiencing a harm—its *probability*—but sometimes they also refer to the severity of the harm if it occurs—its *magnitude*.

Statements of risk are *descriptive* inasmuch as they state the probability that harmful events will occur. However, statements of risk are also *evaluative*, inasmuch as they attach a value to the occurrence or prevention of the events. No statement of risk occurs without a prior negative evaluation of some condition. Thus, risk is both a descriptive and an evaluative concept. At its core, a circumstance of risk involves a possible occurrence of something that has been evaluated as harmful and an uncertainty about its actual occurrence that can be expressed in terms of its probability.

Several types of risks exist: physical, psychological, financial, and legal, among others. The following case illustrates several types of risk: A baby girl suffers from Seckel or "bird-headed" dwarfism, a recessive genetic disease, as well as multiple other medical complications. The child is at risk of starvation if an operation is not performed, but she also is at risk of severe suffering and serious medical complications if the operation is performed. The family is at further risk of psychological harm and economic harm because of the extremely low per capita funding for state institutions that house the mentally retarded. Eventually, the parents decide against the surgery, a decision that, in some jurisdictions, would place them at legal risk.[57]

The term *benefit* sometimes refers to cost avoidance and risk reduction, but, more commonly in biomedicine, it refers to something of positive value, such as life or health. Unlike *risk, benefit* is not itself a probabilistic term. *Probable benefit* is, instead, the proper contrast to risk, and benefits are comparable to harms rather than to risks of harm. Thus, we can best conceive risk–benefit relations in terms of a ratio between the probability and magnitude of an anticipated benefit and the probability and magnitude of an anticipated harm.

Use of the terms *cost, risk,* and *benefit* necessarily involves an evaluation. Values determine *what* will count as costs, harms, and benefits as well as *how much* particular costs, harms, and benefits will count—that is, how much weight they will have in our calculations.

Cost–Effectiveness and Cost–Benefit Analyses

Cost–effectiveness analysis (CEA) and cost–benefit analysis (CBA) are two widely used but controversial tools of formal analysis. They have been increasingly employed in setting and evaluating public policies regarding health, safety, and medical technologies. Some of these policies respond to burgeoning demands for expensive medical care and the need to contain the costs of health care. CEA and CBA are helpful because they present trade-offs in quantified terms.[58] Defenders of these techniques praise them as ways to reduce intuitive weighing of options and to avoid subjective and political decisions. However, critics claim that these methods of analysis are not sufficiently comprehensive, that they fail to include all relevant values and options, that they are often themselves subjective and biased, and that they are sometimes ad hoc. Critics also charge that these techniques concentrate decision-making authority in the hands of narrow, technical professionals who often fail to understand moral, social, legal, and political constraints that legitimately limit use of these methods.

CEA and CBA use different terms to state the value of outcomes. CBA measures both the benefits and the costs in monetary terms, whereas CEA measures the benefits in nonmonetary terms, such as years of life, quality-adjusted life-years, or cases of disease. CEA offers a bottom line such as "cost per year of life saved," whereas CBA offers a bottom line of a benefit–cost ratio stated in monetary figures that express the common measurement. Although CBA often begins by measuring different quantitative units (such as number of accidents, statistical deaths, number of persons treated, and dollars expended), it attempts in the end to convert and express these seemingly incommensurable units of measurement into a common one.

Consider, as an example of these approaches, a debate in the United States in the late 1980s and early 1990s about the use of low-osmolality contrast agents (LOCAs). These agents are used in intravascular radiographic studies, especially in cardiac angiography, because they offer reduced risks of serious adverse reactions, including death. LOCAs also reduce moderate and mild adverse reactions, including nausea. Even though LOCAs do not appear to offer any diagnostic advantage over older, high-osmolality contrast agents, LOCAs would have been universally adopted, either within an institution or the health care system as a whole, because of their superior safety and comfort, if their costs had not been so much greater. At the time, LOCAs cost between ten and 20 times more than alternative agents. Since over ten million intravascular contrast studies are performed in the United States each year, several estimates indicate that the universal use of LOCAs would add a billion dollars to health care costs—by comparison to the use of LOCAs only in high-risk cases.

The relative merits of the available agents were stated in terms of the (monetary) value of life (as appropriate in CBA), but more often in terms of the value of life-years (as is often the case in CEA). Estimates varied greatly, but some studies indicated that the universal use of LOCAs would save lives at the cost of $7.5 million for each death prevented, while others put the cost even higher. Some CEAs found the cost for each year of life saved in the universal use of LOCAs to be approximately $100,000, a figure much higher at the time than, for example, the treatment of hypertension ($30,000) or dialysis for end-stage renal disease ($32,000). However, using LOCAs only for the 15–20% of patients at high risk for serious adverse reactions—for example, because of previous allergy-like reactions—would reduce the cost per death prevented to $1 million and the cost per year of life saved to approximately $31,000 (a figure in line with the other two treatments just identified). Furthermore, the evidence indicated that LOCAs would not fully pay for themselves through reducing the costs of dealing with adverse events. During this period, health care institutions and professionals rarely offered patients the choice of contrast agents (though most would provide LOCAs if patients specifically requested them).

In view of this analysis, controversy raged about whether health care institutions, professionals, and funders should provide LOCAs universally or only selectively. Part of the debate centered on whether sound criteria existed for accurately determining different levels of risk. However, by the mid- to late-1990s, the cost of LOCAs had declined substantially and the cost ratio of LOCAs to high-osmolality contrast agents now, according to some estimates, was closer to 5:1. As a result, LOCAs fared much better in CBAs and CEAs. Their main advantage for low-risk patients is a decrease in discomfort through the reduction of nausea and the like, which, in any event, is transient and can usually be managed (though some commentators describe it as "an hour in hell"—a description that others challenge).[59]

This case illustrates the role and importance of some analytic tools and categories that will be prominent in the remainder of this chapter. Using the common metric of money, CBA permits a comparison of programs that save lives with, for example, programs that reduce disability or accomplish other goals, such as education. By contrast, CEA does not permit an evaluation of the inherent worth of programs or a comparative evaluation of programs with different aims. CEA functions best to compare and evaluate different programs sharing an identical aim, such as saving years of life.

As a result, many CEAs involve comparing alternative courses of action that have similar health benefits in order to determine which is the most cost-effective. A classic example is the use of the guaiac test, an inexpensive test for detecting minute amounts of blood in the stool. Such blood may result from several problems, including hemorrhoids, benign intestinal polyps, or colonic cancer. (The last problem is a major killer, but it may be curable if diagnosed very early.) A guaiac test cannot identify the cause of the bleeding, but if there is a positive stool guaiac and no other obvious cause for the bleeding, physicians undertake other tests. The American Cancer Society in 1974 proposed using six sequential stool guaiac tests to screen for colorectal cancer. This proposal was based on the fact that any single stool guaiac detects only approximately 92% of the colorectal cancers. Two analysts prepared a careful CEA of the six stool guaiac tests. They assumed that the initial test costs four dollars, that each additional test costs one dollar, and that each successive test detects many fewer cases of cancer. They then determined that the marginal cost per case of detected cancer increased dramatically: $1175 for one test; $5492 for two tests; $49,150 for three tests; $469,534 for four tests; $4.7 million for five tests; and $47 million for the full six-test screen.[60]

Such findings do not dictate a conclusion, but the analysis is relevant for a society allocating resources, for insurance companies and hospitals setting policies, for physicians making recommendations to patients, and for patients considering diagnostic procedures. This analysis is a CEA rather than a CBA because it does not attempt to convert the benefit of detection of colorectal cancer into a measure, such as dollars, that can then be compared with the costs. It also does not include other effects that may be hard to measure, such as the reassurance given to patients.

Conceptual confusion surrounds the meaning of CEA. In some cases, when two programs are compared, the cost savings offered by one may be sufficient to view it as more cost-effective than the other. Yet some analysts contend that we should not confuse CEA with either reduced costs or increased effectiveness alone, because it often depends on both together. A program may be more cost-effective than another even if it (1) *costs more*—because it may increase medical effectiveness—or (2) leads to a *decrease in medical effectiveness*—because it may greatly reduce the costs.

For these reasons, some analysts argue that we should use the term *cost-effective* for cases in which "one strategy is . . . (a) less costly and at least as effective; (b) more effective and more costly, its additional benefit being worth its additional cost; or (c) less effective and less costly, the added benefit of the rival strategy not being worth its extra cost."[61] However, many analysts accept only (a), holding that one strategy is more cost-effective than another if it costs less and achieves the same goal. In this conception, CEA presupposes a uniform goal already established by an independent assessment of the benefits of reaching that goal. Diagnostic or therapeutic procedures are then more or less cost-effective in comparison only with others that have the same outcome. That is, if both procedures produce an equal outcome—in, say, life-years—but one is less expensive, then that procedure is more cost-effective.

For an example, consider an early study of leukocyte transfusion during chemotherapy for acute leukemia that showed that prophylactic transfusion costs $2431 more than therapeutic transfusion and increases the patient's life expectancy by 0.0285 years.[62] Whether it is appropriate to say that prophylactic transfusion is more or less cost-effective than therapeutic transfusion depends on the value assigned to the additional benefit relative to the additional cost. Put bluntly, is it worth $85,300 for an additional statistical year of life gained? Without answering this question, one cannot determine whether prophylactic transfusion is cost-effective.

One might think that adopting CEA entails an endorsement of the principle of utility as the moral guideline for such decisions, but the principle of utility does not have the moral power to dictate a particular medical procedure simply because it has the lowest cost-effectiveness ratio (for example, because it provides the greatest benefit for each dollar). To assign priority to the alternative with the lowest cost-effectiveness ratio is to view the possibilities of medical diagnosis and therapy as unduly narrow.[63] For example, such an approach would stop with the first stool guaiac test, because the cost-effectiveness ratio is the lowest for that first test and increases for each subsequent test. This approach to decision analysis excludes from the calculation the value of the additional health benefits, including psychological reassurance, that the additional tests may provide.

Indeed, using CEA alone might yield decisions to forgo very worthwhile costs. For example, preventing accident, disease, and illness has often been touted as the best way to contain the costs of health care, but, from the standpoint of CEA, prevention is not always better than a cure, and it may even be worse. Prevention may produce savings in particular treatments, but it may also add medical expenditures for other health problems.[64] Similarly, successful strategies to reduce risky lifestyles and behavioral patterns generally result in an increase rather than a decrease in social expenditures, because people who live longer often need a wide array of social assistance and services.[65] Nevertheless, preventive strategies, if effective, have the advantage of maintaining health over time, even if they have an increased net cost.

Risk Assessment

Risk assessment is another important analytic technique. As already noted, risk includes the probability and magnitude of negative outcomes. Hence, risk *assessment* involves the analysis and evaluation of probabilities of negative outcomes, especially harms. Risk *identification* involves locating some hazard. Risk *estimation* determines the probability and magnitude of harms from that hazard. Risk *evaluation* determines the acceptability of the identified and estimated risks, often in relation to other objectives. Evaluation of risk in relation to probable benefits is often labeled *risk-benefit analysis* (RBA), which may be formulated in terms of a ratio of expected benefits to risks and may lead to a judgment about the acceptability of the risk under assessment. Risk identification, estimation, and evaluation are all stages in risk assessment. The next stage in the process is risk *management*—the set of individual or institutional responses to the analysis and assessment of risk, including decisions to reduce or control risks. For example, risk management in hospitals includes setting policies to reduce the risk of medical malpractice suits. Some recent discussions hold that society can better interpret and respond to risk by combining risk assessment and risk management into a more holistic approach of "risk characterization," which includes a process of both analysis and deliberation.[66] However, the distinction between risk assessment and risk management remains useful as long as it does not become a rigid distinction or separation.

This section focuses on risk assessment, which frequently undergirds technology assessment, environmental impact statements, and public policies protecting health and safety. The following schema of magnitude and probability of harm is a useful chart for understanding risk assessment:

		Magnitude of Harm	
		Major	*Minor*
	High	1	2
Proba-bility of Harm			
	Low	3	4

For purposes of medical decision-making and public policy, we should determine the acceptability of risks through the most objective estimates of probability and magnitude of harm possible, together with all of the relevant values, including benefits.

As category 4 suggests, a question exists about whether some risks are so insignificant, in terms of either probability or magnitude of harm or both, as not to merit attention. So-called *de minimis* risks are acceptable because they can be construed as effectively zero. For example, according to the Food and Drug Administration (FDA), a risk of less than one cancer per million persons exposed is *de minimis*. Yet the quantitative threshold or cutoff point used in a *de minimis* approach is problematic. For instance, an annual risk of one cancer per million persons for the U.S. population would produce the same number of fatalities (i.e., 275) as a risk of one per 100 in a town with a population of 27,500. Furthermore, in focusing on the annual risk of cancer or death to one individual per million, the *de minimis* approach may neglect the cumulative, overall level of risk created for individuals over their lifetimes by the addition of several one-per-million risks.[67]

Risk assessment also focuses on the acceptability of risks relative to benefits that are sought. With the possible exception of *de minimis* risks, most risks will be considered acceptable or unacceptable in relation to the probable benefits of the actions that carry those risks—for example, the benefits of radiation or a surgical procedure in health care, or the benefits of nuclear power or toxic chemicals in the workplace.[68]

The problem of uncertainty. Although both risk and uncertainty assume a lack of predictability or knowledge of future events, these concepts are distinct. *Risk* refers to the probability and magnitude of a setback to interests. *Uncertainty*, by contrast, refers to a lack of predictability or knowledge because of insufficient evidence. Risk assessment and management are fraught with uncertainty. For example, even though a chemical poses a demonstrable risk of cancer at high dose levels in rodents, inference to its effects on human beings may be quite precarious. A fundamental question, then, is which way to err in situations of uncertainty about how human bodies will react. Whether analysts will resolve uncertainty optimistically or pessimistically will depend on their value judgments and attitudes. Regulators, for example, often assume the most conservative estimate by taking a worst-case scenario.[69]

In efforts to reduce uncertainty, the same standards of evidence—for example, that a particular substance is carcinogenic—often do not apply in all settings. For example, debates arise about where to set evidentiary standards in policies to protect the environment and to protect patients from unsafe drugs, medical devices, and the like. In general, a standard of proof sets forth the risk of error that is acceptable. Acceptance of any confidence level presupposes normative moral, social, and political considerations. For instance, whether a regulatory agency should set a standard of evidence that a substance is toxic or carcinogenic at a 95% confidence level reflects a normative judgment, not merely a scientific judgment, and it will have an impact on both commercial interests and potential victims of the substance.[70]

A common uncertainty is whether and how an agent or technology will interact with other agents or technologies to produce unforeseeable effects.[71] For example, scientists may be uncertain about the effects that simultaneous exposure to several chemicals will have on individuals, because the interaction of the chemicals may produce synergistic rather than additive effects. Other uncertainties about technologies include how people will use them—for example, how physicians will manage them and whether patients will follow instructions. Proposals for safer sex in the AIDS crisis, for instance, hinge not only on the quality of the condoms used but also on the care taken by users. Thus, evidence based on laboratory studies of condoms' effectiveness in preventing HIV transmission is insufficient for a predictive judgment about condoms' effectiveness in actual sexual intercourse.

Other uncertainties stem from the social and cultural context of technological advances. For example, Lynn White has argued that technology assessment requires social analysis, because the impact of a technology is filtered through the society and its culture, often in unpredictable ways. One of his case studies focuses on alcohol, which was distilled from wine as a pharmaceutical in the twelfth century at Salerno, the site of Europe's most famous medical school. Widely heralded initially as a pharmaceutical with beneficial effects for chronic headaches, stomach trouble, cancer, arthritis, sterility, falling or graying hair, bad breath, and a "cold temperament," it gradually led to widespread drunkenness and disorder and then, in the twentieth century, to alcohol-related diseases and automobile accidents, none of which a technology assessment panel in the twelfth century could have predicted.[72]

Risk perception. An individual's perception of risks may differ from an expert's assessment. Variations may reflect not only different goals and "risk budgets," but also different qualitative assessments of particular risks, including whether the risks in question are voluntary, controllable, highly salient, novel, or dreaded.[73] Consider the possible impact of personal life plans and risk budgets on patients' perceptions and assessments of the risks of coronary artery bypass surgery. Of every 100 patients who undergo the operation, one to two die. An active sportsperson might view this risk of death from surgery as insignificant in view of the active life sought; another person might choose medical rather than surgical treatment because of a fear of dying on the operating table.[74] In addition, as we saw in Chapter 3, a patient's perception of risks and benefits may depend in part on how the physician presents them—for example, whether in terms of the probability of dying or the probability of surviving.

Public and professional responses to accidental exposure to the blood of patients infected with HIV provide an illustration. Such exposure produces greater fear than did accidental exposure to the blood of patients with hepatitis B several years ago, even though statistically both exposures carried an approximately equal overall risk of death. The probability of HIV infection is lower (apparently less than 1%), but death from the infection remains close to a certainty over time, despite improved treatments; the probability of infection by the hepatitis B virus is higher, at approximately 25% but, conservatively estimated, the death rate is only five percent. According to one study, the fear of certain death for someone infected with HIV appears to account for the greater fear of HIV infection through accidental exposure.[75] Other factors include the social stigma attached to HIV infection and AIDS. As treatments that delay death from HIV infection improve and social stigma declines, public perceptions of risk will undoubtedly change as well.

Differences in risk perception suggest limitations in attempts to use only objective, quantitative statements of probability and magnitude in reaching conclusions about the acceptability of risk. The public's informed but subjective perception of a harm needs to be considered and given substantial weight when formulating public policy, but the weight will vary with the case. However, the public sometimes inconsistently assumes major risks voluntarily while objecting strenuously to low, externally imposed risks,[76] and experts can helpfully identify different perceptions of risk and collect accurate information about risks. In this way, mistaken public views about these risks can often can be corrected.[77]

Risk–Benefit Analysis (RBA) in the Regulation of Drugs and Medical Devices

Some of the conceptual, normative, and empirical issues in risk assessment and, specifically, RBA are evident in the FDA's regulation of drugs and medical devices. In a rigorous procedure following preclinical animal studies, the FDA requires three phases of human trials. Each stage involves RBA to determine whether to proceed to the next stage and, finally, whether to approve a drug for wider use.

Patients, physicians, and other health care professionals have criticized the process of drug approval in the United States because of the length of time required for approval (an average of eight years from synthesis of the drug, which is several years longer than in European countries). Critics contend that the standard of evidence for a favorable risk–benefit ratio is too high and thus severely limits patients' access to promising new drugs, often in times of dire need created by serious, even fatal, medical conditions.

Society's perception of clinical research has shifted dramatically, in part because of such criticisms. In the 1970s and early 1980s, the emphasis was on protecting individuals from risks associated with research. Beginning in the 1980s, the emphasis shifted to increasing access to participation in research. Particularly in response to the AIDS epidemic and the demands of AIDS activists, the FDA developed mechanisms to provide expanded access to experimental drugs, especially for patients with seriously debilitating or life-threatening conditions and with no satisfactory alternative treatments.[78] In a shift of tradition aimed at insuring access during the conduct of clinical trials, the agency has authorized treatment uses (in contrast to investigational uses) of unapproved experimental drugs for patients with an illness that is serious or poses an imminent threat to life and that has no other satisfactory alternative therapy. Other FDA initiatives include a "fast track" (expedited approval) and a "parallel track." The fast track allows patients with "seriously debilitating" or "life-threatening" conditions to accept greater risks in taking new drugs in the absence of acceptable alternatives.[79] This approach was used in the approval of zidovudine (AZT) to treat AIDS. More specifically, in its medical risk–benefit analysis for expedited approval, the FDA sought to determine first whether the drug's benefits outweighed its risks, both known and unknown, and also whether there was a need for more evidence about those benefits and risks, in view of the disease's "seriously debilitating" or "life-threatening" conditions. The parallel track, by contrast, allows limited access to experimental AIDS drugs that, according to early studies, are reasonably safe and promising, while clinical investigations continue.

These modes of expanded access resulted in part from efforts by AIDS protesters, whose civil disobedience and other dramatic actions drew attention to the needs of patients with AIDS. Such actions have raised questions about the role of advocates in securing access for special groups of patients to new drugs. A tension exists between scientific evidence about risks and benefits and patients' desires for access to certain drugs for certain conditions. Moreover, there are major concerns about the commercial exploitation of these desires if scientific standards of evidence are not maintained. Early and wide access may limit researchers' and the FDA's efforts to complete important double-blind, placebo-controlled clinical trials to establish a firmer RBA of the treatments.

In our view, expanded access to experimental drugs is warranted in response to serious and particularly life-threatening medical conditions, where no effective alternative treatments are available. Such circumstances warrant allowing considerable latitude for patients' values regarding risks and benefits, although not so much as to subvert the FDA's regulation of new drugs to protect the public.

However, the FDA retains a stringency in other areas that continue to stir up controversy. An FDA decision in 1992 to severely restrict the use of silicone-gel breast implants is a well-known example. This decision illustrates societal controversies about RBA and bureaucratic decision-making in the context of health care and medical devices. Women have elected implants for more than 30 years, either to augment their breast size or to reconstruct their breasts following mastectomies for cancer or other surgery. Each year in the United States, prior to this decision, approximately 150,000 implants occurred, 80% for augmentation and 20% for reconstruction. More than two million women in the United States (three million worldwide) have had these implants. Since legislation in 1976,[80] manufacturers have had the burden of proof in establishing that their medical devices are safe and effective before they may be distributed and used, but many manufacturers, including those making silicone-gel breast implants, have had additional time to meet this standard because their products were already on the market.

In April 1992, the FDA appealed to RBA in severely restricting the use of silicone-gel breast implants until additional studies could be conducted to establish their safety. Use was restricted to patients enrolled in clinical studies. Concerns have centered on the implants' longevity, rate of rupture, and link with various diseases. Those who defend *complete prohibition* contend that no woman should be allowed to take a risk of unknown but potentially serious magnitude because her consent could not be informed. However, former FDA Commissioner David Kessler defended a *restrictive policy*, rather than prohibition. He argued that for "patients with cancer and others with a need for breast reconstruction," a favorable risk–benefit ratio could exist in carefully controlled circumstances.[81] Kessler and the FDA distinguished sharply between reconstruction candidates and augmentation candidates, arguing that a favorable risk–benefit ratio exists only for reconstruction candidates.

Kessler insisted that the FDA's decision did not involve "any judgment about values," but simply focused on the "higher risk" presented for women receiving augmentation implants. This controversial claim is based on the fact that women with augmentation implants still have breast tissue. One argument is that, in the presence of an implant, mammography may not detect breast cancer in the breast tissue, and, further, that the use of mammography will create a risk of radiation exposure in healthy young women with breast tissue who have silent ruptures of the gel implant without symptoms. Kessler writes, "In our opinion the risk–benefit ratio does not at this time favor the unrestricted use of silicone breast implants in healthy women."

Critics charge that the government's decision to restrict women's access to silicone-gel breast implants was inappropriately paternalistic, especially when compared to the permissive public decisions reached in European countries. (Europeans have relied heavily on the strong historical evidence indicating a low rate of health problems.) We concur with these critics that the FDA overweighed the unknown risks, in part, because it viewed the benefits of breast implants as either overrated by many women or nonexistent, except in cases of reconstruction. The agency then held these implants to a high standard of safety, instead of allowing women to decide for themselves whether to accept the risks for their own subjectively defined benefits—a clear act of strong paternalism. Regarding the FDA's risk–benefit analysis, Marcia Angell wrote:

> Demonstrating the safety and effectiveness of a drug or device does not, of course, mean showing that there are no side effects or risks. If that were the standard, we would have no drugs or devices, since nearly all of them have possible adverse effects. The issue is the balance between risks and benefits. Greater risks are permitted for greater benefits. In evaluation of the balance, risks and benefits are usually considered separately, then weighed.[82]

The benefits of implants, particularly for women who seek augmentation, cannot be measured in terms of the value of increased life expectancy, but the benefits may still be significant for quality of life. Subjective benefits for many women outweigh the identified risks, and opinion surveys indicate that 90% of women receiving the implants are satisfied with the results. If the evidence had indicated high risk relative to benefit, as well as unwarranted risk-taking by patients, a different conclusion might have been sustained, but evidence available at the time (and since) points in the other direction.[83] Given the considerable range of both scientific and policy disagreement, the FDA policy is unjustifiably paternalistic.

A more defensible policy would permit the continuing use of silicone-gel breast implants, regardless of the users' biological conditions and aims, while requiring adequate disclosure of information about risks (known and unknown). This antipaternalist strategy would allow women to make their own decisions, an approach recommended by the fact that no evidence of major risks to health has appeared in decades of use of silicone-gel implants.[84] Raising the level of disclosure standards is, from this perspective, more appropriate than restraining choice. The FDA itself took a similar course of action subsequent to the 1992 decision when two 1993-released studies confirmed that silicone gel had caused problems in the immune system of laboratory rats. Rather than further upgrading its restrictions on implants, the FDA elected to require breast implant manufacturers to inform women considering implants of the new studies.[85] Similarly, in May 2000, based on completed test results, the FDA ruled that saline-filled breast implants, the only kind still available, could remain on the market but that manufacturers had to undertake a serious effort to warn women of the risks, which include pain, infection, and cosmetic problems, as well as a replacement rate of 20% to 40% over three years.[86]

The FDA's earlier decision about silicone-gel implants also raised disproportionate fears about the risks among the more than one million women now alive with breast implants. Many have sought to have their implants removed. However, some are unable to pay the approximately $5000 required for removal, and at least two women have cut their breasts either to force hospitals to remove the implants or to have their insurance companies pay for explantation.[87] Women's fears are understandable, and the FDA's recommendation to women not to have their implants removed unless they have medical problems rings hollow, because its policy implies that breast implants are dangerous, based on the available evidence regarding their safety.[88]

We reach two general conclusions from our examination of FDA decision-making. First, it is morally legitimate and often obligatory for society to act beneficently through the government and its agencies to protect citizens from harmful medical drugs and devices and those of unproven safety and efficacy. The FDA plays an important role in setting minimum standards of safety and efficacy for drugs and devices. Our conclusion that the FDA should not have severely restricted or prohibited the use of silicone-gel breast implants should not be interpreted as an argument against the role of the FDA as society's guardian. Second, no value-free risk assessments or RBAs exist. Values are evident in the FDA's expanded access to drugs for AIDS and, despite Kessler's disavowal, in its decision to restrict access to silicone-gel breast implants. To hold that risks to women seeking implants for augmentation are significant and more important than subjective cosmetic benefits is a value-laden position, and it raises the question about which moral and nonmoral values should be used.[89]

Both the *value of life* and the *quality of life* are at stake in many controversies about policies and practices to reduce risks and to increase health benefits, as we will now see.

The Value and Quality of Life

We turn in this final section to controversies regarding how to place a value on life—which have centered on CBAs—and to controversies over the value of quality-adjusted life-years (QALYs)—which have centered on CEAs.

Valuing Lives

A dramatic and controversial form of analysis assigns an economic value to human life. Analysts try to determine the monetary value of human life in order to state benefits in terms that can be balanced against the costs. As analysts note, a society may spend amount x to save a life (e.g., by reducing the risk of death from causes such as cancer and mining accidents) in one setting but only spend amount y to save a life in another setting. These different expenditures are inconsistent if life has a certain value and death a certain disvalue that can be compared quantitatively across the two settings. The objective in determining the value of a life, then, is to develop consistency across practices and policies.

Methods for valuing lives. Analysts have developed several methods to determine the value of human life. According to the discounted future earnings (DFE), or human capital approach, we can determine the monetary value of lives by considering what people at risk of some disease or accident could be expected to earn if they survived. (Future income is discounted, because money earned now could be invested and thus is worth more than future income.) On these economic assumptions, those who have no income have no value, and those who drain society's resources (e.g., thieves, the institutionalized mentally ill, the unemployed, and retirees dependent on welfare) have a negative value.

This approach can help measure the economic costs of diseases, accidents, and death, but it biases health policy in favor of classes such as young, adult white men and people with wealth, because they can be expected to earn more. For example, it could support a public health policy to encourage motorcyclists to wear helmets over a cervical cancer detection program. This approach also raises moral questions because it gauges, for policy purposes, the social value of human lives in terms of economic value.

The moral problems associated with the DFE approach have contributed to the popularity of a second, more defensible approach, known as "willingness to pay" (WTP). It considers how much individuals would be willing to pay to reduce the risks of death. One version of WTP focuses on *revealed preferences* by analyzing preferences that are well established in society and that can be identified by empirical research. This research attempts to determine how much risk individuals now assume (e.g., in their decisions about work hazards) in order to obtain certain benefits. Their preferences, as exhibited in their actual balancing of risks and benefits, become the basis for establishing the level of risk that should be permitted in that group when a new technology is introduced or a new hazard is discovered. This approach is reliable only if individuals actually understand the risks and voluntarily assume them. For example, if workers do not understand and appreciate the risks of their work, and if they have few choices in employment, then this version of WTP is unreliable. This approach also takes what is desired or accepted by individuals as the proper measure of what is desirable or acceptable, a normatively flawed assumption.

Another version of WTP focuses on *expressed preferences* by considering how people respond to hypothetical questions designed to determine how much they are willing to pay to reduce the risk of death. One much discussed study asked members of the public how much they would be willing to spend in taxes to put ambulances and other life-saving devices in communities around the country in order to save 20 people from heart attacks each year.[90] A later study attempted to determine whether members of the public would place a priority on allocating medical resources to severely ill patients, even if these patients would benefit less from the treatments than would less ill patients.[91] Such questions are relevant in decisions about developing and funding expensive technologies through community resources. However, individuals' answers to hypothetical questions may not adequately indicate how much they would be willing to spend on an actual program to reduce their (and others') risk of death.

Moral appraisal of valuing lives. An examination of individual risk budgets indicates that people are willing to risk their lives for various possible benefits, including recreation, friendship, fame, and fortune. Religious traditions recognize the moral possibility—in some cases, the obligation—of martyrdom in preserving the faith or integrity of their adherents. These and many other trade-offs suggest that we do commonly place a value on human life. However, we do not always need to place a *monetary* value on human life. In many cases, qualitative factors are more important than the purely economic factors operative in formal analyses. For example, how some deaths occur, by what means they occur, and with what symbolic features may legitimately lead a society to allocate its resources differently in order to reduce various risks of death. Determinations of acceptable risk often derive from subjective perceptions of risk. A society also may justifiably choose to expend time, energy, and money to rescue individuals from peril even when the costs are extremely high. Such unstinting acts of communal beneficence as rescuing trapped coal miners symbolize society's benevolence and affirm the value to society of the victims.

The social value of acts of rescue focuses on "identified lives" in peril, whereas preventive measures to reduce the risk of death aim at "statistical lives"—that is, unknown persons who will be in future danger. Concentrating resources on identified individuals in peril may turn out to be far less efficient than a preventive strategy, but such a priority is not necessarily unwarranted or irrational. Indeed, these policies may be rational *because* they express or symbolize significant values, including moral values.

According to some interpreters, the symbolic value of rescuing identified individuals accounts, in part, for the 1972 U.S. congressional decision—following widespread publicity in the media about particular individuals who were dying of renal failure—to make funds available for virtually all citizens who need renal dialysis or renal transplantation.[92] This decision also reflected the moral importance of equal consideration and treatment. Earlier, hospital committees had decided which identified individuals suffering from end-stage renal failure would receive access to scarce kidney dialysis machines, and thus which ones would live and which ones would die. The end-stage renal disease program is now a multibillion dollar program, and serious questions have emerged about its justifiability from the standpoint of CBA. However, it is not necessarily unreasonable or unethical to violate efficiency criteria in order to express a societal commitment to a precious value.

We also need to consider the probable consequences of using formal analyses such as CBA. For example, putting a price on a nonmarket entity such as human life can reduce its perceived value, and society may choose to value human life more highly in collective decisions than some individuals would in their private decisions.[93] Data gained from CBA and other analytic techniques are relevant to the formation of public policies, but they provide only one set of premises about social beneficence, among others. It is also not necessary in many circumstances to put a specific economic value on human life in order to evaluate possible risk-reduction policies and to compare their costs. Evaluation may reasonably focus on the life-years saved, without attempting to convert them into monetary measures. In the evaluation of health care, CBA has now greatly diminished in importance by comparison to CEA, which often promotes the goal of maximizing quality-adjusted life-years.[94]

Valuing Quality-Adjusted Life-Years

Quality of life and QALYs. In both health policy and health care, everyone is interested not only in saving lives and years of life, but also in the quality of those lives. We agree with the President's Commission for the Study of Ethical Problems in Medicine and Biomedical and Behavioral Research that "quality of life [is] an ethically essential concept that focuses on the good of the individual, what kind of life is possible given the person's condition, and whether that condition will allow the individual to have a life that he or she views as worth living."[95] Improving the quality of a patient's life is an especially important goal in chronic and rehabilitative care. For example, few people appear to be interested in living their life in a persistent vegetative state, and individuals contemplating different modes of treatment for a particular condition commonly trade some life-years for improved quality of life during their remaining life-years.

The basic idea of quality-adjusted life-years or QALYs is that, "if an extra year of healthy (i.e., good quality) life-expectancy is worth one, then an extra year of unhealthy (i.e., poor quality) life-expectancy must be worth less than one (for why otherwise do people seek to be healthy?)."[96] On this scale, if the value of a healthy year of life is one, the value of the condition of death is zero. Various states of illness or disability better than death but short of full health receive a value between zero and one. The value of particular health outcomes depends on the increase in the utility of the health state and the number of years it lasts.[97]

QALYs represent trade-offs between quality and quantity of life and are designed to provide a way to measure the net health effectiveness of different programs, activities, or interventions. That is, QALYs represent an attempt to bring the two dimensions of length of life and quality of life into a single framework of evaluation.[98] Among their various functions, QALYs can be used to monitor the effects of treatments on patients in clinical practice or in clinical trials, to determine what to recommend to patients, and to provide information to patients about the effects of different treatments. In some contexts, it may be sufficient to consider only the net effectiveness of treatments in terms of their QALYs. However, in many contexts, including the allocation of health care resources, we must examine the costs relative to the QALYs provided by different treatments. Only then can we determine efficiency together with effectiveness.

In a widely noted study that illustrates these abstract points, British health economist Alan Williams used QALYs to examine the cost-effectiveness of coronary artery bypass grafting. According to his analysis, bypass grafting compares favorably with pacemakers for heart block. It is also superior to heart transplantation and the treatment of end-stage renal failure, but less cost-effective than hip replacement. He also found that bypass grafting for severe angina and extensive coronary artery disease is more cost-effective than for less severe cases. The rate of survival can be misleading for coronary artery bypass grafting and many other therapeutic procedures that have a major impact on quality of life. On the basis of his analysis, Williams recommended that resources "be redeployed at the margin to procedures for which the benefits to patients are high in relation to the costs.[99]

An underlying question in these proposals is how can we determine quality of life? Analysts often start with rough measures, such as physical mobility, freedom from pain and distress, and the capacity to perform the activities of daily life and to engage in social interactions. Quality of life thus may appear to be one way to talk about the ingredients of a good life. However, this description renders the notion so amorphous and so variable as to be unusable in health policy and health care. It is more promising to identify a certain level of particular goods that are vital for an individual's fulfillment of his or her life plan, and some negative conditions that thwart the realization of individual life plans, whatever their content.[100] These positive and negative conditions provide the needed content for the notion of "health-related quality of life."[101]

For purposes of our discussion here, QALYs will refer only to "health-related quality of life." Despite many methodological variations and limits in current proposals, we will assume that some instruments can be developed and refined to present meaningful and accurate measures of health-related quality of life. Without them, we are likely to operate with implicit and unexamined views about trade-offs between quantity and quality of life in relation to cost.

Ethical Assumptions of QALYs

The ethical assumptions involved in QALY-based CEA require closer attention than the presentation thus far affords. Utilitarianism is CEA's philosophical parent, and some of its problems carry over to its offspring.[102] Implicit in QALY-based CEA is the idea that health maximization is the only relevant objective of health services. But some non-health benefits or utilities of health services also contribute to quality of life. As was evident in our discussion of silicone-gel breast implants, conditions such as asymmetrical breasts may affect a person's subjective estimate of quality of life and may merit inclusion as a source of distress. The problem is that QALY-based CEA attaches utility only to selected outcomes while neglecting values such as how care is provided (e.g., whether it is personal care) and how it is distributed (e.g., whether universal access is provided).[103] Even when QALY-based CEA is conceived as broadly as possible, it will still require supplementation by other values.

Additional questions arise about whether the use of QALYs in CEA is adequately egalitarian. In principle, proponents of QALY-based CEA hold that each healthy life-year is equally valuable for everyone. Thus, a QALY is a QALY, regardless of who possesses it.[104] However, QALY-based CEA may discriminate against older people, because (ceteris paribus) saving the life of a younger person is likely to produce more QALYs than saving the life of an older person. Age will also play a role in considerations of quality of life, which is often more compromised among the elderly.[105]

Other concerns about equality—what some call an "aversion to inequality"— have played a role in some efforts to modify QALY-based CEAs. One modification takes into account the initial severity of illness (even beyond its bearing on the magnitude of the treatment outcome) in order to give greater priority to those who are in greater need. Another modification assigns independent significance to patients' end points in order not to disadvantage patients who have a lower potential for overall health.[106]

QALY-based CEA does not try to realize the greatest good for the greatest number of individuals, or even the greatest medical good for the greatest number of patients. QALY-based CEA also does not consider how life-years are distributed among numbers of patients, and it may not entail efforts to reduce the number of individual victims in its attempts to increase the number of life-years. From this standpoint, no difference exists between saving one person who can be expected to have 40 QALYs and saving two people who can be expected to have 20 QALYs each. Indeed, in principle, CEA will give priority to saving one person with 40 expected QALYs over saving two persons with only 19 expected QALYs each.

This feature of QALY-based CEA suggests that it favors life-years over individual lives, and the number of life-years over the number of individual lives, while failing to recognize societal and professional obligations of beneficence that require rescuing endangered individual lives. John Harris cleverly complains that QALYs are a "life-threatening device," because they suggest that life-years rather than individual lives are valuable.[107]

A tension thus exists between QALY-based CEA and the duty to rescue, even though both are ultimately grounded on beneficence. This tension appears in the widely discussed effort by the Oregon Health Services Commission to develop a prioritized list of health services. More specifically, the State of Oregon wanted to expand its Medicaid coverage to all of its poor citizens, but it could accomplish that goal only by limiting coverage to services considered to have a relatively high priority. (For a fuller explanation, see Chapter 6.) A draft priority list in May 1990 drew vigorous criticism from physicians and other citizens because it ranked some life-saving procedures below some routine procedures. David Hadorn has rightly contended that, "The cost-effectiveness analysis approach used to create the initial list conflicted directly with the powerful 'Rule of Rescue'— people's perceived duty to save endangered life whenever possible."[108]

QALY-based CEA thus faces several questions about the adequacy and value of this tool of analysis for health policy and health care. In particular, we have noted methodological problems in the assignment of priority to life-years over individual lives. The implication of this assignment of priority is that beneficence-based rescue (especially life-saving) is less significant than cost-utility, that the distribution of life-years is unimportant, that saving more lives is less critical than maximizing the number of life-years, and that quality of life is more important than quantity of life. We have rejected some aspect of each of these implications.

Decision-Making Processes: Who Decides and How?

Which and whose values should be included in the calculus of CEA, CBA, and RBA? Those who emphasize decision-making by experts engaged in putatively objective analyses often disagree with those who put a premium on public participation. Experts have an important role to play, particularly in arraying the costs, risks, and benefits involved, but legitimate reasons often exist for not allowing experts to make the final decision. Value judgments pervade the entire process, from risk identification and estimation to risk assessment and management. Furthermore, the source of funds for studies by experts may bias experts toward certain findings. According to one report, some pharmaceutical company-funded studies were eight times less likely to reach unfavorable qualitative conclusions about drugs under investigation than were comparable nonprofit-funded studies.[109] Government-funded studies may suffer from the same problem if government agencies are predisposed to a particular outcome.

Some critics of CEA, CBA, and RBA contend that they are nondemocratic or antidemocratic. By contrast, defenders argue that experts in these techniques respect consumer sovereignty and derive values from expressed, revealed, or implied consumer preferences. Experts then assess costs, risks, and benefits in relation to those values. Defenders of CBA also contend that their methods make it possible for the government to regulate risks "by finding, developing, and legitimating methods for making centralized decisions."[110] They note that the public's perception is sometimes unpredictable and erratic and often reflects whims of the moment.

Our view is that appropriate mechanisms for public participation in decisions that incorporate CEA, CBA, and RBA are at least as socially valuable as the methods themselves. Considerations of justice support specific procedures of public participation, such as adversary hearings and testimony at public forums. A fair and acceptable process of decision-making is defensible because of the principles it embodies, not merely because it will produce a good decision or outcome.[111]

Questions also arise whether the QALYs considered in CEA should reflect the values of the general public or the values of people who have or have had a particular disease, disability, or other condition. Some worry that patients will tend to overstate the disutility of their own condition in an effort to secure additional health care resources and thus distort the CEA. However, current evidence suggests that patients do not make such utility assignments. Perhaps the best approach is to use the reports of patients and ex-patients in determining quality of life, and incorporate them with other social values through representatives of the community.[112]

In practice, analytic techniques tend to attach exaggerated importance to quantifiable values, while ignoring nonquantifiable values, such as relief of pain and suffering and the symbolic significance of actions and policies. For instance, a hospice program caring for dying patients may provide several intangible benefits, such as helping patients die with dignity and without pain and suffering, but a formal CEA/CBA may find little value in these considerations.[113] A related concern is the possible impact of analytic techniques, especially CBA, on personal and social values, perspectives, and attitudes. Legitimate fears exist that economic language, already evident in such terms as "the health care industry," "providers," and "consumers," as well as in CEA and CBA, will corrupt or even replace the traditional moral language of the doctor–patient relationship, especially under pressures of cost containment.[114]

In short, formal analytic techniques cannot serve as methods of decision-making, but they can function as aids to help decision-makers specify obligations of beneficence. It would be misleading in many contexts to view these methods of analysis as more than aids, especially if other interpretations of beneficence or other moral principles point to different conclusions.

Constraints of Distributive Justice

We concentrate on justice in the next chapter, but the above argument leads to a consideration of related problems of justice here. Critics commonly charge that utilitarianism and other analytic techniques fail to take adequate account of problems of justice because they focus on the net balance of benefits over costs without considering their distribution. For example, a study of the costs and benefits of treating mental retardation in small institutions emphasizing advanced individual training might show that costs outweigh the benefits, but justice might nonetheless demand extending special benefits to mentally retarded persons.

Earlier we noted tensions between egalitarian justice and QALY-based CEAs. We may need to modify or limit CEAs to incorporate these egalitarian concerns. Considerations of just distribution also apply to RBAs. Consider four possible patterns of distributing risks and benefits: (1) The risks and benefits may fall on the same party. For example, in most therapy, the patient bears the major risks and stands to gain the major benefits. (2) One party may bear the risks, while another party gains the benefits. For example, one generation may gain the benefits of technologies that will adversely affect future generations. (3) Both parties may bear the risks, but only one party stands to benefit. For example, a nuclear-powered artificial heart would primarily benefit the user, but it would impose risks on persons in close contact with the user. (4) Both parties may gain the benefits, while only one party bears the risks. For example, persons in the vicinity of a nuclear power plant may bear significantly greater risks than other persons who also benefit from the plant.

Nonetheless, principles of distributive justice do not and should not always triumph over social utility and economic efficiency. Here our views stand in contrast to theories that assign principles of justice an absolute priority over consequentialist principles such as utility. As we have maintained in all previous chapters, a practical judgment is required that takes into consideration, specifies, and balances all morally relevant factors, without giving any single one an a priori advantage.

Conclusion

We have reached several conclusions in this chapter that build on conclusions reached in previous chapters. We first distinguished between two principles of beneficence and distinguished both from negative obligations to avoid causing harm. We then defended a version of paternalism that justifies both weak and strong paternalistic actions under some conditions. However, we acknowledged that a policy or rule permitting strong paternalism in professional practice is generally not worth the risk of abuse that it invites. Finally, we argued that formal techniques of analysis—CEA, CBA, and RBA—can be morally unobjectionable ways to implement the principle of utility, but principles of respect for autonomy and justice set limits on uses of these techniques. Chapter 6 further considers the issues of justice that concluded the present chapter.

Notes

1. W. D. Ross, *The Right and the Good* (Oxford: Clarendon Press, 1930), p. 21.
2. Shelly Kagan, *The Limits of Morality* (Oxford: Clarendon Press, 1989), pp. 1–2, 402–03. See also the general theoretical point mode in Peter Singer, "Living High and Letting Die," *Philosophy and Phenomenological Research* 59 (1999): 183–87.

3. One limit is that agents often have discretion about when, where, how, and toward whom to act beneficently. John Stuart Mill argued that we are obligated to practice beneficence, "but not towards any definite person, nor at any prescribed time." Mill, *Utilitarianism*, in vol. 10 of the *Collected Works of John Stuart Mill* (Toronto: University of Toronto, 1969), ch. 5. However, we believe the principles of beneficence create *some* perfect and *some* imperfect obligations.

4. Peter Singer, "Famine, Affluence, and Morality," *Philosophy and Public Affairs* 1 (1972): 229–43.

5. Michael A. Slote, "The Morality of Wealth," in *World Hunger and Moral Obligation*, ed. W. Aiken and H. LaFollette (Englewood Cliffs, NJ: Prentice-Hall, 1977), p. 127. See Slote's later and more theoretical account in "Satisficing Consequentialism," *Proceedings of the Aristotelian Society*, Supp. 58 (1984): 139–64.

6. For a defense of a demanding but restricted maximizing principle, see Michael Otsuka, "The Paradox of Group Beneficence," *Philosophy and Public Affairs* 20 (Spring 1991): 132–49.

7. Peter Singer, *Practical Ethics*, 2d ed. (Cambridge: Cambridge University Press, 1993), p. 246.

8. Our formulation is indebted to Eric D'Arcy, *Human Acts: An Essay in their Moral Evaluation* (Oxford: Clarendon Press, 1963), pp. 56–57. We have added the fourth condition and altered others. See also Ernest J. Weinrib, "The Case for a Duty to Rescue," *Yale Law Journal* 90 (December 1980): 247–93; and Joel Feinberg, *Harm to Others*, vol. I of *The Moral Limits of the Criminal Law* (New York: Oxford University Press, 1984), ch. 4.

9. We here borrow from James S. Fishkin, *The Limits of Obligation* (New Haven, CT: Yale University Press, 1982), esp. pp. 4–9.

10. See Arthur L. Caplan, Robert H. Blank, and Janna C. Merrick, eds., *Compelled Compassion: Government Intervention in the Treatment of Critically Ill Newborns* (Totowa, NJ: The Humana Press Inc., 1992).

11. American Nurses' Association, *Code for Nurses with Interpretive Statements* (Kansas City, MO: American Nurses Association, 1985), sec. 3.1, p. 6.

12. Ludwig Edelstein, *Ancient Medicine*, ed. Oswei Temkin and C. Lillian Temkin (Baltimore, MD: Johns Hopkins University Press, 1967).

13. David Hume, "Of Suicide," in *Essays Moral, Political, and Literary*, ed. Eugene Miller (Indianapolis, IN: Liberty Classics, 1985), pp. 577–89.

14. See David A. J. Richards, *A Theory of Reasons for Action* (Oxford: Clarendon Press, 1971), p. 186; Lawrence Becker, *Reciprocity* (Chicago: University of Chicago Press, 1990); Aristotle, *Nicomachean Ethics*, bks. 8–9.

15. William F. May, "Code and Covenant or Philanthropy and Contract?" in *Ethics in Medicine*, ed. S. Reiser, A. Dyck, and W. Curran (Cambridge, MA: MIT Press, 1977), pp. 65–76.

16. *Epidemics*, 1:11, in W. H. S. Jones, ed., *Hippocrates* (Cambridge, MA: Harvard University Press, 1923), vol. I, p. 165.

17. Edmund Pellegrino and David Thomasma, *For the Patient's Good: The Restoration of Beneficence in Health Care* (New York: Oxford University Press, 1988), p. 29. For subtle instances of apparent paternalism or weakened paternalism that are similar to this model, see Marian Verkerk, "A Care Perspective on Coercion and Autonomy," *Bioethics* 13 (1999): 358–68; and Julian Savulescu, "Rational Non-Interventional Paternalism: Why Doctors Ought to Make Judgments of What is Best for Their Patients," *Journal of Medical Ethics* 21 (1995): 327–31.

18. On the nature of conflict between the autonomy model and the beneficence model, see Mark E. Meaney, "Freedom and Democracy in Health Care Ethics: Is the Cart Before the Horse?" *Theoretical Medicine* 17 (1996): 399–414.

19. Pellegrino and Thomasma, *For the Patient's Good*, pp. 25, 32, 46–47. See also Pellegrino and Thomasma, "The Conflict between Autonomy and Beneficence in Medical Ethics," *Journal of Contemporary Health Law and Policy* 3 (1987): 23–46.

20. Immanuel Kant, *On the Old Saw: That May Be Right in Theory But It Won't Work in Practice*, trans. E. B. Ashton (Philadelphia: University of Pennsylvania Press, 1974), pp. 290–91; John Stuart Mill, *On Liberty, Collected Works of John Stuart Mill*, vol. 18 (Toronto: University of Toronto Press, 1977).

21. See Tom L. Beauchamp and Laurence B. McCullough, *Medical Ethics: The Moral Responsibilities of Physicians* (Englewood Cliffs, NJ: Prentice-Hall, 1984), p. 84.

22. See Donald VanDeVeer, *Paternalistic Intervention: The Moral Bounds on Benevolence* (Princeton, NJ: Princeton University Press, 1986), pp. 16–40; John Kleinig, *Paternalism* (Totowa, NJ: Rowman and Allanheld, 1983), pp. 6–14.

23. National Commission for the Protection of Human Subjects of Biomedical and Behavioral Research, *Report and Recommendations: Research Involving Prisoners* (Washington, DC: DHEW Publication No. OS 76–131, 1976).

24. The term *paternalism* is not wholly felicitous, especially because it is sex-linked. The term *parentalism* might seem preferable, in part because it is gender neutral. See John Kultgen, *Autonomy and Intervention: Parentalism in the Caring Life* (New York: Oxford University Press, 1995). However, the term *paternalism* is now well-established by usage and philosophical discussion. Some feminists in bioethics argue that this usage is a rare case in which society should retain gendered language, because it highlights the link between the privileges of a father in a patriarchical family and the privileges of physicians in an authoritarian medical system. The thesis is that, just as hierarchical arrangements have long been the norm in the family, so paternalism has been the norm in medicine. See Susan Sherwin, *No Longer Patient: Feminist Ethics and Health Care* (Philadelphia: Temple University Press, 1992), ch. 7.

25. L. J. Henderson, "Physician and Patient as a Social System," *New England Journal of Medicine* 212 (1935): 819–23.

26. See Joel Feinberg, "Legal Paternalism," *Canadian Journal of Philosophy* 1 (1971): 105–24, esp. 113, 116. See also, Feinberg, *Harm to Self*, vol. III of *The Moral Limits of the Criminal Law* (New York: Oxford University Press, 1986), esp. pp. 12ff.

27. For the use of illiteracy as a compromising condition, see Florencia Luna, "Paternalism and the Argument from Illiteracy," *Bioethics* 9 (1995): 283–90.

28. Feinberg, *Harm to Self*, p. 14.

29. For interpretations of (strong) paternalism as insult, disrespect, and treatment of individual as unequals, see Ronald Dworkin, *Taking Rights Seriously* (Cambridge, MA: Harvard University Press, 1978), pp. 262–63; and Childress, *Who Should Decide? Paternalism in Health Care* (New York: Oxford University Press, 1982), chap. 3.

30. Robert Harris, "Private Consensual Adult Behavior: The Requirement of Harm to Others in the Enforcement of Morality," *UCLA Law Review* 14 (1967): 585n. Similar complaints in political philosophy are registered in Isaiah Berlin, *Four Essays on Liberty* (Oxford: Oxford University Press, 1969), pp. lxi–lxii, 132–33, 137–38, 149–51, 157.

31. See Jay Katz, Joseph Goldstein, and Alan M. Dershowitz, eds., *Psychoanalysis, Psychiatry, and the Law* (New York: The Free Press, 1967), pp. 552–54, 710–13; and Robert A. Burt, *Taking Care of Strangers: The Rule of Law in Doctor-Patient Relations* (New York: The Free Press, 1979), chap. 2.

32. This case was prepared by Browning Hoffman for a "Medicine and Society," conference at the University of Virginia.

33. Gerald Dworkin, "Paternalism," *The Monist* 56 (January 1972): 64–84; Rosemary Carter, "Justifying Paternalism," *Canadian Journal of Philosophy* 7 (1977): 133–45, esp. 135; and Donald VanDeVeer, *Paternalistic Intervention: The Moral Bounds on Benevolence* (Princeton, NJ: Princeton University Press, 1986), p. 424.

34. Dworkin, "Paternalism," p. 65.

35. See Dworkin, "Paternalism"; and John Rawls, *A Theory of Justice* (Cambridge, MA: Harvard University Press, 1971; revised edition, 1999), pp. 209, 248–49 (1999: 183–84, 218–20).

36. It should be noted that Dworkin himself says, "The reasons which support paternalism are those which support any altruistic action—the welfare of another person." "Paternalism," in *Encyclopedia of Ethics*, ed. Lawrence Becker (New York: Garland Publishing: 1992), p. 940. For a variety of consent and nonconsent defenses of paternalism, see Kleinig, *Paternalism*, pp. 38–73; VanDeVeer, *Paternalistic Intervention, passim*; and Kultgen, *Autonomy and Intervention*, esp. chs. 9, 11, 15.

37. Mary C. Silva, *Ethical Decisionmaking in Nursing Administration* (Norwalk, CT: Appleton and Lange, 1989), p. 64.

38. Compare Kleinig's similar conclusion, *Paternalism*, p. 76.

39. We do not here address the many problems surrounding the definition of suicide. See Tom L. Beauchamp, "Suicide," in *Matters of Life and Death*, 3rd ed., ed. Tom Regan (New York: Random House, 1993), esp. part I; and the articles in John Donnelly, ed., *Suicide: Right or Wrong?* (Buffalo, NY: Prometheus Books, 1991).

40. See James Rachels, "Barney Clark's Key," *Hastings Center Report* 13 (April 1983): 17–19, esp. p. 17.

41. We have adapted this case from Marc Basson, ed., *Rights and Responsibilities in Modern Medicine* (New York: Alan R. Liss, 1981), pp. 183–84.

42. Glanville Williams, "Euthanasia," *Medico-Legal Journal* 41 (1973): 27.

43. See, for example, three articles by psychiatrists Alan L. Berman, Robert E. Litman, and Seymour Perlin in *Non-Natural Death—Coming to Terms with Suicide, Euthanasia, Withholding or Withdrawing Treatment* (Denver, CO: Center for Applied Biomedical Ethics at Rose Medical Center, 1986). See also Douglas Berger, Isao Fukunishi, Mary Alice O'Dowd, et al., "A Comparison of Japanese and American Psychiatrists' Attitudes Towards Patients Wishing to Die in the General Hospital," *Psychotherapy and Psychosomatics* 66 (1997): 319–28.

44. P. M. Marzuk, K. Tardiff, A. C. Leon, et al., "HIV Seroprevalence Among Suicide Victims in New York City, 1991–1993," *American Journal of Psychiatry* 154 (1997): 1720–05; A. L. Dannenberg, J. G. McNeil, J. F. Brundage, et al., "Suicide and HIV Infection: Mortality Follow-up of 4147 HIV-Seropositive Military Service Applicants," *Journal of the American Medical Association* 276 (Dec. 4 1996): 1743–46; R. J. Mancoske, C. M. Wadsworth, D. S. Dugas, et al., "Suicide Risk Among People Living with AIDS," *Social Work* 40 (1995): 783–87; C. A. Alfonso, M. A. Cohen, A. D. Aladjem, et al., "HIV Seropositivity as a Major Risk Factor for Suicide in the General Hospital," *Psychosomatics* 35 (1994): 368–73; M. Marzuk, et al., "Increased Risk of Suicide in Persons with AIDS," *Journal of the American Medical Association* 259 (March 4, 1988): 1333–37.

45. See Richard M. Glass, "AIDS and Suicide," *Journal of the American Medical Association* 259 (March 4, 1988): 1369–70.

46. See President's Commission for the Study of Ethical Problems in Medicine and Bio-medical and Behavioral Research, *Deciding to Forego Life-Sustaining Treatment*, p. 37.

47. Betty Rollin, *Last Wish* (New York: Linden Press/Simon and Schuster, 1985).

48. Childress, *Who Should Decide? Paternalism in Health Care*, ch. 1. On the issues in this section, see Timothy E. Quill and Howard Brody, "Physician Recommendations and Patient Autonomy: Finding a Balance between Physician Power and Patient Choice," *Annals of Internal Medicine* 125 (1996): 763–69; John M. Luce, "Physicians Do Not Have a Responsibility to Provide Futile or Unreasonable Care If a Patient or Family Insists," *Critical Care Medicine* 23 (1995): 760–66; Allan S. Brett and Laurence B. McCullough, "When Patients Request Specific Interventions: Defining the Limits of the Physician's Obligation," *New England Journal of Medicine* 315 (Nov. 20, 1986): 1347–51.

49. We have adapted this case from "The Refusal to Sterilize: A Paternalistic Decision," in *Rights and Responsibilities in Modern Medicine*, ed. Basson, pp. 135–36, where both Tom L. Beauchamp and Eric Cassell discuss it.

50. John D. Lantos, Peter A. Singer, Robert M. Walker, et al., "The Illusion of Futility in Clinical Practice," *The American Journal of Medicine* 87 (July 1989): 82.

51. Robert D. Truog, Allan S. Brett, and Joel Frader, "The Problem with Futility," *New England Journal of Medicine* 326 (June 4, 1992): 1561, which has influenced these paragraphs.

52. Lawrence J. Schneiderman, Nancy S. Jecker, and Albert R. Jonsen, "Medical Futility: Its Meaning and Ethical Implications," *Annals of Internal Medicine* 112 (June 15, 1990): 951; Schneiderman, Jecker, and Jonsen, "Medical Futility: Response to Critiques," *Annals of Internal Medicine* 125 (1996): 669–74.

53. S. E. Bedell, T. L. Delbanco, E. F. Cook, and F. H. Epstein, "Survival after Cardiopulmonary Resuscitation in the Hospital," *New England Journal of Medicine* 309 (September 8, 1983): 569–76.

54. Lantos, et al., "The Illusion of Futility in Clinical Practice," p. 83.

55. J. Chris Hackler and F. Charles Hiller, "Family Consent to Orders Not to Resuscitate," *Journal of the American Medical Association* 264 (September 12, 1990): 1282; Paul E. Marik and Michele Craft, "An Outcomes Analysis of In-hospital Cardiopulmonary Resuscitation: The Futility Rationale for Do Not Resuscitate Orders," *Journal of Critical Care* 12 (1997): 142–46; Louise Swig, Molly Cooke, Dennis Osmond, et al., "Physician Responses to a Hospital Policy Allowing Them to Not Offer Cardiopulmonary Resuscitation," *Journal of the American Geriatrics Society* 44 (1996): 1215–19.

56. This paragraph is indebted to Stuart J. Youngner, "Futility in Context," *Journal of the American Medical Association* 264 (September 12, 1990): 1295–96.

57. This case was prepared by Robert M. Veatch and is used by permission.

58. This paragraph draws on U.S. Congress, Office of Technology Assessment, *The Implications of Cost-Effectiveness Analysis of Medical Technology: Summary* (Washington, DC: U.S. Government Printing Office, 1980); Kenneth E. Warner and Bryan R. Luce, *Cost-Benefit and Cost-Effectiveness Analysis in Health Care* (Ann Arbor, MI: Health Administration Press, 1982); David Eddy, "Cost-Effectiveness Analysis," *Journal of the American Medical Association* 267 (March 25, 1992): 1669–75 (June 24, 1992): 3342–48; and 268 (July 1, 1992): 132–36; and Marthe R. Gold, Joanna E. Siegel, Louise B. Russell, and Milton C. Weinstein, eds., *Cost-Effectiveness in Health and Medicine* (New York: Oxford University Press, 1996).

59. This case study is based on James H. Ellis, Richard H. Cohan, Seema S. Sonnad, and Nina Shafiroff Cohan, "Selective Use of Radiographic Low-Osmolality Contrast Media in the 1990s," *Radiology* 200 (1996): 297–311 (in favor of selective use); Paul W. Radensky and Nanch E. Cahill, "Universal Use of Low-Osmolality Contrast Media for the 1990s," *Radiology* 203 (May 1997): 310–11 (in favor of universal use); Steven M. Palmisano, "Low-Osmolality Contrast Media in the 1990s: Prices Change," *Radiology* 203 (1997): 309; Brendan J. Barrett, Patrick S. Parfrey, and Brian C. Morton, "Safety and Criteria for Selective Use of Low-Osmolality Contrast for Cardiac Angiography," *Medical Care* 36 (1999):1189–97, which argues that clinicans can use guidelines to identify high-risk patients and safely limit LOCAs to them; Elliott C. Lasser, Sandra G. Lyon, and Charles C. Berry, "Reports on Contrast Media Reactions: Analysis of Data from Reports to the U.S. Food and Drug Administration," *Radiology* 203 (1997): 605–10; M. A. Bettmann, T. Heern, A. Greenfield, et al., "Adverse Events with Radiographic Contrast Agents: Results of the SCVIR Contrast Agent Registry," *Radiology* 203 (1997): 611–20; and Peter D. Jacobson and C. John Rosenquist, "The Use of Low-Osmolar Contrast Agents: Technological Change and Defensive Medicine," *Journal of Health Politics, Policy and Law* 21 (Summer 1996): 243–66 (which provides information about the informed consent process). For earlier discussions see Peter D. Jacobson and John Rosenquist, "The Introduction of Low-Osmolar Contrast Agents in Radiology: Medical, Economic, Legal, and Public Policy issues," *Journal of the American Medical Association* 260 (September 16, 1988): 1586–92; Earl P. Steinberg, Richard D. Moore, Neil R. Powe, et al., "Safety and Cost-Effectiveness of High-Osmolality as Compared with Low-Osmolality Contrast Material in Patients Undergoding Cardiac Angiography," *New England Journal of Medicine* 326 (February 13, 1992): 425–30; Brenan J. Barrett, Patrick S. Parfrey, Hilary M. Vasvasour, et al., "A Comparison of Nonionic, Low-Osmolality Radiocontrast Agents with Ionic, High-Osmolality Agents During Cardiac Catherization," *New England Journal of Medicine* 326 (February 13, 1992): 431–436; and John W. Hirshfeld, Jr., "Low-Osmolality Contrast Agents— Who Needs Them?" *New England Journal of Medicine* 326 (February 13, 1992): 482–84; Neil R. Powe, Amy J. Davidoff, Richard D. Moore, et al., "Net Costs From Three Perspectives of Using Low Versus High Osmolality Contrast Medium in Diagnostic Angiocardiography," *Journal of the American College of Cardiology* 21 (June 1993): 1701–09, with editorial comment by Mark A. Hlatky, "Economic Evaluation of Low Osmolality Contrast Media," pp. 1710–11; and A. Michalson, E. A. Franken, Jr., and W. Smith, "Cost-Effectiveness and Safety of Selective Use of Low-Osmolality Contrast Media," *Academic Radiology* 1 (1994): 59–62.

60. Duncan Neuhauser and Ann M. Lewicki, "What Do We Gain from the Sixth Stool Guaiac?" *New England Journal of Medicine* 293 (July 31, 1975): 226–28. See also "American Cancer Society Report on the Cancer-related Checkup," *CA—A Cancer Journal for Clinicians* 30 (1980): 193–240, which recommended the full six stool guaiac tests. Today, issues are focused elsewhere. See J. S. Mandel "Colorectal Cancer Screening," *Cancer Metastasis Review* 16 (1997): 263–79.

61. Peter Doubilet, Milton C. Weinstein, and Barbara J. McNeil, "Use and Misuse of the Term 'Cost Effective' in Medicine," *New England Journal of Medicine* 314 (January 23, 1986): 253–56.

62. M. S. Rosenshein, et al., "The Cost Effectiveness of Therapeutic and Prophylactic Leukocyte Transfusion," *New England Journal of Medicine* 302 (May 8, 1980): 1058–62. For later studies of similar problems, see A. Ortega, G. Dranitsaris, and

A. L. Puodziunas, "What are Cancer Patients Willing to Pay for Prophylactic Epoetin Alfa? A Cost–Benefit Analysis," *Cancer* 15 (1998): 2588–96; and H. Wandt, H. M. Frank, G. Ehninger, et al., "Safety and Cost Effectiveness of a 10 × 10(9)/L Trigger for Prophylactic Platelet Transfusions Compared with the Traditional 20 × 10(9)/L Trigger: A Prospective Comparative Trial in 105 Patients with Acute Myeloid Leukemia," *Blood* 91 (1998): 3601–06.

63. Doubilet, et al., "Use and Misuse of the Term 'Cost Effective in Medicine,' " p. 255.

64. Louise Russell, *Is Prevention Better Than Cure?* (Washington, DC: Brookings Institution, 1986), p. 111.

65. See Howard Leichter, "Public Policy and the British Experience," *Hastings Center Report* 11 (October 1981): 32–39; and *Free to Be Foolish: Politics and Health Promotion in the United States and Great Britain* (Princeton, NJ: Princeton University Press, 1991).

66. See Paul C. Stern and Harvey V. Fineberg, eds., *Understanding Risk: Informing Decisions in a Democratic Society* (Washington, DC: National Academy Press, 1996).

67. Based on the results in Sheila Jasanoff, "Acceptable Evidence in a Pluralistic Society," in *Acceptable Evidence: Science and Values in Risk Management*, ed. Deborah G. Mayo and Rachelle D. Hollander (New York: Oxford University Press, 1991).

68. See Richard Wilson and E. A. C. Crouch, "Risk Assessment and Comparisons: An Introduction," *Science* 236 (April 17, 1987): 267–70.

69. Lester B. Lave, "Health and Safety Risk Analyses: Information for Better Decisions," *Science* 236 (April 17, 1987): 292–93. See also Kristin Shrader-Frechette, *Risk and Rationality: Philosophical Foundations for Populist Reforms* (Berkeley: University of California Press, 1991), ch. 8.

70. See Carl F. Cranor, "Some Moral Issues in Risk Assessment," *Ethics* 101 (October 1990): 123–43, which has influenced this paragraph. See also Shrader-Frechette, *Risk and Rationality*; Mayo and Hollander, eds., *Acceptable Evidence*; and Carl Cranor, *Regulating Toxic Substances: A Philosophy of Science and the Law* (New York: Oxford University Press, 1993). Much recent debate has centered on proposals of a "precautionary principle," particularly in protecting the public health and the environment. According to some interpretations, this principle would reflect a general duty to take reasonable precautions to protect the public health and the environment, even in the absence of clear evidence of harm. See Carolyn Raffensperger and Joel Tickner, eds., *Protecting Public Health and the Environment: Implementing the Precautionary Principle* (Washington, DC: Island Press, 1999), Preface.

71. Ian Hacking, "Culpable Ignorance of Interference Effects," in *Values at Risk*, ed. Douglas MacLean (Totowa, NJ: Rowman and Allenheld, 1986), ch. 7.

72. Lynn White, Jr., "Technology Assessment from the Stance of a Medieval Historian," *Medieval Religion and Technology: Collected Essays* (Berkeley: University of California Press, 1978), pp. 261–76.

73. See Paul Slovic, "Perception of Risk," *Science* 236 (April 17, 1987): 280–85; Slovic, "Beyond Numbers: A Broader Perspective on Risk Perception and Risk Communication," in *Acceptable Evidence*, pp. 48–65, esp. 34–35; and Richard J. Zeckhauser and W. Kip Viscusi, "Risk Within Reason," *Science* 248 (May 4, 1990): 559–64.

74. Lave, "Health and Safety Risk Analyses," p. 291.

75. Lawrence J. Schneiderman and Robert M. Kaplan, "Fear of Dying and HIV Infection vs Hepatitis B Infection," *American Journal of Public Health* 82 (April 1992): 584–89. However, several studies have shown that nurses and surgeons *undervalue* the importance of practices of protection against blood-borne pathogens.

76. Zeckhauser and Viscusi, "Risk Within Reason."

77. For a cultural relativist view, see Mary Douglas and Aaron Wildavsky, *Risk and Culture: An Essay on the Selection of Technology and Environmental Dangers* (Berkeley: University of California Press, 1982); and Aaron Wildavsky and Karl Drake, "Theories of Risk Perception: Who Fears What and Why?" *Daedalus* 119 (Fall 1990): 41–60.

78. On the significant role of AIDS activists, see Steven Epstein, *Impure Science: AIDS, Activism, and the Politics of Knowledge* (Berkeley: University of California Press, 1996); Loretta M. Kopelman, "How AIDS Activists are Changing Research," in *Health Care Ethics: Critical Issues,* ed. John Monagle and David C. Thomasma (Gaithersburg, MD: Aspen Publishers, 1994): 199–209; R. J. Levine, "The Impact of HIV Infection on Society's Perception of Clinical Trials," *Kennedy Institute of Ethics Journal* 4 (1994): 93–98; and Benjamin Freedman, "Suspended Judgement— AIDS and the Ethics of Clinical Trials: Learning the Right Lessons," *Controlled Clinical Trials* 13 (1992): 1–5.

79. At least three states (California, Florida, and Georgia) have enacted legislation to provide for expanded access to investigational drugs. *See* Cal. Welf. & Inst. Code § 14137.8 (West 1997); Fla. Stat. ch. 627.6498 (1996); Ga. Code Ann. § 43–34–42.1 (1997).

80. Medical Device Amendments of 1976, Pub. L. No. 94–295, 90 Stat. 539, a major revision of the Federal Food, Drug, and Cosmetic Act of 1938, Pub. L. No. 75–717, 52 Stat. 1040 (codified as amended at 21 U.S.C. §§ 301-93).

81. David A. Kessler, "Special Report: The Basis of the FDA'S Decision on Breast Implants," *New England Journal of Medicine* 326 (June 18, 1992): 1713–15. All references to Kessler's views are to this article.

82. Marcia Angell, "Breast Implants—Protection or Paternalism?," *New England Journal of Medicine* 326 (June 18, 1992): 1695–96. All direct references to Angell's views are to this article. Angell's criticisms of court decisions in favor of women suing manufacturers of implants appear in her *Science on Trial: The Clash of Medical Evidence and the Law in the Breast Implant Case* (New York: W.W. Norton & Company, 1996). See also Angell, "Evaluating the Health Risks of Breast Implants: The Interplay of Medical Science, the Law, and Public Opinion," *New England Journal of Medicine* 334 (1996): 1513–18.

83. See Lisa S. Parker, "Social Justice, Federal Paternalism, and Feminism: Breast Implantation in the Cultural Context of Female Beauty," *Kennedy Institute of Ethics Journal* 3 (1993): 57–76; and Jack C. Fisher, "The Silicone Controversy: When Will Science Prevail?" *New England Journal of Medicine* 326 (1992): 1696–98.

84. For recent reviews and evaluations of the scientific data, see E. C. Janowsky, L. L. Kupper, and B. S. Hulka, "Meta-analyses of the Relation between Silicone Breast Implants and the Risk of Connective Tissue Diseases," *New England Journal of Medicine* 342 (2000): 781–90; *Silicone Gel Breast Implants: Report of the Independent Review Group* (Cambridge: Jill Rogers Associates, 1998); and S. Bondurant, V. Ernster, and R. Herdman, eds., *Safety of Silicone Breast Implants* (Washington, DC: National Academy Press, 2000). See also P. C. Gerszten, "A Formal Risk Assessment of Silicone Breast Implants," *Biomaterials* 20 (1999): 1063–69. This risk assessment includes a review of the current scientific evidence for the safety of silicone breast implants since the FDA's 1992 decision. A significant body of evidence was also available before the decision.

85. "U.S. Orders Breast Implant Makers to Cite New Studies," *The Washington Post*, March 21, 1993, p. A26.

86. "How Safe Is Safe?" [editorial] *Washington Post*, May 21, 2000, B6.
87. Sandra G. Boodman, "Breast Implants: Now Women Are Having A Hard Time Getting Them Out," *The Washington Post*, June 23, 1992, Health Section, pp. 10–14.
88. Angell, "Breast Implants—Protection or Paternalism?"
89. Controversy about silicone-gel breast implants continues. Dow-Corning decided to file for bankruptcy because of the financial threat impending breast implant litigation posed, despite the lack of clear-cut scientific evidence to support plaintiffs' claims. Scientific evidence in court decisions has played a key role in these controversies. Many have criticized judges' and juries' willingness to permit plaintiffs to recover without adequate scientific data to support causation. However, another interpretation views these rulings as a reasonable and fair response to "implant manufacturers' previous failure to perform adequate safety testing" (which, as we noted, was not legally required because of the time when these implants became available). From this standpoint, the verdicts in favor of the plaintiffs reflected a sense that the poor scientific evidence stems from the manufacturers' decision to sell products without first adequately testing them for safety. In light of the available evidence, then, the question could be framed as, "Which outcome would be more unjust: failure to compensate the women in the event the implants did, in fact, cause systemic disease or throwing a pharmaceutical company into bankruptcy for unwarranted demands for product liability?" Reasonable people have reached different judgments about which outcome best serves justice. However, we do not believe that the scientific evidence warrants either taking breast implants off the market or finding Dow-Corning liable for misconduct. See Rebecca Dresser, "Science in the Courtroom: A New Approach," *Hastings Center Report* 29 (May–June 1999): 26–27; Rebecca S. Dresser, Wendy E. Wagner, and Paul C. Giannelli, "Breast Implants Revisited: Beyond Science on Trial," *Wisconsin Law Review* (1997): 705–76; Rochelle C. Dreyfuss, "Galileo's Tribute: Using Medical Evidence in Court," *Michigan Law Review* 95 (1997): 2055–76. See also Ruth Macklin, "Ethics, Epidemiology, and Law: The Case of Silicone Breast Implants," *American Journal of Public Health* 89 (April 1999): 487. This same issue includes an editorial by Ronald Bayer and articles by Zena Stein and Daniel M. Fox.
90. See Steven E. Rhoads, "How Much Should We Spend to Save a Life?," in *Valuing Life: Public Policy Dilemmas*, ed. Rhoads (Boulder, CO: Westview Press, 1980), p. 293. For recent updating of such a model, including its limitations, see Peter A. Ubel, J. Richardson, and Paul Menzel, "Societal Value, the Person Trade-Off, and the Dilemma of Whose Values to Measure for Cost-Effectiveness Analysis," *Health Economics* 9 (2000): 127–36.
91. Peter A. Ubel "How Stable Are People's Preferences for Giving Priority to Severely Ill Patients?" *Social Science and Medicine* 49 (October 1999): 895–903.
92. Richard Zeckhauser, "Procedures for Valuing Lives," *Public Policy* (Fall 1975): 447–48. Contrast Richard A. Rettig, "Origins of the Medicare Kidney Disease Entitlement: The Social Security Amendments of 1972," in *Biomedical Politics*, ed. Kathi Hanna (Washington, DC: National Academy Press, 1991).
93. For a philosophical critique of CBA, see Elizabeth Anderson, *Values in Ethics and Economics* (Cambridge, MA: Harvard University Press, 1993), esp. ch. 9.
94. The problems we have identified with CBA constitute part of the reason CEA has priority in health care. See Peter A. Ubel, *Pricing Life: Why It's Time for Health Care Rationing* (Cambridge, MA: The MIT Press, 2000), esp. p. 68. See also A. M. Garber, M. C. Weinstein, G. W. Torrance, and M. S. Kamlet, "Theoretical Founda-

tions of Cost-Effectiveness Analysis," in Gold, et al., *Cost-Effectiveness in Health and Medicine*, p. 28.

95. Quoted in John LaPuma and Edward F. Lawlor, "Quality-Adjusted Life-Years: Ethical Implications for Physicians and Policy-Makers," *Journal of the American Medical Association* 263 (June 6, 1990): 2917–21.

96. Alan Williams, "The Importance of Quality of Life in Policy Decisions," in *Quality of Life: Assessment and Application*, ed. Stuart R. Walker and Rachel M. Rosser (Boston: MTP Press Limited, 1988), p. 285.

97. See Erik Nord, *Cost–Value Analysis in Health Care: Making Sense Out of QALY's* (Cambridge: Cambridge University Press, 1999), passim, and Gold, et al., *Cost-Effectiveness in Health and Medicine*, passim.

98. See David Eddy, "Cost-Effectiveness Analysis: Is It Up to the Task?" *Journal of the American Medical Association* 267 (June 24, 1992): 3344.

99. Alan Williams, "Economics of Coronary Artery Bypass Grafting," *British Medical Journal* 291 (August 3, 1985): 326–29. See also M. C. Weinstein and W. B. Stason, "Cost-Effectiveness of Coronary Artery Bypass Surgery," *Circulation* 66, Suppl. 5, pt. 2 (1982): III, 56–66.

100. John Rawls included "health and vigor" as primary natural goods, in contrast to primary social goods. See *A Theory of Justice* (Cambridge, MA: Harvard University Press, 1971), p. 62 (1999: p. 54).

101. Cf. Donald L. Patrick and Pennifer Erickson, "Assessing Health-Related Quality of Life for Clinical Decision Making," in *Quality of Life*, ed. Walker and Rosser, p. 11.

102. See Paul Menzel, Marthe R. Gold, Erik Nord, et al., "Toward a Broader View of Values in Cost-Effectiveness Analysis of Health," *Hastings Center Report* 29 (May–June 1999): 7–15. For a defense of the utilitarian perspective of CEA and QALYs, see John McKie, Jeff Richardson, and Helga Kuhse, *The Allocation of Health Care Resources: An Ethical Evaluation of the 'QALY' Approach* (Aldershot: Ashgate Publishing, 1998). See also the discussion in Joshua Cohen, "Preferences, Needs and QALYs," *Journal of Medical Ethics* 22 (1996): 267–72.

103. Gavin Mooney, "QALYs: Are They Enough? A Health Economist's Perspective," *Journal of Medical Ethics* 15 (1989): 148–52.

104. Alan Williams, "The Importance of Quality of Life in Policy Decisions," in *Quality of Life*, ed. Walker and Rosser, p. 286; Williams, "Economics, QALYs and Medical Ethics—A Health Economist's Perspective," *Health Care Analysis* 3 (1995): 221–26.

105. Some proposals to modify or limit QALY-based CEA by societal values would require even lower weight for the elderly, in line with dominant societal values. See, for example, Nord, *Cost-Value Analysis in Health Care*; Menzel, et al., "Toward a Broader View of Values in Cost-Effectiveness Analysis of Health"; and Ubel, *Pricing Life*.

106. For versions of these two modifications, see the works cited in the previous note. These authors identify these "social values" in various empirical studies, even though they often note that more research is needed to fully establish them. They also recognize that these "social values" have a basis in moral argument. For such research on Australian social values, see Erik Nord, Jeff Richardson, Andrew Street, et al., "Maximizing Health Benefits vs Egalitarianism: An Australian Survey of Health Issues," *Social Science and Medicine* 41 (1995): 1429–37.

107. John Harris, "QALYfying the Value of Life," *Journal of Medical Ethics* 13 (1987): 117. See an expanded discussion of the issue in Peter Singer, John McKie, Helga

Kuhse, and Jeff Richardson, "Double Jeopardy and the Use of QALYs in Health Care Allocation," *Journal of Medical Ethics* 21 (1995): 144–50; John Harris, "Double Jeopardy and the Veil of Ignorance—A Reply," *Journal of Medical Ethics* 21 (1995): 151–57; McKie, Kuhse, Richardson, and Singer, "Double Jeopardy, the Equal Value of Lives and the Veil of Ignorance: A Rejoinder to Harris," *Journal of Medical Ethics* 22 (1996): 204–08; Harris, "Would Aristotle Have Played Russian Roulette?" *Journal of Medical Ethics* (1996): 209–15; and McKie, Kuhse, Richardson, and Singer, "Another Peep Behind the Veil," *Journal of Medical Ethics* (1996): 216–21.

108. David C. Hadorn, "Setting Health Care Priorities in Oregon: Cost-Effectiveness Meets the Rule of Rescue," *Journal of the American Medical Association* 265 (May 1, 1991): 2218. See, further, Peter Ubel, D. Scanlon, and M. Kamlet, "Individual Utilities Are Inconsistent with Rationing Choices: A Partial Explanation of Why Oregon's Cost-Effectiveness List Failed," *Medical Decision Making* 16 (1996): 108–16.

109. See Mark Friedbert, Bernard Saffran, Tammy J. Stinson, et al., "Evaluation of Conflict of Interest in Economic Analyses of New Drugs Used in Oncology," *Journal of the American Medical Association* 282 (October 20, 1999): 1453–57, and Sheldon Krimsky, "Conflict of Interest and Cost-Effectiveness Analysis," *Journal of the American Medical Association* 282 (October 20, 1999): 1474–75. Because of possible bias, some journals refuse to consider CEAs for publication if the analysts have financial relationships with the company. See J. P. Kassirer and Marcia Angell, "The Journal's Policy on Cost-Effectiveness Analysis," *New England Journal of Medicine* 331 (1994): 669–70.

110. Herman B. Leonard and Richard J. Zeckhauser, "Cost–Benefit Analysis Applied to Risks: Its Philosophy and Legitimacy," in *Values at Risk*, ed. MacLean, p. 34.

111. See Stern and Harvey, eds., *Understanding Risk: Informing Decisions in a Democratic Society, passim* and appendix B. See also the discussion in Anderson, *Value in Ethics and Economics*, ch. 9, which stresses democratic alternatives to CBA.

112. See Nord, *Cost-Value Analysis in Health Care*; and Menzel, et al., "Toward a Broader View of Values in Cost-Effectiveness Analysis of Health," pp. 7–15. Contrast Dan Brock, "Justice and the ADA: Does Prioritizing and Rationing Health Care Discriminate Against the Disabled?," *Social Philosophy and Policy* 12 (1995): 159–84.

113. U.S. Congress, Office of Technology Assessment, *The Implications of Cost-Effectiveness Analysis*.

114. See Rashi Fein, "What Is Wrong with the Language of Medicine?" *New England Journal of Medicine* 306 (1982): 863f.

6

Justice

Inequalities in access to health care and in health insurance, combined with dramatic increases in the costs of health care, have fueled debates about what social justice requires in many other countries. But is *inequality* in access to health care a serious problem of justice? Should all age groups, for example, have equal access to health care resources? In attempting to answer such questions, we encounter uncertainty over how to reconcile goals such as equal access to health care, the freedom to choose a health plan, health promotion, a free-market economy, social efficiency, and the beneficent state.

In a short story titled, "The Lottery in Babylon," Jorge Luis Borges depicts a society that distributes all social benefits and burdens solely on the basis of a periodic lottery.[1] Each person is assigned a social role, such as a slave, a factory owner, a priest, or an executioner, purely by the lottery. This random selection system disregards achievement, training, merit, experience, contribution, need, and effort. The ethical and political oddity of the system described in Borges's story is jolting because assigning positions in this way fails so noticeably to cohere with conventional standards. Borges's system appears capricious and unfair, because we expect valid principles of justice to determine how social burdens, benefits, and positions ought to be allocated.

However, if we attempt to expound principles of justice, they seem as elusive as the lottery method seems capricious. The construction of a comprehensive and unified theory of justice that captures our diverse conceptions is even more elusive. Moreover, many principles of justice that have been proposed in biomedical ethics are not distinct from and independent of other principles, such as nonmaleficence and beneficence.[2] We begin to explore these problems in this chapter by analyzing the terms *justice* and *distributive justice*. Later, we will examine substantive principles of justice as well as several problems of social justice that concern how to allocat resources for and within the health care system.

The Concept of Justice

The terms *fairness*, *desert* (what is deserved), and *entitlement* have been used by various philosophers in attempts to explicate *justice*.[3] These accounts interpret justice as fair, equitable, and appropriate treatment in light of what is due or owed to persons. Standards of justice are needed whenever persons are due benefits or burdens because of their particular properties or circumstances, such as being productive or having been harmed by another person's acts. A holder of a valid claim based in justice has a right, and therefore is due something. An injustice thus involves a wrongful act or omission that denies people benefits to which they have a right or distributes burdens unfairly.

The term *distributive justice* refers to fair, equitable, and appropriate distribution determined by justified norms that structure the terms of social cooperation. Its scope includes policies that allot diverse benefits and burdens, such as property, resources, taxation, privileges, and opportunities. *Distributive justice* refers broadly to the distribution of all rights and responsibilities in society, including, for example, civil and political rights. It is to be distinguished from other types of justice, including *criminal* justice, which refers to the just infliction of punishment, and *rectificatory* justice, which refers to just compensation for transactional problems such as breaches of contracts and malpractice.

Problems of distributive justice arise under conditions of scarcity and competition to obtain goods or to avoid burdens. If ample fresh water existed for industrial disposal of waste materials, and no subsequent harm to human beings or other forms of life occurred from this disposal, it would not be necessary to restrict use. Many contemporary discussions of just benefits in prepaid health maintenance programs, just programs of care for the mentally retarded, and appropriate sources of funds for national health insurance similarly involve such trade-offs that have been fashioned under these conditions of society and competition.

A compelling example of distributive justice appears in the recent history of research involving human subjects. Until the 1990s, the paradigm for ethical analysis focused on the *risks and burdens* of research, especially nontherapeutic research, and on the need to protect potential and actual research subjects from harm, abuse, and exploitation. This history in the United States, as Carol Levine notes, "was born in scandal and reared in protectionism."[4] The regulation of research sought to protect vulnerable persons from exploitation in scientific efforts to benefit others. The dominant model in protectionist policies is *nontherapeutic* research, i.e., research that offers no prospect of direct therapeutic benefit to the subject. The concern is about an unfair distribution of *burdens*. However, a paradigm shift recently occurred, in part because of the interest of patients with AIDS in gaining access to new, experimental drugs within as well as outside of clinical trials. The focus shifted to *therapeutic* research and to the possible *benefits* of clinical trials (deemphasizing their risks). As a result, justice as *fair access to research* (both participation in research and access to the results of research) became as important as protection from exploitation.[5] Similar observations apply to the participation of women in research.

Issues concerning the fairness of a distribution generate questions about *principles* of justice. No single principle can address all problems of justice. Somewhat like our division of principles under the heading of beneficence, several principles of justice appear in the common morality and merit acceptance. One principle of justice is *formal*, the others *material*. We indicate in this chapter how to specify and balance these principles in particular contexts. Specifying and balancing promote the coherence that we seek in principles of justice. Sometimes, however, conditions of scarcity force a society to make "tragic choices." In these situations, principles of justice may end up being infringed, compromised, or sacrificed.[6]

The Formal Principle of Justice

Common to all theories of justice is a minimal formal requirement traditionally attributed to Aristotle: Equals must be treated equally, and unequals must be treated unequally. This principle of formal justice (sometimes called the *principle of formal equality*) is "formal" because it identifies no particular respects in which equals ought to be treated equally and provides no criteria for determining whether two or more individuals are in fact equals. It merely asserts that *whatever* respects are relevant, persons equal in those respects should be treated equally.

An obvious problem with this formal principle is its lack of substance. That equals ought to be treated equally does not provoke debate. But how shall we define *equality*, and which differences are relevant in comparing individuals or groups? Presumably all citizens should have equal political rights, equal access to public services, and equal treatment under the law. But how far should equality extend? A typical problem is the following: Virtually all accounts of justice in health care hold that delivery programs and services designed to assist persons of a certain class, such as the poor or the elderly, should be made available to all members of *that class*. To deny benefits to some when others in the same class receive benefits is unjust. But is it also unjust to deny access to equally needy persons outside of the delineated class (e.g., workers with no health insurance)?

Material Principles of Justice

Principles that specify the relevant characteristics for equal treatment are called *material* because they identify the substantive properties for distribution. One such principle is the principle of need, which declares that distribution of social resources based on need is just. To say that a person needs something is to say that, without it, the person will be harmed or at least detrimentally affected. However, we are not required to distribute all goods and services to satisfy all needs, such as needs for bedboards, athletic equipment, and antilock brakes. Presumably our obligations are limited to *fundamental needs*. To say that someone has a fundamental need is to say that the person will be harmed or detrimentally affected in a fundamental way if that need is not fulfilled. For example, the person might be harmed through malnutrition, bodily injury, or nondisclosure of critical information.

If we were to analyze in great detail the notions of fundamental needs, we could progressively specify and shape the material principle of need into a public policy for purposes of distribution. For the moment, however, we are emphasizing only the significance of the step of accepting the principle of need as a valid material principle of justice. This principle is only one material principle of justice. If, by contrast, one were to accept only a principle of free-market distribution, then one would oppose a principle of need as a basis for public policy. All public and institutional policies based on distributive justice ultimately derive from the acceptance (or rejection) of some material principles and some procedures for specifying, refining, or balancing them, and many disputes over the right policy or distribution spring from rival, or at least alternative, starting points with different material principles.

Philosophers and others have proposed each of the following principles as a valid material principle of distributive justice (as well as other principles[7]).

1. To each person an equal share
2. To each person according to need
3. To each person according to effort
4. To each person according to contribution
5. To each person according to merit
6. To each person according to free-market exchanges

No obvious barrier prevents acceptance of more than one of these principles, and some theories of justice accept all six as valid. A plausible moral thesis is that each of these material principles identifies a prima facie obligation whose weight cannot be assessed independently of particular contexts or spheres in which they are applicable.

Most societies invoke several of these material principles in framing public policies, appealing to different principles in different spheres and contexts. For example, unemployment subsidies, welfare payments, and many health care programs are distributed on the basis of need (and to some extent on criteria such as previous length of employment); jobs and promotions in many sectors are awarded on the basis of demonstrated achievement and merit; the higher incomes of some persons are allowed and often encouraged on grounds of free-market wage scales, superior effort, merit, or potential social contribution; and, at least theoretically, the opportunity for a basic education is distributed to all citizens.

Conflicts among the above principles create a serious priority problem as well as a challenge to a moral system that aims for a coherent framework of principles. These conflicts indicate the vital need for both specification and balancing of these principles, as is illustrated by the case of Mark Dalton, a histology technician employed by a large chemical company.[8] Dalton was an excellent worker, but, after a week of sick leave, a company nurse discovered that he had a chronic renal disease. The company determined that the permissible levels of chemical vapor exposure in Dalton's job might exacerbate his renal condition. Management found him another job, with the same salary, but two other employees eligible for promotion were also interested in the job. Both employees had more seniority and better training than Dalton, and one was a woman. In this situation, each of the three employees could legitimately appeal to a different material principle of justice to support his or her claim to the available position. Dalton could cite the material principle of need, arguing that his medical condition required that he either be offered the new position or be dismissed from the company with compensation. With their superior experience and training, the other two employees could invoke material principles of merit, societal contribution, and perhaps individual effort in support of their claims. Considerations of equal opportunity and the past record of promotions in the company also gave the woman valid grounds for claiming that justice entitled her to the position. Without further specification and balancing, such conflicts among general material principles are not resolvable.

Relevant Properties

Material principles identify relevant properties that persons must possess to qualify for a particular distribution, but theoretical and practical difficulties plague the justification of alleged relevant properties. Tradition, convention, moral and legal principles, and public policy can and do function to establish relevant properties. For example, a tennis tournament awards trophies on the basis of achievement (as determined by the tradition-bound rules of tournament tennis) and individuals receive prison terms only if they are found guilty of crimes (as determined by legal and moral norms). However, in many contexts, it is appropriate either to institute a policy establishing relevant properties where none previously existed or to develop a new policy that revises established criteria. For example, it has repeatedly been asked how we should address the question whether nonresident aliens should be allowed on waiting lists for cadaveric organ transplantation in the United States.

Courts often mandate policies that revise entrenched notions about relevant properties. For example, the United States Supreme Court decided, in the case of *Auto Workers v. Johnson Controls, Inc.*,[9] that employers cannot legally adopt "fetal protection policies" that specifically exclude women of childbearing age from a hazardous workplace, because these policies discriminate illegally based on sex. Under the challenged policies, only fertile men could choose whether they wished to assume reproductive risks. The majority of justices held that this gender-based policy used the irrelevant property of being a woman, despite the fact that mutagenic substances affect sperm as well as eggs.

Such problems show us again that abstract principles provide only rough guidelines for forming specific policies or taking concrete actions. We need further moral argument that specifies and balances principles and assesses competing claims in order to determine which concrete aspects of a situation are morally relevant and decisive in forming a reasoned judgment. Agreement will often be difficult to achieve, and, for this reason, some philosophers have concluded that abstract material principles of justice can offer little help until they have been integrated into a systematic framework or theory. But how much help will a general framework or theory of justice provide, and which one(s), if any, should we accept?

Theories of Justice

Theories of distributive justice attempt to connect properties of persons with morally justifiable distributions of benefits and burdens. Philosophers have proposed several theories to determine how to distribute, or, in some cases, redistribute, social burdens and goods and services, including health care. These theories differ with respect to the specific material criteria they emphasize, how they interpret and weight those criteria, the areas or spheres to which they apply them, and the forms of justification they employ.

The following are influential types of theory: *Utilitarian* theories emphasize a mixture of criteria for the purpose of maximizing public utility; *libertarian* theories emphasize rights to social and economic liberty (invoking fair procedures rather than substantive outcomes); *communitarian* theories stress the principles and practices of justice that evolve through traditions and practices in a community; and *egalitarian* theories emphasize equal access to the goods in life that every rational person values (often invoking material criteria of need and equality).

We can expect these theories to succeed only partially in bringing coherence and comprehensiveness to our fragmented visions of social justice. Policies for health care access and distribution, in many countries, provide an example of the problems that confront these theories. People in many countries seek to provide the best possible health care for all citizens, while promoting the public interest through cost-containment programs. They promote the ideal of equal access to health care for everyone, including care for indigents, while maintaining aspects of a free-market competitive environment. These laudable goals of superior care, equality of access, freedom of choice, and social efficiency are extremely difficult to render coherent in a social system. Different conceptions of the just society underlie them, and pursuing one goal is likely to undercut another. Nonetheless, several theories of justice try either to achieve a balance between such competing social goals or to eliminate some health objectives while retaining others.

Utilitarian Theories

Utilitarian theories, which will be treated in more detail in Chapter 8, regard distributive justice as one among several problems of maximizing value. Utilitarians argue that the standard of justice depends on the principle of utility (which demands that we seek to maximize overall good). *Justice* is merely the name for the paramount and most stringent forms of obligation created by the principle of utility. Typically, utilitarian obligations of justice establish correlative rights for individuals that in this theory should be enforced by law, if necessary. These rights are strictly contingent upon social arrangements that maximize net social utility. Rights have no other basis, and disputes even erupt among utilitarians as to whether rights have a meaningful place in moral theory. However, if a system of rights is justified entirely on the grounds that its existence will maximize utility, utilitarians cannot seriously object to rights. The only question is whether any particular system of rights does, in fact, work to maximize social utility.

Many utilitarians favor social programs that protect public health and distribute basic health care to all citizens. However, various questions emerge about rights if utilitarian principles of justice are accepted as solely sufficient. Individual rights, such as the right to health care, have a tenuous foundation when they rest on overall utility maximization, because social utility could change at any time. Furthermore, utilitarian approaches neglect considerations of justice that focus on how benefits and burdens are distributed independently of aggregate welfare. For example, it seems unjust for a society to maximize utility by denying access to health care for some of its sickest and most vulnerable populations.

Principles of utilitarian justice thus present serious problems, but we will see that, when carefully restricted in scope, they do have a legitimate role in forming health policies.

Libertarian Theories

The United States has traditionally, though not exclusively, accepted the free-market ideal that distributions of health care are best left to the marketplace, which operates on the material principle of ability to pay, either directly or indirectly through insurance. In general, under this conception, a just society protects rights of property and liberty, allowing persons to improve their circumstances and protect their health on their own initiative. Health care is not a right under this conception, and the ideal health care system is privatized. A libertarian interpretation of justice focuses not on increasing public utility or meeting the health needs of citizens, but on the unfettered operation of fair procedures.

A major contemporary libertarian theory appears in an influential book by Robert Nozick, who argues for an "entitlement theory" of justice in which government action is justified if and only if it protects citizens' rights.[10] He argues that a theory of justice should affirm individual rights rather than create patterns of economic distribution in which governments redistribute the wealth acquired by persons under the free market. Governments act coercively and unjustly when they tax the wealthy at a progressively higher rate than those who are less wealthy, and then use the proceeds to underwrite state support of the indigent through welfare payments and unemployment compensation.

Nozick accepts a form of procedural justice with three and *only* three principles: justice in acquisition, justice in transfer, and justice in rectification. More specifically, no pattern of just distribution exists independent of free-market procedures of acquiring property, legitimately transferring that property, and providing rectification for those whose property was illegitimately taken or who otherwise were illegitimately obstructed in the free market. Accordingly, justice consists in the operation of just procedures (such as fair play), not in the production of just outcomes (such as an equal distribution of resources). There are no welfare rights and, therefore, no rights or claims to health care can be based on justice.

Libertarians do not oppose utilitarian or egalitarian patterns of distribution if they are freely chosen by participants. Any distribution of goods, including that for health care, is just and justified if (and only if) individuals in the relevant group freely choose it. As a result, libertarians generally support a health care system in which health care insurance is privately and voluntarily purchased. In this system, the state does not coercively take any one's personal property to benefit another. Investors in health care and insured persons have property rights, physicians have liberty rights, and society is not morally obligated to provide health care. Indeed, society is morally obligated to refrain from providing funds by coercive taxation or assigning physicians conscription.

Competing theories of justice reject this uncompromising commitment to liberty and pure procedural justice. In recent years, communitarian and egalitarian theories have offered influential challenges.

Communitarian Theories

Communitarians react negatively to models of society (such as those developed by Mill, Rawls, and Nozick) that base human relationships on rights and contracts and that attempt to construct a single theory of justice by which to judge every society. Communitarians regard principles of justice as pluralistic, deriving from as many different conceptions of the good as there are diverse moral communities. What is due individuals and groups depends on these community-derived standards.[11]

Communitarians emphasize either the responsibility of the community to the individual or, increasingly in contemporary policy, the responsibility of the individual to the community. Some communitarians eschew the language of justice and adopt the language of solidarity, which is both a personal virtue of commitment and a principle of social morality based on the shared values of a group. For example, in the Netherlands, solidarity is sometimes viewed as a collective obligation to take care of citizens. The 1991 report of a Committee for Choices in Health Care, assembled under the Dutch Secretary for Public Health, argued that certain services or procedures are vital to ensure the "adequate functioning of society as a whole," and that their provision should be "consonant with the basic values of Dutch society." The report assigned an "absolute priority . . . to care for the elderly, the handicapped, and psychiatric patients."[12]

Some moderate communitarian writers in biomedical ethics attempt to incorporate aspects of liberal theories into their accounts. For example, Ezekiel J. Emanuel envisions small deliberative democratic communities that develop shared conceptions of the good life and justice.[13] He proposes thousands of community health programs (CHPs), each involving citizen-members who join in a federation. Each family would receive a voucher for participation in their community's CHP, and the CHP would determine democratically which benefits to provide, which care is most important, and whether expensive services, such as heart transplants, will be included or excluded. Justice is located in the guarantee that services will be provided to fulfill a particular community-endorsed conception of social goals.

Michael Walzer's communitarianism, by contrast, focuses on past and present socio-moral practices. According to Walzer, no single principle of distributive justice governs all social goods and their distribution. Rather, several principles constructed by human societies constitute distinct "spheres of justice." Notions of justice do not derive from some rational or natural foundation external to the society, but from standards developed internally, as a political community evolves. Walzer holds that community traditions and practices often include developed commitments of equal access to health care. While conceding that a two-tiered health care system—a decent minimum for all and then liberty of contract for the advantaged—is not unjust in principle, Walzer contends that this system would be unjust in a country such as the United States, where traditions of justice and the "common appreciation of the importance of medical care" have already committed the American people to more in the way of distribtive justice than a two-tier system acknowledges.[14]

Egalitarian Theories

Egalitarian theories of justice hold that persons should receive an equal distribution of certain goods, such as health care, but no prominent egalitarian theory requires equal sharing of all possible social benefits. Qualified egalitarianism re-

234

quires only some basic equalities among individuals, and permits inequalities that redound to the benefit of the least advantaged.

As the major contemporary example of qualified egalitarianism, John Rawls's theory of justice challenges libertarian, utilitarian, and communitarian theories. Rawls argues that "what justifies a conception of justice is not its being true to an order antecedent and given to us, but its congruence with our deeper understanding of ourselves and our aspirations, and our realization that, given our history and the traditions embedded in our public life, it is the most reasonable doctrine for us."[15] A theory of justice therefore matches our commonly accepted judgments of fairness with our general principles.

Although Rawls has not pursued the implications of his theory for health policy, others have. In an influential interpretation and extension, Norman Daniels argues for a just health care system based mainly on a Rawlsian principle of "fair equality of opportunity." Although Daniels offers no explicit defense of this principle, he relies implicitly on the importance of health care needs and on a considered judgment that fair opportunity is central to any acceptable theory of justice. Daniels's thesis is that social institutions affecting health care distribution should be arranged, as far as possible, to allow each person to achieve a fair share of the normal range of opportunities present in that society. The normal range of opportunity reflects the range of life plans that a person could reasonably hope to pursue, given his or her talents and skills. This theory, like Rawls's, recognizes a positive societal obligation to eliminate or reduce barriers that prevent fair equality of opportunity, an obligation that extends to programs to correct or compensate for various disadvantages. It views disease and disability as undeserved restrictions on persons' opportunities to realize basic goals. Health care, then, is needed to achieve, maintain, or restore adequate or "species-typical" levels of functioning (or the equivalents of these levels), so that basic goals can be achieved. A health care system designed to meet these needs should attempt to prevent disease, illness, or injury from reducing the range of opportunity open to the individual. The allocation of health care resources, then, should ensure justice through fair equality of opportunity. Forms of health care that have a significant effect on preventing, limiting, or compensating for reductions in normal species functioning should receive priority in designing health care institutions and allocating health care.[16]

This Rawls-inspired theory has far-reaching egalitarian implications for national health policy. On this account, each member of society, irrespective of wealth or position, would have equal access to an adequate, although not maximal, level of health care—the exact level of access being contingent on available social resources and public processes of decision-making. Better services (e.g., luxury hospital rooms and optional, cosmetic dental work) would be available for purchase at personal expense, including through private insurance.

Daniels and others have used a Rawlsian theory of justice to move beyond access to health care to the social determinants of health outcomes. In doing so, they concentrate on the distribution of welfare, as measured by health indices such as life expectancy, rather than on the distribution of resources.[17] Studies have long indicated that increasing access to health care does not correspondingly reduce inequalities in health among all socioeconomic classes, but Daniels and colleagues contend, in addition, that social justice itself, apart from specific health care services, is "good for our health."[18] They hold that empirical literature on the social determinants of health suggests that societal failures to meet Rawlsian or similar criteria for a just society—protection of equal liberties, provision of equal opportunity in a robust sense, fair distribution of resources, and support for our basic self-respect—contribute to health inequalities. The thesis is that social justice would improve a society's overall health and, at the same time, reduce health inequalities in that society.[19] Policies that stand to improve health by reducing socioeconomic disparities include early childhood intervention and investment, providing basic nutrition, raising the minimum wage, and improving the work environment.[20]

The power of Rawls's theory of justice, together with the political significance of the decent-minimum proposal, have engendered wide support for egalitarianism. As one of their achievements, Rawlsian theories have encouraged discussion of the role of the rule of fair opportunity in a theory of social justice, a topic that merits further discussion.

Fair Opportunity

Daniels's appeal to fair opportunity is only one use of the fair-opportunity rule. To explore this rule further, we need first to consider certain properties that have served as bases of distribution, although, as a matter of justice, they should not be considered relevant properties. These properties include gender, race, IQ, linguistic accent, national origin, and social status. In anomalous contexts, these properties may be relevant. For example, if a script calls for an actor in a male role, then females may be properly excluded (although this example is sometimes contested in contemporary film and theater). But general rules such as "To each according to gender" and "To each according to IQ" are unacceptable material principles. These properties are both irrelevant and discriminatory because they permit differential treatment of persons, sometimes with devastating effects, based on differences for which the affected individual is not responsible and which he or she does not deserve.

The Fair-Opportunity Rule

The fair-opportunity rule says that no persons should receive social benefits on the basis of undeserved advantageous properties (because no persons are responsible for having these properties) and that no persons should be denied social benefits on the basis of undeserved disadvantageous properties (because they also are not responsible for these properties). Properties distributed by the lotteries of social and biological life do not provide grounds for morally acceptable discrimination between persons in social allocations if they are not properties that people have a fair chance to acquire or overcome.

The attempt to supply all citizens with a basic education raises thorny moral problems analogous to those found in health care. Imagine a community that offers a high-quality education to all students with basic abilities, regardless of gender or race, but does not offer a comparable educational opportunity to students with reading difficulties or mental deficiencies. This system seems unjust. The students with disabilities lack basic skills and need special training to overcome their problems; they should receive an education suitable to their needs and opportunities, even if it costs more. The fair-opportunity rule requires that they receive the benefits needed to ameliorate the unfortunate effects of life's lottery.

By analogy, persons with functional disabilities lack capacity and need health care to reach a higher level of function and have a fair chance in life. If they are responsible for their disabilities, they might not be entitled to health care services. But if they are not responsible, the fair-opportunity rule demands that they receive that which will help them ameliorate the unfortunate effects of life's lottery of health.

Mitigating the Negative Effects of Life's Lotteries

Numerous properties might be disadvantaging and undeserved—for example, a squeaky voice, an ugly face, poor command of a language, or an inadequate early education. But which undeserved properties create a right *in justice* to some form of assistance?

One hypothesis is that virtually all abilities and disabilities are functions of what Rawls calls the natural lottery and the social lottery. "The natural lottery" refers to the distribution of advantageous and disadvantageous genetic properties. "Social lottery" refers to the distribution of social assets or deficits through family property, school systems, and the like. It is possible that all talents and disabilities result from heredity, natural environment, family upbringing, education, and inheritance. From this perspective, even the ability to work long hours and the ability to compete are biologically, environmentally, and socially produced. If so, talents, abilities, and successes are not to our credit, just as genetic disease is acquired through no fault of the afflicted person.

Rawls uses fair opportunity as a rule of redress. In order to overcome disadvantaging conditions (whether from biology or society) that are not deserved, the rule demands compensation for those with the disadvantages. The full implications of this approach are uncertain, but the conclusions Rawls reaches are challenging:

[A free-market arrangement] permits the distribution of wealth and income to be determined by the natural distribution of abilities and talents. Within the limits allowed by the background arrangements, distributive shares are decided by the outcome of the natural lottery; and this outcome is arbitrary from a moral perspective. There is no more reason to permit the distribution of income and wealth to be settled by the distribution of natural assets than by historical and social fortune. Furthermore, the principle of fair opportunity can be only imperfectly carried out, at least as long as the institution of the family exists. The extent to which natural capacities develop and reach fruition is affected by all kinds of social conditions and class attitudes. Even the willingness to make an effort, to try, and so to be deserving in the ordinary sense is itself dependent upon happy family and social circumstances.[21]

At a minimum, our social system of distributing benefits and burdens would undergo massive revision if we were to accept this approach. Rather than allowing broad inequalities in social distribution based on effort, contribution, and merit, as some Western nations do, we would achieve justice only if we reduced radical inequalities. Any remaining inequalities would be permissible only if "disadvantaged" persons benefited more from them than from an equal distribution of benefits.

At some point, the process of reducing inequalities introduced by life's lotteries must stop, and occasionally persons who are disadvantaged may not be protected by the fair-opportunity rule.[22] Libertarians rightly stress that the fair-opportunity rule must be constrained by limited resources. However, their principled rationale for this conclusion is questionable. Some disadvantages are merely *unfortunate,* they argue, whereas others are *unfair* (and therefore obligatory in justice to correct). Tristram Engelhardt has argued that society should call a halt to claims of fairness or justice precisely at the point of this distinction between the unfair and the unfortunate: "Where one draws the line between what is unfair and unfortunate will, as a result, have great consequences as to what allocations of health care resources are just or unfair as opposed to desirable or undesirable. If the natural lottery is neutral, in the sense of not creating an obligation to blunt its effects, one does not have [even] prima facie grounds for arguing for a right to health care on the basis of claims of fairness or justice."[23]

We are inclined to think that the problems of rationing addressed later in this chapter create a need for criteria other than the distinction between the unfortunate and the unfair, a criterion that may only beg the central questions of justice. Either way, the implications of the Rawlsian approach and the demands of the fair-opportunity rule remain very uncertain in biomedical ethics and health policy. No bright lines distinguish the unfair and the unfortunate or fair and unfair rationing schemes. It would be inappropriate to explore these theoretical problems further here. The point of exploring them as far as we have is to show that if one accepts the fair-opportunity rule, as we do, it will potentiallly affect many areas of moral reflection and social policy.

Unfair Distributions of Health Care Based on Gender and Race

We can now sketch some implications of the fair-opportunity rule for health care distribution, with particular attention to unfair distributions based on racial and gender properties.

Compelling evidence exists that health care has often been covertly distributed on the basis of these properties, resulting in a differential impact on women and minorities. Several recent studies indicate that African Americans and women have poorer access to various forms of health care by comparison to white males. For example, gender and racial inequities in employment have an impact on job-based health insurance; and the race and gender of physicians often play a role in the quality of patient–physician interaction.[24] An example of the problem of health care distribution appears in at least some parts of the United States in a large difference in the rates of coronary artery bypass grafting (CABG) between white and African-American Medicare patients, as well as between male and female Medicare patients. Differences have been evident since the mid-1980s in many parts of the United States, although differences have been more pronounced in the southeast's rural areas.[25] Differences in need cannot entirely account for the variance, and it remains unclear how far the rates can be explained by physician supply, poverty, awareness of health care opportunities, less willingness among African Americans and women to undergo surgery, and racial prejudice. A recent study found that, after controlling for age, payer, and appropriateness and necessity for CABG, African-American patients in New York State had significant access problems unrelated to patient refusals.[26] Another study found that African-American patients, once their lung cancer had been diagnosed and staged, were 12.7 percent less likely than white patients to have surgical resection.[27]

Evidence suggests that discrimination against African Americans, other minorities, and women occurs at the point of referral to transplantation centers and admission to waiting lists, whose criteria vary greatly. For instance, African Americans are much less likely than whites to be referred for evaluation at transplant centers (a difference of about 23 percentage points) and to be placed on a waiting list or receive a transplant within 18 months of starting dialysis (a difference of about 28 percentage points). These differences cannot be accounted for by patient preferences.[28]

In addition, questions arise about the use of human lymphocyte antigen (HLA) matching for the distribution of kidneys for transplantation. The degree of HLA match between a donor and a recipient influences the long-term survival of the transplanted graft. As a result, the United Network for Organ Sharing (UNOS) revised its criteria for the allocation of donated kidneys to give greater weight to the HLA match, thereby reducing the importance of time on the waiting list, logistics, and urgency of need.[29] However, assigning priority to tissue matching could produce further discriminatory effects for minorities. Most organ donors are white, and certain HLA phenotypes are different in white, African-American, and Hispanic populations. The identification of HLA phenotypes is less complete for African Americans and Hispanics, and yet they have a higher rate of end-stage renal disease. Nonwhite populations are also disproportionately represented on dialysis rolls. African Americans typically wait months longer than whites, almost twice as long, according to some studies, to receive a first kidney transplant.[30] It also appears to be the case that if organs are allocated on the basis of tissue match, whites gain an advantage.[31]

Justice minimally requires careful monitoring of point systems to determine whether discriminatory effects occur. In the case of transplantation, it may be justified to sacrifice some probability of success in order to take action, based on the fair-opportunity rule, to protect minorities. Defenders of the primacy of tissue matching argue that allocation rules can be constructed to reflect the natural lottery (which determines the spread of HLA types in the population), but the social context may still cause problems of injustice. For example, there are legitimate worries about the exploitation of minorities as sources of organs for others. Social factors also play a role in the higher rate among African Americans of medical conditions, such as hypertension, that contribute to end-stage kidney failure and the need for both dialysis and transplantation.[32]

Problems plaguing minority patients are parallel to those facing women patients. The Council on Ethical and Judicial Affairs of the American Medical Association has examined data that raise concerns about whether women are disadvantaged because of inadequate attention to research, diagnosis, and treatment of their health problems.[33] Some studies indicate that women have more physician visits per year than men and receive more services per visit, yet gender disparities still appear in three critical areas: (1) diagnosis of lung cancer, (2) diagnosis and treatment of cardiac disease, and (3) access to kidney transplantation. Biological differences alone do not account for these disparities. The Council notes that gender bias need not be manifest in an overt manner. Social attitudes involving stereotypes, prejudices, and gender–role attributions may be present, including the attribution of women's health complaints to emotional rather than physical causes.

In the use of diagnostic and therapeutic procedures for patients with coronary heart disease, for example, evidence exists that men and women are treated differently for reasons that appear unrelated to their medical conditions. One study found that women reported more cardiac disability than men before myocardial infarction, but that they were less likely than men to have procedures recommended that were known to reduce symptoms and improve cardiac function.[34] There is ongoing debate about whether these procedures are overused in men, underused in women, or both. However, at least for heart disease and perhaps for lung disease as well, many health care professionals and public officials still appear to have a biased view of these diseases as male diseases.[35]

The Right to a Decent Minimum of Health Care

We have seen that questions about whom shall receive what share of society's scarce resources generate controversies about a national health policy, unequal distributions of advantages to the disadvantaged, and rationing health care. These questions of distributive justice recur for problems of access to and distribution of health insurance, expensive medical equipment, artificial organs, and other goods and services. Ultimately, the primary economic barrier to health care access in many countries—notably the United States when compared with the other 28 industrialized nations—is the lack of adequate insurance. More than 40 million U.S. citizens (approximately 18% of the nonelderly population) lack health insurance of any kind. Inadequate insurance affects persons who are uninsured, uninsurable, underinsured, or only occasionally insured. Although each year, the United States spends more resources on health care than any country in the world, it is the only industrialized nation with less than half of its population eligible for public health insurance.[36]

More than 60% of the U.S. population has employer-based health insurance coverage (although the share of Americans with job-based health benefits declined from 69% in 1987 to 64% in 1996). Another 25% has either private health insurance unconnected to employment or some form of publicly supported health insurance programs (Medicaid, Medicare, and the like, which have grown in recent years). The remainder of the population has no health insurance: More than 50 million nonelderly adults in the U.S.—approximately one-third of that population—experience a gap in coverage within a two-year period; approximately two-thirds of these same uncovered adults have no insurance for at least one full year. Many uninsured persons are employed, but by companies offering no health insurance benefits. This situation is common with employees of small firms for whom the costs of maintaining insurance are much higher than for large employers. Many employee-benefit packages also provide no coverage for dependents or for part-time employees.[37]

Other U.S. citizens are uninsurable, although many of them are employed by firms offering health coverage, and some could afford standard health insurance. The problem for them is that forms of insurance other than open-enrollment group plans typically require physical examinations as well as family and personal medical histories as a condition of eligibility. Those with poor health or preexisting conditions or family histories that suggest the potential for expensive future claims are often denied coverage under exclusion clauses (or are offered only inferior and more expensive coverage). Insurers exempt certain illnesses, treatments, or conditions from coverage, and refuse to accept persons in specified occupations or with certain lifestyles. The AIDS crisis has presented dramatic instances of these problems of uninsurability and underwriting practices.

This morally shameful circumstance needs redress. Justice in access to health care depends on maintaining fair-opportunity rules, which, in turn, requires sharing financial risks in an insurance scheme. A deep flaw in the U.S. system is that both legislators and insurers act as if the uninsured are the responsibility of the other party, while neither assumes the responsibility for rectifying the moral unfairness that results from an actuarially fair system.[38] As a result, many, including persons in employer-based plans, are denied coverage for the primary condition for which they need coverage. They constitute one subgroup of those who, though insured, are underinsured. Exclusionary clauses deny access for various types of treatment and exclude coverage for specific diseases, injuries, organ systems, and preexisting conditions.

Many parts of the system in the United States are unfair because of the extraordinary reliance on employers for financing the system. Persons who work for medium- to large-size employers are not only better covered, but are, in part, subsidized by tax breaks in the system. When employed persons who are not covered become ill, taxpayers rather than free-riding employers usually pick up the bill. The financing of health care is also regressive. Low-income families pay premiums comparable to and often higher than the premiums paid by high-income families, and many individuals who do not qualify for group coverage pay dramatically more for the same coverage than those who qualify in a group. Finally, eligibility for Medicaid varies dramatically from state to state, and not one state covers all citizens who are below the poverty line.

Health care for the needy in former eras was handled through institutions, such as charity hospitals. But in the new era of high technology and commensurately high costs, virtues of charity and moral ideals have proved inadequate to the task of meeting many health care needs. The older models of voluntary assistance have gradually given way to a controversial model of an *enforceable right* to health care based in justice.

In this circumstance, and despite various controversies, a broad social consensus appears to be emerging that all citizens should be able to secure equitable access to health care, including insurance coverage without temporal gaps and unjust exclusionary clauses. The problem with this consensus is its thinness: Citizens disagree sharply on a range of political solutions proffered to improve access, on the role of government in these solutions, and on methods of financing them. It is unclear whether such a fragile consensus favoring equitable access can generate a secondary consensus about implementing equal access in an appropriate and meaningful public policy. We will now address these problems as moral issues, beginning with arguments in support of a moral right to health care.

Arguments Supporting a Right to Health Care

The debate about the right to health care has been characterized more by political rhetoric than careful analysis. The primary question is whether the government should be involved in health care allocation and distribution, rather than leaving these matters to the marketplace. Society has often allowed a rule of ability to pay to determine the distribution of health goods and services, but we will argue that this rule should not serve as our only principle of distributive justice.

A right to health care can be general or specific. Before concentrating on a general right to health care, we need to say why specific moral and legal rights to health care contrast sharply with a general right. Many societies recognize a "patchwork" of specific rights. For example, it is widely acknowledged that it is morally obligatory, based on fairness, to provide health care to military veterans. A similar claim supports the provision of health care and compensation to subjects who were injured in research undertaken on behalf of society. However far such "patchworking" or "spot zoning" of rights extends, it will not by itself amount to a general right to health care.[39]

Two main arguments support a general moral right to health care: (1) an argument from collective social protection and (2) an argument from fair-opportunity.[40] The first argument focuses on the similarities between health needs and other needs that government has conventionally protected. Threats to health are relevantly similar to threats presented by crime, fire, and pollution. We conventionally use collective actions and resources to resist the latter threats, and many collective schemes to protect health are present in virtually all societies, including programs of environmental protection and sanitation. Consistency suggests that essential health care assistance in response to threats to health should likewise be a collective responsibility. This argument, by analogy, makes a critical appeal to coherence: If government has an obligation to provide one type of essential service, then it must have an obligation to provide another.

One can dismiss this argument by maintaining that such government responsibilities are nonobligatory, nonessential, and expendable. This perspective will be favored by few beyond those who accept a libertarian account of justice. On each of the nonlibertarian theories of justice previously explicated, the argument from government services does successfully generate a public obligation to provide some level of goods and services to protect health, at least in the circumstances of most contemporary societies. Relevant *dissimilarities*, it must be admitted, do exist between health care and other public programs, especially those designed to protect health.[41] These programs pertain to social goods, such as public health, whereas health care is largely a matter of the individual's private good. The argument from collective social protection, therefore, might seem to fail. But additional premises could be found in society's right to expect a decent return on the investment it has made in physicians' education, funding for biomedical research, and other parts of the medical system that pertain dominantly to health care. The return we expect on this taxed investment is health care protection for ourselves and our families. We legitimately expect the scope of protection to extend beyond public health measures, because we fund even more training and research in medicine than in public health.

Nevertheless, we cannot reasonably expect a direct individual return on all collective investments. Some investments seek only the discovery of cures or treatments, not the provision of cures and treatments once discovered. Even if the government funds drug research and regulates the drug industry, this activity does not justify the expectation that the government will subsidize or reimburse individuals' drug purchases (although, in fact, many governments do reimburse for drugs in some cases). In the instance of physician education, some might argue that society invests in training physicians and protecting the public health, not in health care services themselves. This first argument in support of a moral right to health care, then, can secure only a *decent return* on our investment, not a *full return or refund*. We consider this problem of a decent basic minimum in the next section.

A second argument buttresses this first argument by appeal to the fair-opportunity rule. This argument gauges the justice of social institutions by their tendency to counteract lack of opportunity caused by unpredictable bad luck and misfortune over which the person has no meaningful control. The need for health care is far greater among the seriously diseased and injured, because the costs of health care for them can be uncontrollable and overwhelming, particularly as their health status worsens. Insofar as injury, disability, or disease creates profoundly significant disadvantages and reduces agents' capacity to function properly, justice requires that we use societal health care resources to counter these effects and to restore to persons a fair chance to use their capacities.[42]

One additional argument for a *legal* right to health care appeals to the role of governmental coordination in effecting *charitable goals*. According to the "enforced beneficence argument," as Allen Buchanan calls it, beneficent citizens who do not believe that the needy have a *moral* right to health care could still establish health programs for the needy while coercively taxing others to sustain those programs.[43] This argument challenges libertarian and egalitarian assumptions that coercive transfers of social resources are justified only if the persons to whom they are transferred have moral *rights* to the resources. But if the goals are sufficiently fundamental and important, Buchanan argues that coercion can be morally justified to realize these broad social goals, even in the absence of a moral right.

A contemporary example of the need for a scheme of enforcement and coordination appears in the aforementioned private health insurance coverage that forms the hub of the payment system in the United States. Employers are not obligated to provide insurance, and no enforceable scheme of contributions exists, although states are permitted to regulate certain activities of insurance companies. As health care costs and other costs increase, employers find it more difficult to offer insurance to employees. Many employers provide no health care benefits, and firms that do provide their employees insurance suffer a competitive disadvantage and resent competitor firms who, in effect, refuse to shoulder the burden of paying a fair share of the insurance costs. The noncontributing firms are competitively advantaged free-riders in the system of funding health care, and for this reason, firms that supply health insurance for their employees increasingly favor mandatory contributions by all firms in an enforceable system of health care insurance.

This so-called *mandating* is one way to level the playing field by not allowing free-riders to avoid paying a fair share while shifting costs to others. Many firms are now willing to give up their control to contract for employee health care benefits and to promote a more efficient and equitable system.[44] This argument need not move to the conclusion that firms should be required to supply private health insurance. Economic realities, such as wage levels, corporate finance, and various costs might make this approach to mandating inefficient and unfair. The appropriate conclusion is that a more efficient and equitable system is needed, but not necessarily a system exclusively featuring either public or private insurance, and not necessarily an egalitarian system.

The Scope of the Right to Health Care

An intractable, and very important, problem about the right to health care is how to specify the precise entitlements and limits of the right. Two broad views have attracted wide support: a right of *equal access* to health care and a right to a *decent minimum* of health care. Both are egalitarian. The former promotes equal access to all bona fide health care resources. The latter incorporates a weak egalitarian point of view that entails equal access only to fundamental health care resources.

"Access to health care" has several meanings. Sometimes it means only that one is not legitimately prevented from obtaining health care. In this sense, having a right of access does not entail that others must provide health care or equitably distribute care. The system of access turns ultimately on freedom of choice and financial responsibility. Libertarians favor this interpretation and limit one's rights to this form of access. More commonly, however, a right of access to health care refers to a right to obtain specified goods and services to which every entitled person has an equal claim. Here values of equality and solidarity are prominent. A very inclusive understanding of this right requires that everyone have equal access to every treatment that is available to anyone.

Those who promote access to a decent minimum or adequate level of care usually do not specify precisely where to set limits on expenditures for health care. Their first concern is that basic health care must be universally accessible. The decent-minimum approach entails acceptance of a two-tiered system of health care: enforced social coverage for basic and catastrophic health needs (tier 1), together with voluntary private coverage for other health needs and desires (tier 2). The first tier distributes health care based on need, and meets needs by universal access to basic services. This tier would presumably cover at least public health protections and preventive care, primary care, and acute care, as well as special social services for those with disabilities. In this conception, society's obligations are not limitless but fall under a general model of a safety net for everyone.[45]

The decent minimum, so understood, offers a possible compromise among libertarians, utilitarians, communitarians, and egalitarians, because it incorporates some moral premises that each theory stresses. It guarantees basic health care for all on a premise of equal access, while allowing unequal additional purchases by individual initiative and contract. It mixes private and public forms of distribution and it affirms collective as well as free-market methods of delivering health care. Utilitarians should find the proposal attractive because it serves to minimize public dissatisfaction and to maximize social utility, without demanding unduly burdensome taxation. It also permits allocation decisions based in part on formal techniques, such as cost-effectiveness analysis. The egalitarian finds an opportunity to use an equal access principle and to see fair opportunity embedded in the distributional system. The communitarian perspective, too, is not neglected. A societal consensus about values, even if only rough and incomplete, is required for a practicable system. The common good is a basic point of reference for public deliberation about how to establish the decent minimum. Finally, the libertarian sees an opportunity for free-market production and distribution. The two-tiered system provides indigent persons with opportunities for health care that would otherwise not be available to them, but leaves a tier for free choice and charity. In addition, various forms of competition and incentives may be used as tools to increase the system's productivity and the quality of health care.

A health care system that finds pockets of support from each of these four types of theory could also turn out to be the fairest approach to democratic reform of the system.[46] We do not now have—and are not likely ever to have—a single viable theory of social justice.[47] Each theory has its attractive and unattractive features, and many citizens appropriately fear the social consequences of adopting one of these philosophical systems as the sole basis for justice in health policy. Experience suggests that, while appeals to one of these accounts of justice works well in some contexts, each can yield disastrous results in others.

Despite these attractions, the decent-minimum proposal has proved difficult to explicate and implement. It raises questions about whether society can fairly, consistently, and unambiguously devise a public policy that recognizes a right to care for primary needs without creating a right to exotic and expensive forms of treatment, such as liver transplants. Such coverage might provide what many deem to be marginal benefits in quality-adjusted life-years (see Chapter 5). In truth, the model is purely programmatic until society delineates the decent minimum in operational terms. In light of the current flux in national health systems, this task is, we believe, the major problem confronting health policy in many, perhaps all, countries today.[48]

Fair public participation is indispensable in the process of setting the threshold of a decent minimum. When substantive standards are contested—for example, regarding a decent or sufficient level of health care—a democratic society tends to resort to democratic procedures. This tendency is understandable and frequently warranted, but it also may lead to unjust outcomes. The President's Commission rightly concluded: "It is reasonable for a society to turn to fair, democratic political procedures to make a choice among just alternatives. Given the great imprecision in the notion of adequate health care, however, it is especially important that the procedures used to define the level be—and be perceived to be—fair."[49] Careful cost-effectiveness analysis (CEA) and cost–benefit analysis (CBA), as we discussed in Chapter 5, can aid deliberations and decisions within these procedures. (See the section below on "Strategies for Setting Priorities.") However, we need to recognize that much of the debate also concerns which values should determine what will count as benefits and costs, how much the identified benefits and costs will count, and how to handle uncertainty—all within appropriate constraints of social justice.

Public preferences can also play a role in setting the decent minimum, as Ronald Dworkin proposes in this hypothetical test of what "ideal prudent insurers" would choose under stated conditions. Dworkin rightly criticizes what he perceives as an undue use of the "rescue principle." This principle asserts that it is intolerable when a society allows people to die who could have been saved by spending more money on health care.[50] He argues that this principle grows out of an "insulation model" that treats health care as different from and superior to all other goods and that calls for its equal distribution, even if society distributes no other goods equally. Yet this model may not capture the way in which we do rank goods. In place of this model, Dworkin proposes that we try to imagine a "prudent insurance" ideal, which envisions health care under "a free and unsubsidized market," without all the deficiencies that currently characterize markets in health care. Thus ideal market presupposes a fair distribution of wealth and income, full information about the benefits, costs, and risks of various medical procedures, and ignorance about the likelihood that any particular person will experience morbidity, either life threatening or non-life threatening, from diseases and accidents. Under such circumstances, whatever aggregate amount a well-informed community decides to spend on health care is just, as is the distribution pattern it chooses.

These assumptions about prudent choices under fair conditions may help us to determine what a universal health care system should ensure that everyone has. If most prudent buyers with average means in a free market would buy a certain level of health coverage, then there must be "unfairness" in the current system if it prevents them from obtaining this level. This strategy presumably allows one to determine what justice would require in the way of a decent minimum.[51] Establishing precise entitlements will nonetheless invariably involve trade-offs, and no right to health care will trump all competing claims of social utility or the common good when larger questions of macroallocation are at stake.

These issues are too complex for ethical theory to resolve. We cannot fix an entitlement to health care or a comprehensive public policy in this book, but we can further explore intimately connected conceptual and moral problems, including the place of individual responsibility for ill health and the moral foundations of allocation decisions.

Forfeiting the Right to Health Care

If we assume that all citizens enjoy a right to a decent minimum of health care, can particular individuals forfeit that right even when they wish to preserve it? The question is not whether a person loses the full range of entitlements under the right to health care, but whether he or she forfeits the right to certain forms of care through actions that result in personal ill health and that generate health care needs (or, alternatively, through antisocial behavior, such as criminal conduct). Examples include patients who acquired AIDS as a result of unsafe sexual activities or intravenous drug use, smokers with lung cancer, and alcoholics who develop liver disease. It is unfair, some charge, for individuals to pay higher premiums or taxes to support people who voluntarily engage in risky actions, and it is fair to withhold societal funds from needy individuals whose medical needs resulted from voluntary risk-taking.[52] This conclusion does not conflict with the rule of fair-opportunity, they would argue, because risk-takers' voluntary actions reduced their opportunity.

However, compelling questions of justice raise issues about how far society can fairly exclude risk-takers from coverage. First, it must be possible to identify and differentiate various causal factors in morbidity, such as natural causes, the social environment, and personal activities. Once these factors have been identified, solid evidence must establish that a pertinent disease or illness resulted from personal activities, rather than some other cause. Second, the personal activities in question must have been autonomous, in the sense that the actors were aware of the risks and accepted them. If the risks are unknown at the time of action, individuals cannot be justly held responsible for them, and if an individual is unaware of a particular risk known to other people, questions arise about whether it is fair to use the standard of what a reasonable person should have known.

Regarding the first condition, it is virtually impossible to isolate causal factors in many cases of ill health because of complex causal links and our limited knowledge. Medical needs often result from the conjunction of genetic predispositions, personal actions, and environmental and social conditions. The respective roles of these different factors will often be impossible to establish with reasonable certainty. It is not possible to determine with certainty whether a particular individual's lung cancer resulted from personal cigarette smoking, passive smoking, environmental pollution, occupational conditions, or heredity (or some combination of these causal conditions). If, as many argue, ill health is broadly rooted in socially induced causes, such as environmental pollutants and infant feeding practices, then the class of diseases covered by the right to a decent minimum will presumably expand as evidence about the causal roles of these factors increases.

Problems in policing the system are also relevant. To determine accurately the causal conditions of particular health problems and to locate voluntary risk-takers, officials would need broad investigative powers. In the worst-case scenario, these officials would invade privacy, break confidentiality, and keep detailed records in order to document health abuses that could result in a forfeiture of the right to a particular type of health care. Such enforcement would carry heavy financial costs in addition to its morally unattractive features.

A major reason for debates about forfeiture of rights to health care is rising costs, but prevention of risks through alterations in lifestyle and conduct often leads to counterintuitive outcomes. Some risk-taking involves less rather than more medical care, because it results in earlier and quicker deaths than might occur if individuals lived longer and developed chronic debilitating conditions. For example, Louise Russell used cost-effectiveness analysis to compare health care costs in groups of men of the same age who had the same blood serum cholesterol levels. She found that "low-risk," nonsmoking men with low blood pressure consistently generate far higher health care costs *per year of life* than "high-risk" men who smoke and have high blood pressure.[53] When extended to include programs for the elderly, the cost–benefit case for denying care to individual risk-takers may disappear altogether, because risk-takers may cost less. As noted earlier, we should expect an increase rather than a decrease in overall expenditures for both health care and social security as a result of controlling health risks.[54]

It would, nonetheless, be fair to require individuals to pay higher premiums or taxes if they accept well-documented risks that may result in costly medical attention. Risk-takers might be required to contribute more to particular pools, such as insurance plans, or to pay a tax on their risky conduct, such as an increased tax on cigarettes. These requirements may fairly redistribute the burdens of the costs of health care and, at the same time, deter risky conduct without disrespecting autonomy. Questions about individual responsibility and the just allocation of health care have emerged with special poignancy for patients with alcohol-related end-stage liver failure who need liver transplants. Liver transplantation has recently improved such patients' chances of survival and a higher quality of life. By 1997, more than 87% of liver transplant recipients survived at least a year, and, over the previous eight years, almost 74% had a five-year survival rate.[55] However, despite dramatic increases in the number of liver transplants, from 15 in 1980 to 2946 in 1991 to 4339 (72 from living donors) in 1998, donated livers are scarce, and many patients suffering from end-stage liver failure (ESLF) die before they can obtain transplants. A major cause of ESLF is excessive use of alcohol that causes cirrhosis of the liver. As a result, the question arises whether patients who have alcohol-related ESLF should be excluded from waiting lists for liver transplants or should be given lower priority ratings. Arguments for their lower priority or total exclusion often appeal to the probability that they will resume a pattern of alcohol abuse and again experience ESLF, thereby wasting the transplanted liver. However, studies have demonstrated that patients with alcohol-related ESLF who receive a liver transplant and abstain from alcohol do as well as patients whose ESLF resulted from other causes.[56] Liver transplantation can be a sobering experience, and some centers and funding agencies already require waiting periods of a year to establish abstinence. Thus, a good case exists for not excluding alcohol-related ESLF patients, but rather for introducing conditions that require demonstrated and extended abstention from alcohol.

Nonetheless, Alvin Moss and Mark Siegler propose that patients with alcohol-related ESLF (more than 50% of the patients with ESLF) automatically receive a lower priority ranking in the allocation of donated livers than patients who develop end-stage liver disease through no fault of their own.[57] Their argument appeals to fairness, fair opportunity, and utility. They contend that it is fair to hold people responsible for their decisions, and then to allocate organs with a view to utilitarian outcomes. Assigning lower priority to patients with alcohol-related ESLF is unfortunate, Moss and Siegler argue, but not unfair: "It is fairer to give a child dying of biliary atresia an opportunity for a first normal liver than it is to give a patient with [alcohol-related ESLF] who was born with a normal liver a second one."[58] In addition, Moss and Siegler use the utilitarian argument that public support is indispensable for liver transplantation, both for securing funds and for securing organ donations. Giving patients with alcohol-related ESLF equal priority for donated livers could reduce public support for liver transplantation, and this consequence could be devastating for transplant programs and patients needing transplants.

Despite these ongoing debates, a consensus currently exists among transplant professionals that patients with alcohol-related ESLF should not be totally excluded.[59] Ideally, such patients should be evaluated on a case-by-case basis (considering medical need and probability of successful transplantation), rather than automatically receiving a lower priority. An individual can then receive a lower priority rating, as warranted. The following two examples illustrate conditions under which personal responsibility can and should affect priorities and lead to a lower rating: (1) For the alcoholic who fails to seek effective treatment for alcoholism and develops alcohol-related ESLF, a lower priority is clearly justified (although total exclusion needs a stronger argument than has yet been produced). (2) If a transplant recipient fails through personal negligence to take his or her immunosuppressant medication and the transplant then fails, it would be just for the transplant team to give that person a lower priority for a second transplant or even to deny him or her a second transplant. Individual responsibility is in these ways relevant from the standpoint of justice.

The issues raised by this debate will intensify when lung transplantation becomes more common and more cigarette smokers seek transplants, often in competition with patients who have lethal genetic conditions, such as cystic fibrosis.

The Allocation of Health Care Resources

Specification of the right to a decent minimum of health care encounters theoretical and practical difficulties of just and justified social allocations. We cannot here address specific issues, such as cost containment in hospitals, methods of reducing infant mortality rates, tax deductions for medical care, and incentives to employers and third-party payers. We can, however, present and assess general arguments for and against different systems of setting priorities and allocating health care.

To allocate is to distribute by allotment. Such distribution does not presuppose either a person or a system that rations resources. A criterion of ability to pay in a competitive market, for example, is a form of allocation. "Macroallocation" decisions determine the funds to be expended and the goods made available, as well as the methods of distribution. "Microallocation" decisions determine who will receive particular scarce resources. This distinction between the macro and the micro levels of allocation is useful, but the line between them is not sharp, and they often interact.

Norman Daniels correctly argues that the scope and design of basic health care institutions involve allocation decisions to determine the following:

1. What kinds of health care services will exist in a society?
2. Who will receive them, and on what basis?
3. Who will deliver them?
4. How will the burdens of financing them be distributed?
5. How will the power and control of those services be distributed?[60]

These decisions about the allocation of funds determine how much health care to provide and what kind of health care to provide for which problems. These decisions have far-reaching effects on other patterns of allocation. For example, the funds allocated for medical and biological research may affect the availability of training programs for physicians. Specific monetary allocations also can affect a physician's choice of a profession, institution, location, and the like.

Problems of allocation are classifiable by types, each of which involves competition among desirable programs or alternatives. We will identify four distinct, yet interrelated types. The third and fourth are particularly important for the remainder of this chapter.

1. Partitioning the Comprehensive Social Budget

Every large political unit operates with a budget, which includes allocations for health and for other social goods, including housing, education, culture, defense, and recreation. Health is not our only value or goal, and expenditures for other goods inevitably compete for limited resources with health-targeted expenditures. Some commentators argue that these problems are political rather than moral and should be resolved through political processes, as long as those processes contain morally just procedures that reflect the values, preferences, and priorities of the entire society. Their thesis is that only in such a forum can we determine whether public funding for health care is adequate. From this perspective, a citizen cannot complain of injustice if society uses a morally justified procedure to allocate more money to space programs or defense programs than to health programs.[61]

2. Allocating Within the Health Budget

The next type of allocation decision concerns funds from within the budget segment devoted to health. We protect and promote health in many ways besides the provision of medical care. Health policies and programs for occupational safety, environmental protection, injury prevention, consumer protection, and food and drug control are all parts of society's effort to protect and promote the health of its citizens. The term "health resources," then, is not a substitute for "medical resources," and the budget for health vastly exceeds the specific portion for health care. Many policy implications follow. For example, equalizing medical care is not the most effective strategy for equalizing the opportunity for health, in view of the impact of the standard of living, housing, sanitation, and the like on health.

3. Allocating Within the Health Care Budget

Once society has determined its budget for health care, it still must allocate its resources within health care, by selecting certain projects and procedures for funding. Many decisions must be made, including whether priority should go to prevention or treatment.[62] Expenditures for treatment, rather than prevention, are far higher in the current health care systems of most industrialized nations, but government officials might choose, for example, to concentrate on preventing heart disease rather than on rescuing individuals by heart transplants or artificial hearts. In many cases, preventive care is more effective and more efficient in saving lives, reducing suffering, raising levels of health, and lowering costs. How society might appropriately mix preventive and treatment strategies will depend, in part, on knowledge of causal links, such as those between disease and environmental and behavioral factors. Polio vaccination and preventive dentistry are standard examples of success in preventive care, but these models do not work well for kidney failure and heart failure, where preventive care is more speculative, in part because numerous medical problems can cause these organs to fail.

Preventive care typically reduces morbidity and premature mortality for unknown, "statistical lives," whereas critical interventions concentrate on known, "identifiable lives."[63] Many societies have historically been more likely to favor identified persons and to allocate resources for critical care, even if evidence exists that preventive care is more effective and efficient. Sometimes the public becomes alarmed by its allocation patterns when it becomes aware, for example, that public funds are available and that sufficient private funds cannot be raised for a person in need of an expensive medical procedure. Yet good evidence exists to show that public health expenditures targeted at poorer communities for preventive measures, such as prenatal care, save many times that amount in future care. Accordingly, our moral intuitions often drive us in two conflicting directions: Allocate more to rescue persons in medical need and allocate more to prevent persons from falling into such need.

Determining which categories of injury, illness, or disease (if any) should receive a priority ranking in the allocation of health care resources is another aspect of allocation. For example, should heart disease have priority over cancer? In trying to determine priorities among medical needs, policymakers must examine various diseases in terms of factors such as their communicability, frequency, cost, associated pain and suffering, and impact on length of life and quality of life. It might be justified, for instance, to concentrate less on killer diseases, such as some forms of cancer, and more on widespread disabling diseases, such as arthritis.

4. Allocating Scarce Treatments for Patients

Because health needs and desires are virtually limitless, every health care system faces some form of scarcity, and not everyone who needs a particular form of health care can gain access to it. At one time or another, medical resources and supplies, such as penicillin, insulin, kidney dialysis, cardiac transplantation, and space in intensive care units, have been allocated for specific patients or classes of patients. These decisions are more difficult when an illness is life-threatening and the scarce resource potentially life-saving. The question can become, "Who shall live when not everyone can live?" Such allocation occurs in the United Kingdom by several means, including queuing and the use of restrictive criteria for services,[64] and health care has often been nonsystematically allocated in the United States by ability to pay for health care and adequacy of health insurance.

Allocation decisions of type 3 (the health care budget) above and allocation decisions of type 4 (scarce treatments for patients) interact. Type 3 decisions partially determine the necessity and extent of patient selection by determining the availability and supply of a particular resource. In contrast, distress at making difficult choices through explicit decisions of type 4 sometimes leads society to modify its macroallocation policies at the level of type 1 to increase the supply of a particular resource. For example, in the face of difficult allocation decisions about dialysis machines, the U.S. federal government decided to provide funds to ensure near-universal access to kidney dialysis and kidney transplantation without regard for ability to pay.

In the remaining two major sections of this chapter, we discuss the types of allocation decision categorized above as types 3 and 4. Both are often discussed under the topic of *rationing,* and related terms, such as *triage.*[65] The choice of terms is not unimportant, because each term has a different history involving changes in meaning. *Rationing,* for example, originally did not suggest harshness or an emergency. It meant a form of allowance, share, or portion, as when food is divided into rations in the military. Only recently has *rationing* been linked to limited resources, crisis management, and the setting of priorities in the health care budget.

Rationing now has three primary meanings. The first is closely related to "denial from lack of resources." In a market economy, for example, all types of goods, including health care, are to some extent rationed by ability to pay for it. A good is denied if one lacks the resources to pay for it. A second sense of *rationing* derives not from market limits but from social policy limits: The government determines an allowance or allotment, and individuals are denied access beyond the allotted amount. Rationing gasoline and certain types of food during a war is a well-known example, but a national health system that does not allow purchases of goods or insurance beyond an allotted amount is an equally good example. Finally, according to a third meaning of *rationing*, an allowance or allotment is determined and distributed equitably, but those who can afford additional goods are not denied access beyond the allotted amount. In this third form, rationing involves elements of each of the first two forms: Public policy fixes an allowance, and those who cannot afford additional units are thereby effectively denied access beyond the allowance.

We will use "rationing" in each of the three senses, while concentrating on the third sense.

Rationing and Setting Priorities

Many people now believe that the primary task in macroallocation of health care is to establish priorities in the health care system (type 3 above). Structuring clear priorities has been difficult in many countries, and health care costs continue to rise dramatically as a result of several conditions—in particular, good insurance, new technology, and longer life-expectancy in an aging population. Insured patients typically pay between ten percent and 25% of the costs of their covered health care; insurance pays the rest. When parties who are insured pay far less than the actual value of what they consume, they will consume more than they otherwise would. Physicians and patients alike have an incentive to use any service, irrespective of cost, as long as it is covered.

These problems of contemporary health policy are extraordinarily complicated, and we can here consider only three substantive issues: (1) allocating funds for expensive treatments, in particular heart transplants, (2) setting priorities (as occurred in Oregon's health care budget), and (3) rationing by age.

Allocating Funds for Heart Transplants

Controversies over funding heart transplants began shortly after cardiac transplantation became increasingly effective in the 1980s as a result of medical improvements that included immunosuppressant medication. In 1980, only 36 heart transplants occurred in the United States, but the numbers increased dramatically in the next decade. By 1990, the figure was close to 2100; in the 1990s, it stablized in the range of 2100 to 2375.[66] Changing medical and political circumstances have led to alterations of policy that close one gap in equity only to open another.

Despite the high cost of coverage for heart transplants and other expensive forms of health care, arguments have been offered for funding them. For instance, the federal Task Force on Organ Transplantation (appointed by the U.S. Department of Health and Human Services) recommended that "a public program should be set up to cover the costs of people who are medically eligible for organ transplants but who are not covered by private insurance, Medicare, or Medicaid and who are unable to obtain an organ transplant due to the lack of funds."[67] The task force limited its proposed policy to the financially needy.

The Task Force grounded its recommendation on two arguments from justice. The first argument emphasizes the continuity between heart and liver transplants and other forms of medical care (including kidney transplants) that are already accepted as part of the decent minimum of health care that society should provide. The Task Force argued that heart and liver transplants are comparable to other funded procedures in terms of their effectiveness in saving lives and enhancing the quality of life. According to the National Heart Transplantation Study, which provided data relevant to these deliberations, 80% of heart transplant recipients survived for one year, and 50% were alive after five years, with a good quality of life according to both objective and subjective criteria. By 1998, almost 86% of heart transplant recipients survived for one year and, in the most dramatic improvement, almost 70% survived at least five years.[68] In response to the charge that heart and liver transplants are too expensive, the Task Force argued that the burden of saving public health funds should be distributed equitably rather than imposed on particular groups of patients, such as those suffering from end-stage heart or liver failure. Under the assumption that society is committed to providing funds to meet a wide variety of health care needs, "it is arbitrary to exclude one life-saving procedure while funding others of equal life-saving potential and cost."

The Task Force offered a second argument for the federal government's role in guaranteeing equitable access to organ transplants, this time focusing on practices of organ donation and procurement. Various public officials, including the President of the United States, participate in efforts to increase the supply of donated organs by appealing to all citizens to donate their organs and their dead relatives' organs. They aim their appeals at all segments of society. However, the Task Force argued, it is unfair and sometimes exploitative to solicit people, rich and poor alike, to donate organs if those organs are then distributed on the basis of ability to pay.[69] Furthermore, it is inconsistent to prohibit the sale of organs, and then to distribute donated organs according to ability to pay. Moreover, it is morally problematic to distinguish buying an organ for transplantation from buying an organ transplant procedure when a donated organ is the centerpiece of the procedure.

Despite their attractive features, these arguments do not establish that justice requires the government to provide health care irrespective of its cost or that it is arbitrary to use a reasonably structured system of rationing. Once a society has achieved a fair threshold of funding, it may select some procedures while excluding others when they are of equal life-saving potential and of equal cost, as long as it can identify relevant differences through a fair procedure involving substantial public participation. It would, ceteris paribus, be unfair to solicit people to make gifts of organs and then distribute them on the basis of ability to pay, but it would also be unfair to spend in excess of a fairly established level of funding merely because of such gifts.

Potential donors need to understand the limits built into the system of procurement and distribution, but assuming this understanding by donors and a fair system for allocating collected organs, a government could legitimately encourage donation, even if it could not pay for transplantation. In the end, we must situate recommendations about funding heart transplants and all other expensive treatments in the larger context of a social policy of macroallocation (types 1–3 discussed above).

Setting Priorities

Background history of the Oregon Health Plan. Legislators and citizens in the State of Oregon have engaged in a closely watched and pioneering effort to establish priorities in allocating health care by extending health insurance coverage to uninsured state residents below the poverty line. As the first effort to ration health care funds systematically in the United States, Oregon's plan became a focal point for discussion of every major aspect of national health policy, including access to care, cost-effectiveness, rationing, and the decent minimum. Many believed and even hoped that the Oregon plan would mark the beginning of a new era in American medical care that would bring it closer to the more systematic approaches to rationing adopted in many other countries.[70]

Faced with escalating costs and demands for more efficient and fairer access to quality health care, the Oregon legislature passed a Basic Health Services Act in July 1989 designed to ensure that all citizens with a family income below the federal poverty level would receive a decent minimum of health care coverage. This act created the Oregon Health Services Commission (OHSC), which was charged with producing a ranked priority list of services that would define what could constitute a decent minimum of coverage by Medicaid (the state/federal program that provides funds to cover medical needs for financially impoverished citizens). The goal was to fund as many top priority-ranked services as possible for all eligible citizens. In 1990, the OHSC issued a preliminary list of 1600 ranked medical procedures ranging "from the most important to the least important" services, based in part on data about quality of well-being after treatment and cost effectiveness analysis. The ranking was widely criticized as unjust and arbitrary. For example, tooth-capping was ranked above appendectomies. Later, the list was reduced to 709 ranked services, as it abandoned cost-effectiveness analysis and appealed to citizen values (gathered at community meetings). The goal became to rank items on the prioritized list by *clinical effectiveness* and *social value*. Such spare categories obviously need greater specificity, and much ingenuity has gone into these efforts in Oregon.

The following policy has been a stable part of the plan: If predetermined spending levels are insufficient to fund all desirable services when the plan is set in motion, services with the lowest priority will be eliminated from coverage. Medicaid funding will be provided for all eligible persons needing procedures as far down the list as possible, giving priority to the higher-ranked procedures. The plan does not eliminate anyone's eligibility for Medicaid coverage, and in this respect, treats everyone equally.

The Oregon Health Plan was formally implemented in 1994 as a "demonstration program" (under a waiver from the Health Care Financing Administration). The eligible population grew dramatically—from 10,000 eligibles in March 1994 to nearly 100,000 by December 1994—vastly exceeding all expectations in numbers. As a result, the number of eligibles had to be reduced, and Oregon initiated an assets test as well as eliminating all full-time students (though some students were reinstated as of 1998). Oregon had hoped to ration services, not people, but its goal was soon thrown into question. Within the state, there was initially a strong endorsement of the list of covered services, because it did succeed in expanding access. However, many procedures (e.g., incapacitating hernias, tonsillectomy, and adenoidectomy) still fell below the cut-off line of the priority list.[71]

A basic question has haunted the Oregon Plan: How high can the cutoff line be set and still constitute a decent minimum package in accordance with the demands of social justice? The history of the plan demonstrates that the priority list may be an inadequate way to manage budget short falls, which have occurred in every year.

Critics have contended that the Oregon Plan contains serious defects because it (1) fosters an "us versus them" conception of health care through its focus on benefits to the poor and (2) lacks specificity about the conditions and treatments that will and will not be covered. The sensitive issue of who would fare poorly under the Oregon Plan has also proved troublesome to resolve. Clearly some groups, such as extremely premature infants, would not do well under the plan (because treatments offer minimal to no improvement in quality of life), and some persons would fare well by being guaranteed coverage. For example, the plan ensures that the disabled and the elderly will always be eligible, and these groups should continue to receive the same benefits as they did before the revised plan.

Some have argued that Oregon's rating of net benefit by *category of treatment* is intrinsically unfair, because some patients needing any given treatment will do far better on the treatment than some other patients needing the identical treatment. If Medicaid recipients who were already being served by public programs in Oregon were made worse off, this fact would constitute a serious objection to the plan, even if the plan achieved a net reduction of inequality in the treatment of the poor. Accordingly, the fairness of the plan depends on whether, as a result of its provisions, indigent persons suffer harms (setbacks to their interests), whether the state is doing enough for indigent persons in the state, and whether alternative policies might further improve the position of indigent persons.[72]

Strategies for setting priorities.[73] In light of Oregon's experience and recent literature in biomedical ethics, the topic of *setting priorities* has emerged as the most pressing issue about justice and health policy. Several strategies have been proposed to guide policymakers.

Even before the developments in Oregon, an influential literature for setting priorities had emerged from health economics, as we saw in Chapter 5. This literature urged use of cost-effectiveness analysis (CEA), the most important version being cost–utility analysis (CUA). In this strategy, health benefits are measured in terms of anticipated health gains, whereas costs are measured in terms of expenditures of resources. The goal is utilitarian: the greatest health benefits for the money expended. Health benefits are quantified, and an attempt is made to incorporate the outcome directly into public policy by measuring the impact of interventions on both the length and quality of life. QALYs has become a generic name for such measures (see Chapter 5, pp. 206–214).

Libertarians, egalitarians, and communitarians have all raised significant objections to this strategy for setting limits. Charges of discrimination against infants, the elderly, and the disabled (especially those with permanent incapacitation and the terminally ill), as well as uncertainties about how to judge gains in quality of life, have led many to conclude that appeals to QALYs sometimes allow impermissible trade-offs in setting priorities. This literature has generated many puzzle cases. For example, will life-saving interventions (e.g., heart transplantation) lose out altogether in the competition for priority if other interventions (e.g., arthritis medication) prove to provide a greater improvement in quality of life?

Attempts to resolve such problems are numerous, and no consensus now appears on the horizon, either in health policy or in biomedical ethics. However, many now seem open to the use of utility-driven strategies to generate *data* that the public and policymakers could weigh, together with other considerations. Public preferences, sound arguments for various policy options, and knowledge of the literature of ethics and health policy could replace or constrain any morally offensive trade-offs suggested by economic analysis.[74]

One strategy proposed by some writers on this theme is to abandon direct appeals to theories of justice and instead to use a finely honed understanding of the democratic process and democratic legitimacy to reach decisions about priorities. The hope is to develop an account of fair deliberative mechanisms capable of supporting democratic procedures. For example, in the context of setting priorities in managed care, Norman Daniels and James Sabin suggest that we adopt a system of publicly accessible decision-making (and justification), together with backup processes of review and appeal.[75]

The problem with all strategies of setting limits by democratic procedure is that majority preferences, no matter how well informed and fair, will sometimes eventuate in unjust outcomes. Even if understood as a method for use primarily when all else fails, a purely procedural solution will return us to the same failures of justice that we have already encountered in health care. This literature remains relatively unclear about what makes democratic procedures fair, how to protect against unfair outcomes, whether citizen deliberators could ever satisfy the demands of true deliberative democracy, and how much real agreement they could reach. Such a system may only reflect the deep disagreements already evident in different theories of justice. Deliberative democracy in action will almost certainly express conflicting principles of justice, as well as different choices of principles for particular contexts. Accordingly, deep suspicion is warranted about purely procedural strategies for setting priorities.

Other contemporary writers have proposed that we supplement economic and utilitarian strategies of setting priorities by introducing *citizen preferences* directly into the strategies themselves. For example, Erik Nord has proposed that we replace CUA and QALYs with what he calls cost–value analysis. He suggests that we make a direct appeal to the public's preferences whenever questions of interpersonal trade-offs arise in health care. His commitment is to give the public what it wants by asking questions directly to citizens. Nord maintains that the answers given by the public are often starkly different from those found in cost–utility analyses, because the public will weigh factors such as severe incapacity and life-saving technologies more heavily than will cost–utility strategies.[76]

This approach raises several questions. It is unclear how to solicit and aggregate preferences—as well as why preferences alone should count in the public policy process. The problem of how to frame a question fairly, so that the question does not itself determine the outcome (as we discussed in Chapter 3), looms large in this method. Related issues arise about how to ask a question so that a respondent actually understands what is at stake in treating a particular disease or injury (e.g., a deadly disease that afflicts only a small number of people in a particular minority group). No less important are the problems of how to assess the validity of preferences. Any attempt to eliminate biased preferences seems to invoke some form of appeal to justice that is beyond the method itself. Yet, biases and invalid preferences are often what need to be addressed through public policy processes.

These problems with contemporary approaches to setting limits indicate that we are far from finding an acceptable strategy. Perhaps we are headed for a mixed use of these methods—and, as some libertarians have suggested,[77] to a return to the free market for solutions to some problems. The libertarian proposal is that individuals should set their own priorities in health benefits packages (perhaps through distributed vouchers) rather than to have priorities set for them by the public, even through democratic processes. Only in this way, libertarians maintain, will the market in health care become efficient and make persons accountable for their lifestyles.

This important debate over how to set priorities manifests the deep conflicts between libertarians and those who emphasize utility, equality, or community. Though some thinkers today are ready to forsake traditional theories of justice, these theories likely have staying power. What now seems *unlikely,* however, is that one of these theories will oust the others in the bid to capture fully our sense of justice in the distribution of health care.

Age-Based Rationing

A third issue focuses not on rationing by excluding services, such as heart transplants, but on rationing by excluding persons in a particular age group or at least by giving these persons lower priority. Sometimes policies provide advantages for the elderly—for example, in Medicare entitlements—but at other times policies disadvantage the elderly because of their age. For example, in the United Kingdom implicit rationing policies have excluded elderly, end-stage kidney patients from kidney dialysis and transplantation because of their age and/or expected quality of life.[78] Policies for allocating transplantable kidneys in the United

States give explicit priority to patients under 18 years of age, by starting their waiting time immediately upon registration on the waiting list of the United Network for Organ Sharing, rather than requiring that they meet certain other medical criteria, and by assigning candidates under 11 years of age four additional points and candidates 11 through 17 years of age three additional points.

Several arguments attempt to justify the explicit use of age in allocation policies, both in assigning priorities for research and treatment and in selecting particular patients for a treatment, such as dialysis. These proposals sometimes rest on judgments about the probability of successful treatment (i.e., medical utility). For instance, age may be an indicator of the probability of surviving a major operation; age could therefore be made a relevant consideration in selecting patients for major transplant procedures. Judgments of the probability of success also can include the length of time that the recipient of an organ is expected to survive, a period that is usually shorter for an older patient than for a younger patient. If anticipated QALYs is a criterion, younger patients will typically do far better than older patients.

Some philosophers have mounted other impressive arguments to justify age-based allocation of health care, both in principle and in practice. Their arguments have a particular resonance in societies in which elderly citizens (65 and older) receive a very large percentage of national annual health care expenditures, although they represent a far smaller percentage of the population. The proportion of the elderly continues to increase in most industrialized nations, particularly those 85 years old and older. In these nations, a greater percentage of health care resources is spent on the elderly over age 65 than on the entire population under age 65. For example, Belgium (the lowest) spends 1.7 times more and Finland 5.5 times more on health care for citizens over 65 than for citizens under age 65.[79] Daniels offers one influential argument for viewing age as different from race and gender for purposes of health care allocation.[80] He appeals to prudential individual decisions about health care from the perspective of an entire lifetime rather than a particular moment in time. Each age group represents a stage in a person's life span. The goal is to allocate resources prudently throughout the stages of life within a social system that provides a fair lifetime share of health care for each citizen. As prudent deliberators, we would choose (assuming conditions of scarcity) to distribute health care over a lifetime in a way that improved our chances of attaining a normal life span. We would, Daniels argues, reject a pattern that reduced our chances of reaching a normal life span but increased our chances of living beyond a normal life span if we did become elderly. Instead, we would choose to shift resources that might otherwise be consumed in prolonging the lives of the elderly to the treatment of younger persons. In this way, we would maximize each person's chances of living a normal life span.

Other arguments that focus on distribution over a lifetime appeal to principles of justice and fairness with less attention to individual prudence.[81] One argument

holds that the young should have priority for life-extending medical care because
the old have had an opportunity to live more years and, on grounds of fairness,
the young deserve chance to live those additional years. For instance, Alan
Williams approaches intergenerational equity through a "fair innings" argument.
This argument builds on the intuition that everyone is entitled to some "normal"
span (typically in a number of years) and that those who fall short are somehow
cheated, whereas those who get more live on "borrowed time." This "fair innings"
argument focuses on outcomes rather than processes or resources. It considers a
person's whole lifetime experience, and it seeks equality. Williams stresses that
this conception of intergenerational equity would *require*, not merely *permit*,
"greater discrimination against the elderly than would be dictated simply by efficiency objectives."[82]

Another approach to age-based health care rationing, proposed by Daniel Callahan, takes a communitarian perspective.[83] He argues that society should guarantee decent and basic care to all individuals, but not unlimited efforts to conquer
illness and death. Society should help the elderly live out a full and natural life
span in which life's possibilities have "on the whole been achieved" and after
which death is a "relatively acceptable event." When individuals reach the natural life span in their late seventies or early eighties, we should seek to relieve
their suffering rather than extend their lives; and we should provide long-term
care and support services as part of the basic minimum of care.[84] Callahan's age
cutoff has the advantage of practicability, but it has the disadvantage of appearing arbitrary.

All of these calls for age-based rationing face moral, political, and practical
problems.[85] Ageist attitudes and practices in some countries are probably too en-
grained to implement strong age-based rationing while also achieving solidarity
and equity. Proposals for age-based rationing could perpetuate injustice by stereo-
typing the elderly, by treating them as scapegoats because of increases in health
care costs, and by creating unnecessary conflicts between generations. Elderly
persons in each generation will complain that they did not have access to new
technologies that were developed (often using their taxes for funding) after they
passed through their earlier years, and they will claim that it would be unfair to
deny them those technologies now. These complaints would exist at the beginning of age-based allocation and would persist through new technological developments.

Some critics contend that age-based rationing of life-extending technologies
would not save substantially on resources, in part because the provision of care,
including long-term care and support services, is expensive and cannot always
be sharply differentiated from the care that prolongs life. For instance, although
six percent of the enrollees in Medicare who die within a year cost the program
28% of its budget during that year, some experts argue that saving the costs of
the last few weeks of life would not produce large reductions of costs overall,

and they note difficulties in predicting the final weeks of life for many patients. Others claim that population *aging* may be contributing far less to health care expenditures than many observers have claimed.[86]

Even if we agree that age-based allocations of health care do not necessarily violate the fair-opportunity rule, they would generally be unjust in many countries at this time. Only if a society takes a systematic approach to ensure equitable access to health care can it fairly decide the issues surrounding age-based rationing, and even then difficult questions would remain.

The Need for a Comprehensive and Coherent System

Countries lacking a comprehensive and coherent system of health care financing and delivery are destined to continue on the same trail of higher costs and larger numbers of unprotected citizens, unless they make significant changes. They must improve both utility (efficiency) and justice (fairness). Although justice and utility may appear to be opposed values, both are indispensable in shaping a health care system. Creating a more efficient system by cutting costs and providing appropriate incentives can conflict with the goal of universal access to health care, but justice-based goals of universal coverage (as well as autonomy-based goals of informed consent) also may make the system inefficient. The solution is to design or redesign a health care system that incorporates both justice and utility.

An essential part of any acceptable solution involves specifying the plan's primary objectives, together with the conditions of any morally acceptable system. Four objectives should be primary. The first objective is unobstructed access to a decent minimum of health care through some form of universal insurance coverage that operationalizes the right to health care. The forms and sources of coverage might be pluralistic (see below), but public providers will have to insure some vulnerable parties by providing a safety net.

The second objective is to develop acceptable incentives for physicians and consumer-patients. Society seeks to allocate services as efficiently as possible, whereas patients and physicians seek to optimize individual patients' care. Decision-making from one perspective conflicts with decision-making from the other perspective, creating tensions and inefficiencies.[87] To avoid these problems, some constraints will be required in order to meet the goal of a decent minimum. Unless cost consciousness and cost controls are introduced and maintained, expenditures will spiral out of control, and the necessity for rationing at the first tier will threaten the goal of providing a decent minimum.

The third objective is to construct a fair system of rationing that will not violate the decent minimum standard. Rationing at the first tier would sabotage the moral foundations of the enterprise.

Finally, the fourth objective is to implement a system that can be put into effect incrementally, without drastic disruption of basic institutions that finance and deliver health care. For example, even if a system of universal access with a single payer were adopted, some existing private and public insurance agencies could be retained for some period of time.

Several carefully reasoned proposals attempt, at least partially, to meet these objectives. Despite many differences, these proposals fall into two families: (1) unified systems and (2) pluralist systems. Plans of the first type look primarily to egalitarian justice, with utility a secondary consideration. Plans of the second type look primarily to utility (efficiency and broad coverage), with egalitarian justice a secondary consideration. Typically, pluralist systems incorporate greater freedom of choice for consumers, patients, and providers. Although we cannot here consider the details of any one plan or develop an ideal plan, we can outline these two families of plans and suggest the primary considerations that should guide us (1) in choosing one type of plan over another or (2) in attempting to render the two types coherent by employing them in different areas—for example, the first (a unitary system) at the first tier of health care and the second (a pluralist system) at the second tier in a two-tier system. A society's history, established institutions, and cultural traditions, as well as stages of technological development, will obviously affect both the desirability and feasibility of any particular proposal, including the balance among efficiency, equality, and liberty.

Unified systems. Universal access is often modeled on socialized systems, such as those in the United Kingdom, Canada, and the Scandinavian countries. In these countries, a unified national system in principle covers all citizens without reference to age, health status, medical condition, or employment status. The justification for the system is that only government can provide universal coverage and bring increases in health care expenditures in line with the gross domestic product. One proposal to implement such a system in the United States is the Physician's National Health Plan (PNHP), which would be funded by the federal government and administered by the states. The plan is that each person receives a national health card, pays no charges for services, is free to choose a provider, and is eligible to receive covered services, which include long-term and chronic care services. Physicians are free to work on a salaried basis or to practice privately. Regional boards establish private fees, and no physician would be allowed to bill the government more than the amount established by the boards. A single public payer replaces the hundreds of private insurers (including Medicaid and Medicare) that provide insurance in the United States.[88]

Although Canadians have done well with such a system, many people in the United States believe that the Canadian system cannot be successfully adapted in the United States. Many U.S. citizens and the majority of its politicians believe such a system would be bureaucratic, inefficient, and perfunctory—eventuating in long queues for poorly delivered services. Among the controversial features of the unified strategy is the elimination or near elimination of competitive aspects of the financing system. Private health insurers would have no significant function, and no incentives would be provided for consumer choice of plans. The public-sector monopoly in unified plans has been vigorously attacked on grounds of disutility. Many people question the credibility of a unified plan on grounds that that no industrialized nation that has adopted such a system has been able to create incentives to reduce waste while efficiently organizing and managing the delivery of care.

Pluralist systems. Pluralist approaches to financing health care allow for a diverse array of health plans, both profit and nonprofit, as well as both private and public. Consumers have a choice of plans, and, ideally, each plan will be responsive to consumers because all plans, with the exception of safety-net government plans, must compete for subscribers. Virtually all of these plans would rely on a mixture of tax incentives and disincentives that encourage employers to provide coverage, as well as on some form of public assistance in coverage. However, not all pluralist approaches seek universal coverage.

Pluralist approaches aim to increase both utility and justice in the system, but their overriding goal is usually to produce a wider and deeper social utility. Rarely do proponents of pluralist approaches seriously entertain a principle such as Rawls's difference principle, which holds that basic inequalities are justified only if they work to the advantage of the socially worst-off group. And few plans propose a safety net or a floor below which no citizens would be allowed to fall. This weak egalitarian strategy contrasts sharply with unified-system plans, which often make strong appeals to egalitarian principles of justice.

Neither a unified nor a pluralist strategy is disqualified as such. Both could be made ethically acceptable in particular social and historical circumstances. The major issue is how well and how fully any system realizes the four objectives listed above in a coherent package. In light of the dual values of utility and justice, the best plan is likely to be the one that most coherently promotes both values and that insists on universal access to a decent minimum of health care. Any system that can meet these conditions should be morally justifiable and should serve society well in addressing questions of macroallocation.

Rationing Scarce Treatments to Patients

Health care professionals and policymakers often must decide who will receive an available scarce medical resource that cannot be provided to all needy people. In discussing this form of rationing, often called *microallocation*, we will concentrate on priority schemes for selecting recipients of scarce health care (often in urgent circumstances). We will assess policies of rationing beyond ability of pay, according to norms of justice. Two broad approaches vie for primacy: (1) a *utilitarian* strategy that emphasizes social efficiency and maximal benefit to patients and (2) an *egalitarian* strategy that emphasizes the equal worth of persons and fair opportunity. We will argue that these approaches can be coherently combined through specification and balancing.

We will defend a system that uses two sets of substantive standards and procedural rules for rationing scarce medical resources. First, the system needs criteria and procedures to determine a qualifying pool of potential recipients, such as patients eligible for heart transplantation. Second, it requires criteria and procedures for final selection of recipients, such as the patient to receive a particular heart. We will use several examples from organ transplantation, where genuine scarcity exists and where the two-stage process is illuminating.

Screening Potential Recipients

We can arrange criteria for screening potential recipients of care in three basic categories that were originally proposed by Nicholas Rescher: constituency, progress of science, and prospect of success.[89] We will use arguments from justice to fill in critical gaps in this structure.

The constituency factor. The first criterion uses social rather than medical factors. In particular, it is determined by clientele boundaries (e.g., veterans served by medical centers that were constructed for veterans), geographic or jurisdictional boundaries (e.g., citizens of a legal jurisdiction served by a publicly funded hospital), and ability to pay (e.g., the wealthy). These criteria are entirely nonmedical, and they involve moral judgments that often are not impartial (e.g., excluding noncitizens or including only veterans). Such clientele boundaries are sometimes acceptable, but often they are indefensible. For example, some use accidents of geography to distribute organs donated for transplantation. Local use of donated organs is a poor system for assuring that the most suitable candidates receive available organs, but geographical factors do become relevant if the donated organs cannot be shipped long distances or across certain borders or institutions without risk to their viability.

The Task Force on Organ Transplantation in the United States proposed that donated organs be considered national, public resources to be distributed, within limits, according to both the needs of patients and the probability of successful transplantation.[90] In a controversial recommendation, the Task Force acknowledged that foreign nationals do not have the same moral claim on organs donated in the United States as its own citizens and residents do. In claiming that national citizenship and residency are morally relevant properties for distribution, the Task Force acknowledged that compassion should lead to the admission of some nonresident aliens. In a split vote, it recommended that nonresident aliens comprise no more than ten percent of the waiting list for cadaver kidneys donated for transplantation and that all patients on the waiting list, including nonresident aliens, have access to organs, according to the same criteria of need, probability of success, and time on the waiting list.[91]

Progress of science. The second criterion, advancement of scientific knowledge, is relevant during an experimental phase in the development of a treatment. For example, physician-investigators may justifiably exclude patients who have other diseases that might obscure the research result in order to determine whether an experimental treatment is effective and how it can be improved. This criterion of scientific progress is research-oriented, and its use rests on moral and prudential judgments about the most efficient use of resources. The factors used to select patients for participation in such research will require reassessment when a treatment becomes accepted.

Prospect of success. Whether a treatment is experimental or routine, likelihood of success is a relevant criterion because a scarce medical resource should be distributed only to patients who have a reasonable chance of benefit. Ignoring this factor is unjust, because it wastes resources, as in the case of organs that can be transplanted only once. For example, although heart-transplant surgeons sometimes list their patients as urgent priority candidates for an available heart because the patients will soon die if they do not receive a transplant, some of these patients are virtually certain to die even if they do receive the heart. High quality candidates are passed over in the process. A classification and queuing system that permits urgent need to determine priority exclusively is as unjust as it is inefficient.

The prospect of success commonly reflects judgments of medical suitability, as formulated by medical experts. However, "medical" suitability can covertly include undefended criteria, such as social worth. In 1980, the U.S. government withheld funding for heart transplants because of this problem. The criteria at Stanford—then the major cardiac transplantation center in the country—excluded patients with "a history of alcoholism, job instability, antisocial behavior, or psychiatric illness," while requiring "a stable, rewarding family and/or vocational environment to return to post-transplant." Critics held that these social criteria were inappropriate for programs receiving public funds.

Judgments of *medical utility* focus on maximizing the welfare of patients, whereas judgments of *social utility* focus on maximizing society's welfare.[92] For example, in distributing scarce organs for transplantation, medical utility requires that the organs be used in an effective and efficient way to maximize the welfare of patients suffering from end-stage organ failure. In judgments of social utility, decision-makers consider which recipient(s) of health care would contribute the most to society. Judgments of medical utility implicitly assume that the social value of all lives is equal, a dubious assumption, whereas judgments of social utility require comparative assessments of the social worth of lives, a dubious enterprise.

Controversy persists about whether current operational criteria for allocating organs, among other forms of health care, are designed to realize medical utility, social utility, or both.[93] The Task Force on Organ Transplantation excluded criteria such as race and sex as unjust, but it did not categorically exclude criteria such as age, lifestyle, and a social network of support, holding instead that these criteria require constant public scrutiny through a fair and open process.[94] Because we have already discussed age and lifestyle, we will concentrate on the social network of support, but we note in passing that age and lifestyle can help to predict medical utility or to indicate social utility.

In admitting patients to waiting lists, heart transplant programs commonly consider the existence and quality of a support network, including the family, in their judgments about the prospect of success of heart transplantation. For example, Loma Linda University explicitly noted that Baby Jesse's parents were unmarried when it initally declined to admit that child to its heart transplant waiting list. A network of support is often medically important in the overall success of the transplantation, particularly in post-transplant care, and it can have an impact on medical utility in the sense of an effective and efficient use of a donated organ. However, rules of justice, including fair opportunity, suggest that society seek alternative support systems rather than using the absence of such a network as a reason for excluding a patient from transplantation.[95]

Selecting Recipients

Standards proposed for final selection of patients have often been more controversial than those for initial screening. However, lack of consensus about screening criteria (e.g., how sick patients should be prior to admission to a waiting list) can also create problems in final selection. Debate about final selection has centered on medical utility, social utility, and impersonal mechanisms, such as lotteries and queuing. All have been used in the selection of patients.

Medical utility. We assume, as an unargued premise, that judgments about medical utility should figure into decisions to ration scarce medical resources. Differences in patients' needs and in their prospects for successful treatment are relevant considerations. If the resource is not reusable, as in the case of transplanted organs, avoidance of waste is paramount. We should also gauge selection procedures to save as many lives as possible.

Appeals to medical utility do not necessarily violate principles of justice, but some difficulties already mentioned recur here. Both need and prospect of success are value-laden concepts, and uncertainty commonly exists about likely outcomes and about the factors that contribute to success. For example, kidney transplant surgeons dispute the importance of having a good tissue match, because minor tissue mismatches can be managed by immunosuppressant medications that reduce the body's tendency to reject transplanted organs. Insisting on the seemingly objective criterion of tissue type in distributing organs can also disadvantage persons with a rare tissue type.

Furthermore, medical need and prospect of success sometimes come into conflict. For example, in intensive care units, trying to save a patient whose need is medically urgent sometimes inappropriately consumes resources that could be used to save more people.[96] Giving priority to the sickest patients or those with the most urgent medical needs may itself be unfair, because it may be a poor use of resources.[97]

Rationing schemes that altogether exclude considerations of medical utility in using resources are indefensible. However, judgments of medical utility are not sufficient by themselves if utility is roughly equal among candidates or if an unjust distribution occurs. This problem takes us to the subject of chance and queuing.

Impersonal mechanisms of chance and queuing. Both equality and fair opportunity sometimes justify the use of chance and queuing in allocating of benefits and burdens. We began this chapter by noting the oddity and unacceptability of using a lottery to distribute all social positions. However, a lottery or another system of chance is not always odd and unacceptable. If medical resources are scarce and not divisible into portions, and if no major disparities exist in medical utility for patients (particularly when selection determines life or death), then considerations of fair opportunity and equal respect may justify queuing, a lottery, or randomization—depending on which procedure is the most appropriate and feasible in the circumstances.

Similar judgments have supported the use of lotteries several times in recent years to determine who would gain access to new drugs that were available only in limited supply, either because they had only recently been approved or because they remained experimental. For instance, Berlex Laboratories held a lottery to distribute Betaseron, a new genetically engineered drug that appeared to slow the deterioration caused by multiple sclerosis, and several drug companies held lotteries to distribute a new class of compounds (protease inhibitors) to AIDS patients. In the latter case, Dr. Alberto Avendano of the National Association of People with AIDS proposed a lottery as "closest to the fairest way." At one point in the summer of 1994, more than 18,500 patients competed for about 3600 slots. Although some argued that patients with AIDS who had participated in clinical trials should have priority, others stressed the symbolic value of the lotteries: "Lotteries say that after you meet medical criteria, all persons should have an equal shot at the good of society. Lotteries celebrate an understanding that all humans are endowed with equal dignity."[98]

Yet some critics of random selection contend that the use of impersonal mechanisms reflects an irresponsible refusal to make a decision, but different reasons can be invoked to support these procedures, depending on the circumstances. Barbara Goodwin finds their justification in impartiality together with "the moral judgment that people should be treated as absolutely equal where basic life chances (chances of life or survival) are involved."[99] In addition to promoting fair opportunity and equal treatment, random methods make the selection with little investment of time and financial resources and thus provide utilitarian benefits. Lotteries can also create less stress for all involved, including patients.[100] A random system makes selections efficiently, and by-passed candidates may feel less distress at being rejected by chance than by judgments of comparative social worth.

However, both theoretical and practical problems with random selection merit consideration. One question concerns the weight of the rule "first come, first served." Under some conditions, a patient already receiving a particular treatment has a severely limited chance of survival, whereas other patients who need the treatment have a far better chance of survival. Does "first come, first served" imply that those already receiving treatment have absolute priority over those who arrive later but have either more urgent needs or better prospects of success?

One example of this problem arises in intensive care units (ICUs). Although admission to the ICU establishes a presumption in favor of continued treatment, it does not give a person an absolute claim for continuing priority, regardless of changing medical circumstances. An example appears in decisions in neonatal intensive care about the use of extracorporeal membrane oxygenation (ECMO), a form of cardiopulmonary bypass used to support newborns with life-threatening respiratory failure. ECMO qualifies as a truly scarce resource, because it is not widely available and requires the full-time presence of well-trained personnel. Robert Truog argues, rightly in our judgment, that ECMO should be withdrawn from a newborn with a poor prognosis in favor of another with a good prognosis if the latter is far more likely to survive requires the therapy and cannot be safely transferred to another facility.[101] Such displacement of a child from the ICU requires justification, but it does not constitute abandonment or injustice if other forms of care are provided.

Accordingly, our arguments for the use of mechanisms of chance or queuing in rationing health care to patients apply only if no major disparities in medical utility exist. Which mechanism, queuing or chance, is preferable will depend largely on practical considerations, but queuing appears to be feasible and acceptable in many health care settings, including emergency medicine, ICUs, and organ transplant lists. A complicating factor is that some people do not enter the queue (or the lottery) in time because of factors such as slowness in seeking help, inadequate or incompetent medical attention, delay in referral, or overt discrimination. A system is unfair if some people gain an advantage in access over others because they are better educated, better connected, or have more money for frequent visits to physicians. A regular lottery would reduce this problem, but it also might introduce other forms of unfairness unless carefully controlled for medical utility.

Social utility. Although criteria of social utility are controversial, the comparative social value of potential recipients is, under some conditions, a relevant and even decisive consideration. An analogy often used to show the importance of such judgments is that of giving priority to some sailors familiar with the dangers of a crowded lifeboat to increase the chances of saving more people than would otherwise be saved. Another familiar (though more disputed) example comes from World War II, when the scarce resource of penicillin was distributed to U.S. soldiers suffering from venereal disease rather than to those suffering from battle wounds. The rationale was military need: The soldiers suffering from venereal disease could be restored to battle more quickly.[102]

An argument in favor of social–utilitarian selection is that medical institutions and personnel are trustees of society and must consider the probable future contributions of patients in need of scarce lifesaving resources. However, we might keep such judgments of social worth separate from medical care in order to protect the relationship of personal care and trust between patients and physicians, which would be seriously threatened if physicians were trained to look beyond their patients' needs to society's needs. Other problems center on reduction of persons to their social roles and functions, and violation of equal respect for persons.[103]

We acknowledge the merit of all the above criticisms of social worth criteria. However, we argue below that, in certain rare and exceptional cases involving persons of critical social importance, criteria of social value are appropriately overriding.

Triage. Defenders of social–utilitarian calculations in rationing health care sometimes invoke the model of triage, which has become increasingly common in health care facilities. The French term *triage* means "sorting," "picking," or "choosing." It has been applied to sorting items, such as wool and coffee beans, according to their quality. In the delivery of health care, triage is a process of developing and using criteria for prioritization. It has been used in war, in community disasters, and in emergency rooms where injured persons have been sorted for medical attention, according to their needs and prospects. Decisions to admit and to discharge patients from ICUs often involve some form of triage. The objective is to use available medical resources as effectively and as efficiently as possible. The traditional and contemporary rationale has been utilitarian: Do the greatest good for the greatest number.[104]

Triage decisions often appeal to medical utility rather than social utility in determining the maximal utilitarian outcome. For example, disaster victims are generally sorted according to medical need. Those who have major injuries and will die without immediate help, but who can be salvaged, are ranked first; those whose treatment can be delayed without immediate danger are ranked second; those with minor injuries are ranked third; and those for whom no treatment will be efficacious are ranked fourth. This priority scheme is fair and does not involve judgments about individuals' comparative social worth.

However, judgments of comparative social worth are inescapable and acceptable in some situations. For example, in an earthquake when some injured survivors are medical personnel who suffer only minor injuries, they justifiably receive priority of treatment if they are needed to help others. Similarly, in an outbreak of infectious disease, it is justifiable to inoculate physicians and nurses first to enable them to care for others. Under such conditions, a person may receive priority for treatment on grounds of social utility if and only if his or her contribution is indispensable to attaining a major social goal. As in analogous lifeboat cases, we should limit judgments of comparative social value to the specific qualities and skills that are essential to the community's immediate protection, without assessing the *general* social worth of persons. If we limit exceptions based on social utility to emergencies involving necessity, they do not threaten the ordinary moral universe or imply the general acceptability of social–utilitarian calculations in distributing health care.

Our contention, then, is that principles and rules of justice, in conjunction with other principles, mandate attention to medical utility, followed by the use of chance or queuing for scarce resources when medical utility is roughly equal for eligible patients. Considerations of utility may be legitimately invoked in cases in which the favored individuals, when treated, can contribute to a better overall outcome. This nexus of standards should prove to be both coherent and stable despite mixed appeals to egalitarian justice and utility.

The contrast between our proposals and a system such as Nicholas Rescher's is significant. His system relies on social utility until no major disparities in social value appear among the candidates for a scarce resource. At this point, he resorts to chance. By contrast, our approach starts with medical need and probability of successful treatment (medical utility), and then uses chance and queuing as ways to express fairness and equality, unless major disparities exist in potential recipients' specific social responsibilities and probable social contributions in an emergency.

This structure of ethical considerations requires careful monitoring because of evidence that nonethical and even unethical factors play roles in rationing health care. For example, some studies have suggested that in ICUs the number of cases of severely ill patients denied admission would increase as bed availability decreased. To investigate an operative assumption that medical condition and suitability controlled admission, researchers used retrospective chart review to determine the factors that actually influenced patient-selection decisions in a surgical ICU. The study occurred during a temporary nursing shortage that resulted in the closure of two to six of the unit's 16 beds over a three-month period. The researchers discovered that considerations other than medical suitability and severity of illness decisively influenced bed allocation: "political power [in the institution], medical provincialism [one service pitted against another], and income maximization overrode medical suitability in the provision of critical care services."[105]

Conclusion

In this chapter we have examined several philosophical theories and approaches to justice, including egalitarian, communitarian, libertarian, and utilitarian theories. We have maintained that no single theory of justice or system of distributing health care is necessary or sufficient for constructive reflection on health policy. Our discussions in Chapter 1 (and in Chapters 8 and 9) expose several limitations in the use of general ethical theories, and those limitations are particularly prominent in debates about what justice implies for allocation decisions. Each influential theory of justice provides a philosophical reconstruction of a valid perspective on the moral life, but one that only partially captures the range and diversity of that life.

The richness of our moral practices, traditions, and theories helps explain why diverse theories of justice have all received skillful defenses in recent philosophy. In the absence of a social consensus about these competing theories of justice, we can expect that public policies will shift ground, now emphasizing one theory, later emphasizing another. The existence of these rival theories does not justify the piecemeal approach that many countries, including the United States, have taken to their health care systems. A piecemeal approach avoids asking larger questions of justice about what the people of a nation should expect from their health care system and how the nation can address citizens' needs for increased insurance, long-term care, and the like.

Policies of just access to and financing of health care, together with strategies of efficiency in health care institutions, dwarf in social importance every other issue considered in this book. Many barriers exist to achieving access to health care. For millions who encounter those barriers, a just health care system remains a distant goal. Even though every society must ration access to health care through some mechanism(s), many societies can close gaps in access more conscientiously than they have to date. We have suggested a general perspective from which to approach these problems. In particular, we have proposed that society recognize an enforceable right to a decent minimum of health care within a framework for allocation that incorporates both utilitarian and egalitarian standards.

Notes

1. Jorge Luis Borges, *Labyrinths* (New York: New Directions, 1962), pp. 30–35.
2. For example, Onora O'Neill construes justice in terms of universal principles that require avoidance of action that "injures either systematically or gratuitously." See her *Towards Justice and Virtue: A Constructive Account of Practical Reasoning* (Cambridge: Cambridge University Press, 1996).
3. In addition to Robert Nozick's emphasis on *entitlement* and John Rawls's emphasis on justice as *fairness* (see below), Brian Barry interprets justice as *impartiality* in his *Justice as Impartiality* (Oxford: Clarendon Press, 1995). For attention to justice as *desert*, see Alasdair MacIntyre, *Whose Justice, Which Rationality?* (Notre Dame, IN: University of Notre Dame Press, 1988).
4. See Carol Levine, "Changing Views of Justice after Belmont: AIDS and the Inclusion of 'Vulnerable' Subjects," in *The Ethics of Research Involving Human Subjects: Facing the 21st Century,* ed. Harold Y. Vanderpool (Frederick, MD: University Publishing Group, 1996), p. 106.
5. For valuable essays, see Jeffrey P. Kahn, Anna C. Mastroianni, and Jeremy Sugarman, eds., *Beyond Consent: Seeking Justice in Research* (New York: Oxford University Press, 1998).
6. See, for example, Guido Calabresi and Philip Bobbitt, *Tragic Choices* (New York: W.W. Norton, 1978).
7. See, for example, Nicholas Rescher, *Distributive Justice* (Indianapolis, IN: Bobbs-Merrill, 1966), ch. 4. Rescher's list stems in part from John A. Ryan, *Distributive Justice: The Right and Wrong of Our Present Distribution of Wealth* (New York: The Macmillan Company, 1922), ch. XV, "The Principal Canons of Distributive Justice."
8. This case was reported by Robert E. Stevenson in *Hastings Center Report* 10 (December 1980): 25.
9. *International Union, UAW v. Johnson Controls,* 111 S.Ct. 1196 (1991).
10. Robert Nozick, *Anarchy, State, and Utopia* (New York: Basic Books, 1974), esp. pp. 149–82.
11. See Alasdair MacIntyre, *Whose Justice? Which Rationality?*, pp. 1, 390–403. For a strong (but problematic) communitarian approach to health promotion, see David R. Buchanan, *An Ethic for Health Promotion: Rethinking the Sources of Human Well-Being* (New York: Oxford University Press, 2000).
12. See Henk Ten Have and Helen Keasberry, "Equity and Solidarity: The Context of Health Care in the Netherlands," *Journal of Medicine and Philosophy* 17 (August 1992): 463–77, esp. 474–76.
13. Ezekiel J. Emanuel, *The Ends of Human Life: Medical Ethics in a Liberal Polity* (Cambridge, MA: Harvard University Press, 1991).
14. Michael Walzer, *Spheres of Justice: A Defense of Pluralism and Equality* (New York: Basic Books, 1983), esp. pp. 86–94.
15. Rawls, "Kantian Constructivism in Moral Theory" (The Dewey Lectures), *Journal of Philosophy* 77 (1980): 519. Rawls has progressively emphasized Kantian conceptions of rationality less and traditions in modern constitutional democracies more. See his *Political Liberalism* (New York: Columbia University Press, 1996).
16. Daniels, *Just Health Care* (New York: Cambridge University Press, 1985), pp. 34–58.
17. For the distinction between equality of welfare and equality of resources, see Ronald Dworkin, "What is Equality? Part I: Equality of Welfare," *Philosophy and Public Affairs* 10 (Summer 1981): 185–246; Dworkin, "What is Equality? Part 2: Equality of Resources," *Philosophy and Public Affairs* 10 (Fall 1981): 283–345. See also

G. A. Cohen, "Equality of What? On Welfare, Resources and Capabilities," in *The Quality of Life*, ed. Martha Nussbaum and Amartya Sen (Oxford: Clarendon Press, 1992).

18. See Norman Daniels, Bruce Kennedy, and Ichiro Kawachi, "Justice Is Good for Our Health," *Boston Review* 25 (February/March 2000): 4–19 (with responses), from which this discussion draws, unless otherwise indicated. A related version of the essay by Daniels and colleagues appears in "Why Justice Is Good for Our Health: The Social Determinants of Health Inequalities," in "Bioethics and Beyond," *Daedalus* 128 (Fall 1999): 215–51. See further Ichiro Kawachi and Bruce P. Kennedy, "Income Inequality and Health: Pathways and Mechanisms," *HSR: Health Services Research* 34 (April 1999, Part II): 215–27; and Ichiro Kawachi, Bruce Kennedy, and Richard G. Wilkinson, eds., *Income Inequality and Health: A Reader* (New York: New Press, 1999).

19. Daniels and colleagues draw on Goran Dahlgren and Margaret Whitehead, *Policies and Strategies to Promote Social Equality in Health* (Stockholm: Institute of Future Studies, 1991).

20. Critics of this line of argument contend that the problem within wealthier societies is still largely one of pockets of poverty, rather than one of social inequality itself. Some critics charge that focusing on income redistribution rather than on increased access to health care is a mistake in countries where universal access to health care has a significant chance of successful implementation. See further Ezekiel Emanuel, "Political Problems," *Boston Review* 25 (2000): 14–15.

21. Rawls, *A Theory of Justice* (Cambridge, MA: Harvard University Press, 1971; revised edition, 1999), pp. 73f (1999: pp. 63–65) (italics added).

22. See Bernard Williams, "The Idea of Equality," as reprinted in *Justice and Equality*, ed. Hugo Bedau (Englewood Cliffs, NJ: Prentice-Hall, 1971), p. 135; Jeff McMahan, "Cognitive Disability, Misfortune, and Justice," *Philosophy and Public Affairs* 25 (1996): 3–35; and Janet Radcliffe Richards, "Equality of Opportunity," *Ratio* 10 (1997): 253–79.

23. H. Tristram Engelhardt, Jr., "Health Care Allocations: Responses to the Unjust, the Unfortunate, and the Undesirable," in *Justice and Health Care*, ed. Earl Shelp (Dordrecht, Holland: Kluwer Press, 1981), pp. 126–27; Engelhardt, *The Foundations of Bioethics*, 2nd ed. (New York: Oxford University Press, 1996), ch. 8; and Gert Jan Van Der Wilt, "Health Care and the Principle of Fair Equality of Opportunity," *Bioethics* 8 (1994): 329–49.

24. Nancy S. Jecker, "Can an Employer-Based Health Insurance System Be Just?" *Journal of Health Politics, Policy and Law* 18 (1993): 657–73; Lisa Cooper-Patrick, et al., "Race, Gender, and Partnership in the Patient–Physician Relationship," *Journal of the American Medical Association* 282 (August 11, 1999): 583–89; and Kim Lutzen and Conny Nordin, "The Influence of Gender, Education and Experience on Moral Sensitivity in Psychiatric Nursing: A Pilot Study," *Nursing Ethics* 2 (1995): 41–50.

25. Kenneth C. Goldberg, Arthur J. Hartz, Steven J. Jacobsen, et al., "Racial and Community Factors Influencing Coronary Artery Bypass Graft Surgery Rates for All 1986 Medicare Patients," *Journal of the American Medical Association* 267 (March 18, 1992): 1473–77; and Lucian L. Leape, et al., "Underuse of Cardiac Procedures: Do Women, Ethnic Minorities, and the Uninsured Fail To Receive Needed Revascularization?" *Annals of Internal Medicine* 130 (February 2, 1999): 183–92. In the latter study, no differences were found in use rates by sex, ethnic group, or payer status in 13 New York city hospitals.

26. See Edward L. Hannan, et al., "Access to Coronary Artery Bypass Surgery by Race/Ethnicity and Gender Among Patients Who Are Appropriate for Surgery," *Medical Care* 37 (1999): 68–77. See also Eric D. Peterson, et. al., "Racial Variation in the Use of Coronary-Revascularization Procedures: Are the Differences Real? Do They Matter?" *New England Journal of Medicine* 336 (February 13, 1997): 480–86; and Wayne H. Giles, et al., "Race and Sex Differences in Rates of Invasive Cardiac Procedures in U.S. Hospitals: Data from the National Hospital Discharge Survey," *Archives of Internal Medicine* 155 (February 13, 1995): 318–24. The latter studies contrast sharply with the findings in Leape, et al. (see previous note).

27. See P. B. Bach, et al., "Racial Differences in the Treatment of Early-Stage Lung Cancer," *New England Journal of Medicine* 341 (1999): 1198–1205; and Talmadge E. King, Jr., and Paul Brunetta, "Racial Disparity in Rates of Surgery for Lung Cancer," *New England Journal of Medicine* 341 (1999): 1231–33. See also M. A. Haynes and B. D. Smedley, eds., *The Unequal Burden of Cancer: An Assessment of NIH Research and Programs for Ethnic Minorities and the Medically Underserved* (Washington, DC: National Academy Press, 1999).

28. See John Z. Ayanian, et al., "The Effect of Patients' Preferences on Racial Differences in Access to Renal Transplantation," *New England Journal of Medicine* 341 (November 25, 1999): 1661–69; see also Norman G. Levinsky, "Quality and Equity in Dialysis and Renal Transplantation," *New England Journal of Medicine* 341 (November 25, 1999): 1691–93.

29. UNOS, "Heart Allocation Policy," *UNOS Update* 5 (1989): 1–2; see James F. Childress, "Fairness in the Allocation and Delivery of Health Care," in *A Time to Be Born and a Time to Die: The Ethics of Choice*, ed. Barry S. Kogan (New York: Aldine de Gruyter, 1991), ch. 11, and in Childress, *Practical Reasoning in Bioethics* (Bloomington, IN: Indiana University Press, 1997), ch. 12.

30. See Office of the Inspector General, *The Distribution of Organs for Transplantation: Expectations and Practices*, OEI-01-89-00550 (Washington, DC: U.S. Department of Health and Human Services, Office of Analysis and Inspection, 1991). A follow-up study found that from 1988 to 1994, the median waiting time for whites for a kidney transplant increased from 11.3 months to 20.1 months (78%), while the median waiting time for blacks increased from 20.1 months to 39.7 months (98%). See Office of Inspector General, *Racial and Geographic Disparity in the Distribution of Organs for Transplantation*, OEI-01-98-00360 (Washington, DC: U.S. Department of Health and Human Services, June 1998). Another study covering a slightly longer period than the 1991 report found only a 29% increase in waiting time for blacks and attributed the overall disparity in waiting time to various factors, including the fact that more whites were likely to be on multiple waiting lists, a fact that raises other issues of justice. See Fred P. Sanfilippo, et al., "Factors Affecting the Waiting Time of Cadaveric Kidney Transplant Candidates in the United States," *Journal of the American Medical Association* 267 (January 8, 1992): 247–52.

31. See Robert M. Veatch, "Allocating Organs by Utilitarianism Is Seen as Favoring Whites over Blacks," *Kennedy Institute of Ethics Newsletter* 3 (July 1989). Contrast Sanfilippo, et al., "Factors Affecting the Waiting Time of Cadaveric Kidney Transplant Candidates in the United States," which found that the changes in UNOS policy to emphasize HLA match "did not worsen the disparity in waiting time for black or presensitized patients" (p. 247).

32. Considerations of justice played a role in the UNOS decision in the mid-1990s to alter the point system for the allocation of cadaveric kidneys by eliminating points for some levels of match and increasing the role of time on the waiting list. See *1994*

Annual Report of the U.S. Scientific Registry for Transplant Recipients and the Organ Procurement and Transplantation Network-Transplant Data: 1988–1993 (Richmond, VA: UNOS, and Bethesda, MD: Divison of Organ Transplantation, Bureau of Health Resources Development, Health Resources and Services Administration, U.S. Department of Health and Human Services, 1994), V–6–7.

33. Council on Ethical and Judicial Affairs, American Medical Association, "Gender Disparities in Clinical Decision Making," *Journal of the American Medical Association* 266 (July 24, 1991): 559–662.

34. Richard M. Steingart, et al., "Sex Differences in the Management of Coronary Artery Disease," *New England Journal of Medicine* 325 (July 25, 1991): 226–30. See also John Z. Ayanian and Arnold M. Epstein, "Differences in the Use of Procedures between Women and Men Hospitalized for Coronary Heart Disease," *New England Journal of Medicine* 325 (July 25, 1991): 221–25.

35. Bernadine Healy, a former Director of the National Institutes of Health, noted that "the problem is to convince both the lay and medical sectors that coronary heart disease is also a women's disease, not a man's disease in disguise. [As in Isaac B. Singer's story, *Yentl the Yeshiva Boy*] being 'just like a man' has historically been a price women have had to pay for equality." Bernadine Healy, "The Yentl Syndrome," *New England Journal of Medicine* 325 (July 25, 1991): 274–76. See, further, R. Strauss, et al., "Effects of Morbidity, Age, Gender, and Region on Percutaneous Transluminal Coronary Angioplasty Utilisation," *Public Health* 113 (1999): 79–87; and Evelyne Shuster, "For Her Own Good: Protecting (and Neglecting) Women in Research," *Cambridge Quarterly of Healthcare Ethics* 5 (1996): 346–61.

36. Gerard F. Anderson, "In Search of Value: An International Comparison of Cost, Access, and Outcomes," *Health Affairs* 16 (1997): 163–71. This study shows that the United States is frequently in the bottom quartile of industrialized nations in indicators such as life expectancy and infant mortality.

37. The Kaiser Commission on Medicaid and the Uninsured, *Uninsured in America: A Chart Book*, prepared by Catherine Hoffman (Kaiser Family Foundation, 1998) esp. Sect. 1, Figure 10; Kenneth E. Thorpe, "Expanding Employment-Based Health Insurance: Is Small Group Reform the Answer?" *Inquiry* 29 (1992): 128–36; and Employee Benefit Research Institute, *Issue Brief*, No. 104 (July, 1990).

38. See Norman Daniels, "Insurability and the HIV Epidemic: Ethical Issues in Underwriting," *The Milbank Quarterly* 68 (1990): 497–525; and Office of Technology Assessment, U.S. Congress, *AIDS and Health Insurance* (Washington, DC: OTA, 1988).

39. We do not suppose that these examples are uncontroversial. They are intended to illustrate specific rights to health care and the kinds of arguments that may support them. For some of these examples, see Allen E. Buchanan, "The Right to a Decent Minimum of Health Care," *Philosophy and Public Affairs* 13 (Winter 1984): 66–67. For another example, see our discussion below of the debate about funding organ transplants.

40. For more detail regarding these and other arguments, see Tom L. Beauchamp, "The Right to Health Care in a Capitalistic Democracy," in *Rights to Health Care*, ed. T. J. Bole III and W. B. Bondeson (Boston: D. Reidel, 1992); and James F. Childress, *Practical Reasoning in Bioethics,* Chapter 13.

41. See Loren E. Lomasky, "Medical Progress and National Health Care," *Philosophy and Public Affairs* 10 (1980): 72–73; and Gary E. Jones, "The Right to Health Care and the State," *Philosophical Quarterly* 33 (1983): 278–87.

42. See Daniels, *Just Health Care*, ch. 3 and 4.

43. Allen Buchanan, "Health-Care Delivery and Resource Allocation," in *Medical Ethics,* 2nd ed., ed. Robert M. Veatch (Boston: Jones and Bartlett Publishers, 1997), esp. pp. 355–59.

44. See Brown, "The Medically Uninsured;" Allen Buchanan, "Health-Care Delivery and Resource Allocation;" and Gerald M. Oppenheimer and Robert A. Padgug, "AIDS: The Risks to Insurers, the Threat to Equity," *Hastings Center Report* 16 (October 1986): 18–22.

45. See Mary Ann Baily, "Defining the Decent Minimum," in *Health Care Reform: A Human Rights Approach,* ed. Audrey Chapman (Washington, DC: Georgetown University Press, 1994), pp. 167–85; Robert M. Veatch, "Single Payers and Multiple Lists: Must Everyone Get the Same Coverage in a Universal Health Plan?" *Kennedy Institute of Ethics Journal* 7 (1997): 153–69; Alastair V. Campbell, "Defining Core Health Services: The New Zealand Experience," *Bioethics* 9 (1995): 252–58.

46. A study that supports this conclusion is Peter A. Ubel, et al., "Cost-Effectiveness Analysis in a Setting of Budget Constraints—Is It Equitable?" *New England Journal of Medicine* 334 (May 2, 1996): 1174–77.

47. The immense difficulties of reforming the U.S. system, or "nonsystem," were never more evident than in the controversy about and subsequent defeat of the Clinton health plan. For discussion, see Norman Daniels, "The Articulation of Values and Principles Involved in Health Care Reform," *Journal of Medicine and Philosophy* 19 (1994): 425–33; Wendy K. Mariner, "Patients' Rights to Care under Clinton's Health Security Act: The Structure of Reform," *American Journal of Public Health* 84 (1994): 1330–35; H. Tristram Engelhardt, "Health Care Reform: A Study in Moral Malfeasance," *Journal of Medicine and Philosophy* 19 (1994): 501–16.

48. A two-tiered conception has been under discussion in many countries. See, for example, Ruud H. J. ter Meulen, "Limiting Solidarity in the Netherlands: A Two-Tier System on the Way," *Journal of Medicine and Philosophy* 20 (1995): 607–16; Lars F. Hansson, Ole Frithjof Norheim, and Knut W. Ruyter, "Equality, Explicitness, Severity, and Rigidity: The Oregon Plan Evaluated from a Scandinavian Perspective," *Journal of Medicine and Philosophy* 19 (1994): 343–66; Gert Jan van der Wilt, "Towards a Two-Tier Health System in the Netherlands: How to Put Theory into Practice," *Journal of Medicine and Philosophy* 20 (1995): 617–30; Gwen Gray, "Access to Medical Care Under Strain: New Pressures in Canada and Australia," *Journal of Health Politics, Policy and Law* 23 (1998): 905–47; Soren Holm, " 'Socialized Medicine,' Resource Allocation and Two-tiered Health Care—The Danish Experience," *Journal of Medicine and Philosophy* 20 (1995): 631–37; Octavi Quintana and Alberto Infante, "Setting Priorities in the Spanish Health Care System," *Journal of Medicine and Philosophy* 20 (1995): 595–606.

49. *Securing Access to Health Care*, vol. I, p. 42.

50. This discussion of Dworkin's position draws from his "Will Clinton's Plan Be Fair?" *New York Review of Books*, January 13, 1994, pp. 20–25; and "Justice in the Distribution of Health Care," *McGill Law Journal* 38 (1993): 883–98. His position combines an argument for a right to health care with a limitation on that right, both based on the ideal prudential insurer. For an appeal to actual, in contrast to hypothetical, prudence (influenced by David Hume), see Larry R. Churchill, *Self-Interest and Universal Health Care: Why Well-Insured Americans Should Support Coverage for Everyone* (Cambridge, MA: Harvard University Press, 1994).

51. For a careful analysis and critique of Dworkin's and other hypothetical choice models, see Madison Powers, "Hypothetical Choice Approaches to Health Care Alloca-

tion," in *Allocating Health Care Resources, Biomedical Ethics Reviews*, ed. James
M. Humber and Robert F. Almeder (Totowa, NJ: Humana Press, 1995), pp. 55–84.

52. Robert M. Veatch, "Voluntary Risks to Health: The Ethical Issues," *Journal of the
American Medical Association* 243 (January 4, 1980): 50–55.

53. Louise B. Russell, "Some of the Tough Decisions Required by a National Health
Plan," *Science* 246 (Nov. 17, 1989): 892–96.

54. See, for example, Howard Leichter, *Free to Be Foolish: Politics and Health Promotion in the United States and Great Britain* (Princeton, NJ: Princeton University
Press, 1991), p. 38.

55. These data are from the United Network for Organ Sharing (UNOS), which is the
source of other data about transplantation in this chapter unless otherwise indicated.
See, in particular, *1999 Annual Report of the U.S. Scientific Registry of Transplant
Recipients and the Organ Procurement and Transplantation Network: Transplant
Data: 1989–1998* (Rockville, MD: U.S. Department of Health and Human Services,
Health Resources and Services Administration, Office of Special Programs, Divi-
sion of Transplantation; and Richmond, VA: UNOS, 1999).

56. T. E. Starzl, D. Van Thiel, A. G. Tzakis, et al., "Orthotopic Liver Transplantation for
Alcoholic Cirrhosis," *Journal of the American Medical Association* 260 (November
4, 1988): 2542–44; and A. DiMartini, et al., "Outcome of Liver Transplantation in
Critically Ill Patients with Alcoholic Cirrhosis: Survival According to Medical Variables and Sobriety," *Transplantation* 66 (1998): 298–302.

57. Alvin H. Moss and Mark Siegler, "Should Alcoholics Compete Equally for Liver
Transplantation?" *Journal of the American Medical Association* 265 (March 13,
1991): 1295–98.

58. Robert Veatch argues that we should consider justice in giving fewer points in the
allocation system to patients with a history of alcoholism, because individuals are
entitled to opportunities for health and have a duty not to squander those opportunities. See Robert M. Veatch, *The Ethics of Organ Transplantation* (Washington, DC:
Georgetown University Press, 2000). See also Walter Glannon, "Responsibility, Alcoholism, and Liver Transplantation," *Journal of Medicine and Philosophy* 23 (1998):
31–49, which adopts a personal control and responsibility model.

59. An argument based on justice against the total exclusion of alcoholics from liver
transplantation appears in Carl Cohen, Martin Benjamin, and the Ethics and Social
Impact Committee of the [Michigan] Transplant and Health Policy Center, "Alcoholics and Liver Transplantation," *Journal of the American Medical Association* 265
(March 13, 1991): 1299–1301.

60. Daniels, *Just Health Care*, p. 2.

61. This line of argument is reasonable, but a proviso is essential. If a society did not
allocate sufficient funds to provide a decent minimum of health care, the system itself would be unjust. Questions about the justice or injustice of particular allocation
decisions—for example, to fund or not to fund heart transplants—cannot be adequately processed or resolved without a prior guarantee of a decent minimum.

62. An illuminating discussion of this issue is found in Paul T. Menzel, *Medical Costs,
Moral Choices* (New Haven, CT: Yale University Press, 1983), ch. 7.

63. A classic article on this now commonplace distinction is Thomas C. Schelling, "The
Life You Save May Be Your Own," in *Problems in Public Expenditure Analysis*, ed.
Samuel B. Chase, Jr. (Washington, DC: Brookings Institution, 1966), pp. 127–76.

64. Henry J. Aaron and William B. Schwartz, *The Painful Prescription: Rationing Hospital Care* (Washington, DC: The Brookings Institutions, 1984); and "Rationing Hos-

pital Care: Lessons from Britain," *New England Journal of Medicine* 330 (January 5, 1984): 52–56. For a critical response to their interpretation of the situation in Great Britain, see Frances H. Miller and Graham A. H. Miller, *"The Painful Prescription*: A Procrustean Perspective?" *New England Journal of Medicine* 314 (1986): 1383–86. For an examination of allocation decisions of type 3 in the U.K., see Rudolf Klein, Patricia Day, and Sharon Aedmayne, *Managing Scarcity: Priority Setting and Rationing in the National Health Service* (Buckingham, England: Open University Press, 1996).

65. For a valuable discussion of "rationing," and a defense of its broad use, see Peter A. Ubel, *Pricing Life: Why It's Time for Health Care Rationing* (Cambridge, MA: The MIT Press, 2000).

66. *UNOS Transplant Patient Data Sources* (as of Oct. 22, 1999); *1999 Annual Report of the U.S. Scientific Registry for Transplant Recipients and the Organ Procurement and Transplantation Network: Transplant Data: 1989–1998*. For an overview of the developments into 1986, see U.S. Department of Health and Human Services, Report of Task Force on Organ Transplantation, *Organ Transplantation: Issues and Recommendations* (Washington, DC: DHHS, 1986). See also Institute of Medicine, "Improving the Nation's Organ Transplantation System" (http://www.iom.edu/iom/iomhome.nsf/pages/1999+reports).

67. Task Force, *Organ Transplantation*, pp. 11, 105.

68. Roger W. Evans, et al., *The National Health Transplantation Study* (Seattle: Battelle Human Affairs Research Centers, 1984), vols. I–V; and Evans, *Executive Summary: The National Cooperative Transplantation Study*, BHARC-100-91-020 (Washington, DC: U.S. Department of Commerce, June 1991). See also *1999 Annual Report of the U.S. Scientific Registry of Transplant Recipients and the Organ Procurement and Transplantation Network: Transplant Data: 1989–1998*, pp. 179–88.

69. Contrast Norman Daniels, "Comment: Ability to Pay and Access to Transplantation," *Transplantation Proceedings* 21 (June 1989): 3434. For a sharp criticism, see F. M. Kamm, "The Report of the U.S. Task Force on Organ Transplantation: Criticisms and Alternatives," *Mount Sinai Journal of Medicine* 56 (May 1989): 207–20.

70. Oregon Senate Bill 27 (March 31, 1989). See also Lawrence Jacobs, Theodore Marmor, and Jonathan Oberlander, "The Oregon Health Plan and the Political Paradox of Rationing: What Advocates and Critics Have Claimed and What Oregon Did," *Journal of Health Politics, Policy and Law* 24 (1999): 161–80; David M. Eddy, "What's Going on in Oregon?" *Journal of the American Medical Association* 266 (July 17, 1991): 417–20.

71. Health Economics Research, Inc., for the Health Care Financing Administration, *Evolution of the Oregon Plan* (Washington: NTIS No. PB98-135916 INZ, Dec. 12, 1997, as updated Jan. 19, 1999). Oregon Department of Administrative Services, *Assessment of the Oregon Health Plan Medicaid Demonstration* (Salem, OR: Office for Oregon Health Plan Policy and Research, 1999).

72. See Norman Daniels, "Is the Oregon Rationing Plan Fair?" *Journal of the American Medical Association* 265 (May 1, 1991): 2232–35. In early 2000, Oregon Announced a new public outreach initiative to evaluate "the appropriateness and effectiveness of the process used to prioritize health services." *Oregon Health Policy Quarterly* (January 21, 2000): 1.

73. This section is indebted to Madison Powers and Ruth Faden, "Inequalities in Health, Inequalities in Health Care: Four Generations of Discussion about Justice and Cost-Effectiveness Analysis," *Kennedy Institute of Ethics Journal* 10 (2000): 109–27.

74. L. B. Russell, et al., "The Role of Cost-Effectiveness Analysis in Health and Medicine," *Journal of the American Medical Association* 276, no. 14 (1996): 1172–77; see also Frances M. Kamm, *Morality, Mortality: Death and Whom To Save From It*, vol. 1 (New York: Oxford University Press, 1993).

75. Norman Daniels and James E. Sabin, "Last Chance Therapies and Managed Care: Pluralism, Fair Procedures, and Legitimacy," *Hastings Center Report* 28, (March/April 1998): 27–41. See also the widely discussed work on deliberative democracy by Dennis Thompson and Amy Gutmann, *Democracy and Disagreement* (Cambridge: The Belknap Press of Harvard University Press, 1996).

76. Erik Nord, *Cost-Value Analysis in Health Care: Making Sense out of QALY's* (Cambridge: Cambridge University Press, 1999). See similar issues raised in Paul Menzel, "How Should What Economists Call 'Social Values' Be Measured?" *Journal of Ethics* 3 (1999): 249–73; and Christopher Murray and Arnab Acharya, "Understanding DALYs," *Journal of Health Economics* 16 (1997): 703–30.

77. See John C. Goodman and Gerald L. Musgrave, *Patient Power: Solving America's Health Care Crisis* (Washington, DC: Cato Institute, 1992).

78. John McKenzie, et al., "Dialysis Decision Making in Canada, the United Kingdom, and the United States," *American Journal of Kidney Diseases* 31 (1998): 12–18; Adrian Furnham and Abigail Ofstein, "Ethical Ideology and the Allocation of Scarce Medical Resources," *British Journal of Medical Psychology* 70 (1997): 51–63; A. J. Wing, "Why Don't the British Treat More Patients with Kidney Failure?" *British Medical Journal* 287 (1983): 1157; and V. Parsons and P. Lock, "Triage and the Patient with Renal Failure," *Journal of Medical Ethics* 6 (1980): 173–76.

79. See Binstock and Post, eds., *Too Old for Health Care?, passim;* and Organization for Economic Co-operation and Development, *Financing and Delivering Health Care* (Paris: OECD, 1987), esp. p. 90; Erik Nord, et al., "The Significance of Age and Duration of Effect in Social Evaluation of Health Care," *Health Care Analysis* 4 (1996): 103–11.

80. See especially Daniels, *Just Health Care*, ch. 5, and *Am I My Parents' Keeper?* (New York: Oxford University Press, 1988). Our discussion is drawn from the latter unless otherwise indicated.

81. See, for example, Robert M. Veatch, "How Age Should Matter: Justice as the Basis for Limiting Care to the Elderly," in *Facing Limits: Ethics and Health Care for the Elderly*, ed. Gerald R. Winslow and James W. Walters (Boulder, CO: Westview Press, 1993), pp. 211–29; and F. M. Kamm, *Morality, Mortality: Death and Whom to Save from It*. Both Kamm and Veatch argue that priority for the young is morally required.

82. Alan Williams, "Intergenerational Equity: An Exploration of the 'Fair Innings' Argument," *Health Economics* 6 (1997): 117.

83. See especially Daniel Callahan, *Setting Limits*, *What Kind of Life* (New York: Simon & Schuster, 1990), and *False Hopes: Why America's Quest for Perfect Health Is a Recipe for Failure* (New York: Simon & Schuster, 1998). Most of our discussion is based on *Setting Limits*.

84. Callahan, "Afterward," in *A Good Old Age? The Paradox of Setting Limits*, ed. Paul Homer and Martha Holstein (New York: Simon & Schuster, 1990), p. 301; "Old Age and New Policy," *Journal of the American Medical Association* 261 (February 10, 1989): 905–06.

85. For a comparison and modest criticism of both, see Dan W. Brock, "Justice, Health Care, and the Elderly," *Philosophy and Public Affairs* 18 (1989): 297–312.

86. See P. Zweifel, S. Felder, and M. Meiers, "Ageing of Population and Health Ex-

penditure: A Red Herring," *Health Economics* 8 (1999): 485–96; Dennis W. Jahnigen and Robert H. Binstock, "Economic and Clinical Realities: Health Care for Elderly People," in *Too Old For Health Care?*, ed. Binstock and Post, ch. 2; J. M. O'Connell, "The Relationship Between Health Expenditures and the Age Structure of the Population in OECD Countries," *Health Economics* 5 (1996): 573–78.

87. See David M. Eddy, "The Individual vs. Society," *Journal of the American Medical Association* 265 (May 8, 1991): 2399–2401, 2405–06.

88. See Kevin Grumbach, et al., "Liberal Benefits, Conservative Spending: The Physicians for a National Health Program Proposal," *Journal of the American Medical Association* 265 (May 15, 1991): 2549–54.

89. Nicholas Rescher, "The Allocation of Exotic Medical Lifesaving Therapy," *Ethics* 79 (1969): 173–86.

90. Task Force, *Organ Transplantation*. A valuable discussion of the evolution of U.S. organ transplant policies appears in Jeffrey Prottas, *The Most Useful Gift: Altruism and the Public Policy of Organ Transplants* (San Francisco: Jossey-Boss Publisher, 1994).

91. Task Force, *Organ Transplantation*, p. 95. The task force recommended that hearts and livers not be allocated to nonimmigrant aliens, unless it was clear that no U.S. citizen or resident could use the organs. The different recommendations for renal and for extrarenal organs were based, in part, on the fact that there is no alternative or backup treatment for heart or liver failure, whereas dialysis is available for most cases of end-stage kidney failure. Over time UNOS's policies have evolved to require transplant centers to use the same standards in transplanting nonresident aliens and U.S. citizens and residents, to charge nonresident aliens the same fees as domestic patients, and to establish a mechanism for community participation and review if they admit nonresident aliens to their waiting list. Furthermore, a UNOS committee will review the activities of any member transplant center whose proportion of nonresident alien recipients of each organ type exceeds 5% of the total number of transplants of that organ type at that center over the calendar year. *1999 Annual Report of the U.S. Scientific Registry of Transplant Recipients and the Organ Procurement and Transplantation Network: Transplant Data: 1989–1998*, p. 420.

92. See James Childress, "Triage in Neonatal Intensive Care: The Possibilities and Limitations of a Metaphor," in *Practical Reasoning in Bioethics*, ch. 11.

93. For a study of this underexamined problem that emphasizes the German context, see Volker H. Schmidt, "Selection of Recipients for Donor Organs in Transplant Medicine," *Journal of Medicine and Philosophy* 23 (1998): 50–74.

94. Task Force, *Organ Transplantation*, ch. 5.

95. See *Report of the Massachusetts Task Force on Organ Transplantation* (October 1984).

96. Contrast Robert M. Veatch, "The Ethics of Resource Allocation in Critical Care," *Critical Care Clinics* 2 (January 1986): 73–89. See also Gerald Winslow, *Triage and Justice: The Ethics of Rationing Life-Saving Medical Resources* (Berkeley: University of California Press, 1982); and John Kilner, *"Who Lives? Who Dies?" Ethical Criteria in Patient Selection* (New Haven, CT: Yale University Press, 1990).

97. Controversy has raged over the last several years about UNOS allocation criteria for organs, especially livers. The Department of Health and Human Services, which awards the contract for the Organ Procurement and Transplantation Network that UNOS has held, has proposed greater attention to urgency of need in the allocation

point system, whereas UNOS has paid more attention to probability of successful outcomes. However, the major problem stems from the priority assigned to local and regional use of livers, i.e., their use where they are retrieved. Thus, patients in some geographical areas receive liver transplants even though their needs are less urgent than those of patients in nearby areas, and waiting times vary greatly from one area to another. In our judgment, the best arrangement would be to distribute organs as broadly as possible, in accordance with an appropriate balance of urgency of need and probability of successful outcome and within unavoidable logistical constraints in order to prevent damage to those organs. Of course, various transplant centers have economic interests at stake, and these economic interests may not match patients' interests. For a recent discussion, see Institute of Medicine, Committee on Organ Procurement and Transplantation Policy, Division of Health Sciences Policy, *Organ Procurement and Transplantation: Assessing Current Policies and the Potential Impact of the DHHS Final Rule* (Washington, DC: National Academy Press, 1999). UNOS' statement of general principles for organ allocation appears in "The UNOS Statement of Principles and Objectives of Equitable Organ Allocation," *UNOS Update* (August 1994): 20–30. For a critique of UNOS's criteria for allocating organs, with particular attention to kidneys, see Council on Ethical and Judicial Affairs, American Medical Association, "Ethical Considerations in the Allocation of Organs and Other Scarce Medical Resources Among Patients," *Archives of Internal Medicine* 155 (January 9, 1995): 29–40.

98. The statement derives from Evan DeRenzo. It appeared in Diane Naughton, "Drug Lotteries Raise Questions: Some Experts Say System of Distribution May Be Unfair," *Washington Post, Health Section*, September 26, 1995, pp. 14–15. See also Tamar Lewin, "Prize in an Unusual Lottery: A Scarce Experimental Drug," *New York Times*, January 7, 1994, pp. A1 and A17.

99. Barbara Goodwin, *Justice by Lottery* (Chicago: University of Chicago Press, 1992), p. 178.

100. In Seattle, members of a closely watched committee that selected patients for dialysis felt intense pressure and stress, often accompanied by guilt. See John Broome, "Selecting People Randomly," *Ethics* 95 (1984): 41.

101. Robert D. Truog, "Triage in the ICU," *Hastings Center Report* 22 (May/June 1992): 13–17.

102. See Ramsey, *The Patient as Person*, pp. 257–58. For the controversy about this example, see Robert Baker and Martin Strosberg, "Triage and Equality: An Historical Reassessment of Utilitarian Analyses of Triage," *Kennedy Institute of Ethics Journal* 2 (1992): 101–123.

103. See James F. Childress, "Who Shall Live When Not All Can Live?" *Soundings* 53 (1970): 339–55; also in Childress, *Practical Reasoning in Bioethics*, ch. 10, which updates the argument in response to criticism.

104. Winslow, *Triage and Justice*; but contrast Baker and Strosberg, "Triage and Equality: An Historical Reassessment." See also Robert A. Gatter and John C. Moskop, "From Futility to Triage," *Journal of Medicine and Philosophy* 20 (1995): 191–205; Society of Critical Care Medicine—Ethics Committee, "Consensus Statement on the Triage of Critically Ill Patients," *Journal of the American Medical Association* 271 (April 20, 1994): 1200–03.

105. Mary Faith Marshall, et al., "Influence of Political Power, Medical Provincialism and Economic Incentives on the Rationing of Surgical Intensive Care Unit Beds," *Critical Care Medicine* 20 (March 1992): 387–94.

7

Professional–Patient Relationships

The previous four chapters presented moral principles relevant to medicine, health care, and research with human subjects. In this chapter we further specify these principles by presenting moral rules of veracity, privacy, confidentiality, and fidelity as they apply to health care professionals or researchers and their patients or subjects. Some rules specify a single principle, and others specify more than one principle.

Veracity

Surprisingly, codes of medical ethics have traditionally ignored obligations and virtues of veracity. The Hippocratic Oath does not recommend veracity, nor does the Declaration of Geneva of the World Medical Association. The Principles of Medical Ethics of the American Medical Association (AMA) in effect from its origins until 1980 made no mention of an obligation or virtue of veracity, giving physicians unrestricted discretion about what to divulge to patients. In its 1980 revision, the AMA recommended simply and without elaboration that physicians "deal honestly with patients and colleagues."[1] By contrast to this traditional disregard of veracity, virtues of candor, honesty, and truthfulness are among the most widely praised character traits of health professionals and researchers in contemporary biomedical ethics.

In both traditional codes and current literature, significant uncertainties and ambiguities exist about the nature and status of norms and virtues of veracity. We can say now, as Henry Sidgwick observed in the nineteenth century, that "It does not seem clearly agreed whether Veracity is an absolute and independent obligation, or a special application of some higher principle."[2] G. J. Warnock included veracity as an independent principle and virtue that ranked in importance with beneficence, nonmaleficence, and justice.[3] We will argue that obligations of veracity are best understood as specifications of more than one principle and that conscientious adherence to these specifications is vital for a strong patient–professional relationship.

Obligations of Veracity

Veracity in the health care setting refers to comprehensive, accurate, and objective transmission of information, as well as to the way the professional fosters the patient's or subject's understanding. Three arguments contribute to the justification of obligations of veracity. First, the obligation of veracity is based on respect owed to others. As we saw in Chapter 3, respect for autonomy provides the primary justificatory basis for rules of disclosure and consent. Even if consent is not at issue, the obligation of veracity still depends on respect owed to others. Second, the obligation of veracity has a close connection to obligations of fidelity and promise keeping.[4] When we communicate with others, we implicitly promise that we will speak truthfully and that we will not deceive our listeners. By entering into a relationship in therapy or research, the patient or subject enters into a contract or covenant that includes a right to the truth regarding diagnosis, prognosis, procedures, and the like, just as the professional gains a right to truthful disclosures from patients and subjects. Third, relationships between health care professionals and their patients and between researchers and their subjects ultimately depend on trust, and adherence to rules of veracity is essential to foster trust.[5]

Like other obligations in this volume, veracity is prima facie binding, not absolute. Careful management of medical information—including nondisclosure, deception, and lying—will all occasionally be justified when veracity conflicts with other obligations. Although the weight of various obligations of veracity is difficult to determine outside specific contexts, some generalizations may be tendered: Deception that does not involve lying is usually less difficult to justify than lying, in part because it does not threaten as deeply the relationship of trust between deceiver and deceived. Underdisclosure and nondisclosure are also usually less difficult to justify. By contrast to obligations not to lie and deceive, the obligation to disclose information in health care depends on special relationships. For example, the patient entrusts care to the clinician and thereby gains a right to information that the clinician would not otherwise be obligated to provide.[6]

Disclosing Bad News to Patients

Withholding a diagnosis of cancer or a prognosis of imminent death from patients has been widely discussed, and various views exist in different cultures about when, if ever, nondisclosure can be justified.[7] In a striking case that illustrates the problem, Mr. X, a 54-year-old male patient, consented to surgery for probable malignancy in his thyroid gland. After the surgery, the physician told him that the diagnosis had been confirmed and that the tumor had been successfully removed, but did not inform him of the likelihood of lung metastases and death within a few months. However, the physician informed Mr. X's wife, son, and daughter-in-law about the fuller diagnosis and about the prognosis for Mr. X, but all of them, including the physician, agreed to conceal the diagnosis and prognosis from Mr. X. The physician told Mr. X only that he needed "preventive" treatment, and Mr. X consented to irradiation and chemotherapy. The physician did not inform Mr. X of the probable causes of his subsequent shortness of breath and back pain. Unaware of his impending death, Mr. X died three months later.[8]

Shifts in policies of disclosure. Over a couple of decades, a dramatic shift occurred in U.S. physicians' stated policies of disclosure of the diagnosis of cancer to patients. In 1961, 88% of the physicians surveyed indicated that they sought to avoid disclosing a diagnosis of cancer to patients, but by 1979, 98% of those surveyed reported a policy of disclosure to cancer patients. The reasons for the changes include the availability of more treatment options for cancer, improved rates of survival from some forms of cancer, fear of malpractice suits, involvement of team members in hospitals, altered societal attitudes about cancer, greater attention to patients' rights, and physicians' increased recognition of communication as an effective means of enhancing patients' understanding and compliance.[9]

In the 1979 survey, physicians identified the "four most frequent factors considered in the decision to tell the patient" as age (56% of respondents), a relative's wishes regarding disclosure to the patient (51%), emotional stability (47%), and intelligence (44%). It is unfortunate that—as in the case of Mr. X—familial preferences often unjustifiably influence clinicians' decisions about disclosure of diagnosis and prognosis to patients. Some physicians might counter that the family can help the physician determine whether the patient is autonomous and capable of receiving information about serious risk. Although true, this criticism begs the most important question: By what right does a physician initially disclose information to a family without the patient's consent? The family provides desirable care and support for many patients, but an autonomous patient has the right to veto familial involvement. If veracity is a primary rule or virtue in the physician's moral orientation, it is unethical for the physician to first disclose information to a family, even if the family requests it. The best policy is to ask the patient both at the outset and as the illness progresses about the extent to which he or she wants to involve others. (See our discussion of disclosure in Chapter 3.)

Cases of cautious disclosure. Despite what we have just said about the role of the family, many complexities and nuances in particular cases suggest a legitimate need to qualify this rule. For example, some complexities of physician–patient communication about cancer appear in the following case. Over the years, a 90-year-old patient, who as a young man had been decorated for his courageous actions in battle, had become greatly fearful that he would develop cancer, which, for him, meant a shameful, painful, and fatal disease that would spread inexorably. He was referred for an ulcer on his lip; a biopsy established the diagnosis of squamous cell carcinoma, which would require only a short course of radiotherapy to cure, without any need for surgery or even admission to the hospital. The elderly patient, tears in his eyes, asked, "It's not cancer, is it?" The physician responded emphatically that it was not cancer.[10]

The physician in this case justified his action on several grounds. First, he stressed the patient's need for "effective reassurance." Second, he contended that it was "more truthful" to tell this patient that he did not have cancer than to tell him that he did, because it would have been impossible to say that he had cancer but that it was curable "without leaving him with a false and untrue impression," given his particular, and unchangeable beliefs. Third, speaking to this patient and his concerns in his own language expressed not paternalistic arrogance but respect for him. Implicit in these justifications is a conviction that, because of his false beliefs, this patient lacked the capacity to understand the diagnosis of cancer, which, *for him*, entailed the prognosis of death. (See our discussion of false belief in Chapter 3 and of weak paternalism in Chapter 5.)

Nicholas Christakis has observed that professional norms in the United States generally support frankness and directness in sharing information about diagnosis and about therapeutic options, but discourage bluntness in sharing prognostic information.[11] For prognosis, professional norms reflect the values of truthfulness, accuracy, and empathy, along with the therapeutic value of hope for patients. Virtues of compassion, gentleness, and sensitivity are prominent. These norms and virtues tend to support disclosure of "bad news" over time rather than at once. In one study, half of the U.S. physicians interviewed indicated that when they deliver bad news to patients, they emphasize treatment possibilities and leave out the worst part (the full prognosis).[12] Disclosing information over time avoids what has been called "truth dumping" and "terminal candor." It attempts to achieve truthfulness within constraints set by principles of beneficence, nonmaleficence, and respect for patient autonomy. In addition to dispensing information gradually, clinicians following these professional norms present the information optimistically, building on indeterminancy and ambiguity, and appealing to statistics about patients with similar conditions.

An example of justified staged-disclosure and cautious language about prognosis, with a view toward maintaining a patient's hope, appears in a case in rehabilitation medicine.[13] For close to a month, a physician in a stroke rehabilitation unit carefully managed information and made ambiguous statements in his interactions with a patient who had suffered a stroke and who asked at their first session how long it would be before his arm improved. From the beginning, the doctor knew that the patient was unlikely to recover significant use of his arm, but he couched his answer carefully, replete with caveats and uncertainty that did not fully match what he believed or felt. He stressed the limitations of prognostication, the unpredictability of recovery, and the need to allow the brain a chance to heal. The patient accepted those answers for the time being, apparently preferring the physician's "ambiguous statements about the future to the alternative judgment of the permanent paralysis he fears." This indefinite, but caring and supportive, exchange continued, with the physician praising the patient's progress in walking and in performing daily activities despite residual weakness. After two weeks, when the patient was enthusiastic about his progress but asked again "How about my arm?" the physician responded, "The arm may not recover as much as the leg." Although this statement confirmed the patient's fears, he focused on his overall progress in the hope that the physician might be mistaken, especially in light of the latter's repeated emphasis on his inability "to accurately prognosticate."

Commenting on this case later, the physician noted that, having been trained in the era of "patient autonomy," he once felt that he "should share all available information [he] could provide about prognosis as early as possible," trying to temper unfavorable news, for instance, about arm recovery, with positive predictions of restored walking and independent living. However, because his patients hoped for a return to their earlier lives, the bad news tended to overwhelm the good news. Thus, he became convinced that most of his "patients were not ready for the cold hard facts the minute they arrived at the rehabilitation hospital. They needed time to come to terms with the reality of their disabilities, while simultaneously regaining lost function. This is a process that shouldn't be rushed." Further stressing that patients with such severe illnesses seek a mixture of hope and reality, the physician contended that "providing either one alone is a disservice. Hope is a fragile commodity, easily crushed by careless provision of the 'facts.' . . . In our zeal for patient autonomy, we should not forget the importance of nurturing that hope."

Arguments for limited disclosure. Implicit in many physicians' justifications for their actions are three arguments for limited disclosure and for some measure of deception in health care. These arguments all assume that breaches of obligations of veracity are prima facie wrong, but that they can sometimes be justified. The first argument rests on what Henry Sidgwick and many after him have called "benevolent deception." Such deception has long been a part of medical tradition. Its defenders holds that disclosure, particularly of a prognosis of death, sometimes violates obligations of beneficence and nonmaleficence by causing the patient anxiety, by destroying the patient's hope, by retarding or erasing a therapeutic outcome, by leading the patient to commit suicide, and the like.

This first line of argument—"What you don't know can't hurt and may help you"—is consequentialist. One objection to this argument rests on the uncertainty of predicting consequences. Samuel Johnson stated this objection sharply: "I deny the lawfulness of telling a lie to a sick man for fear of alarming him. You have no business with consequences; you are to tell the truth. Besides, you are not sure what effects your telling him that he is in danger may have."[14] As Tolstoy once wrote, lies may add to rather than relieve suffering: "What tormented Ivan Ilych most was the pretense, the lie—which for some reason they all kept up . . . that he was merely ill and not dying, and that he only need stay quiet and carry out the doctor's orders and then some great change for the better would result."[15]

Another objection to benevolent deception focuses on deception's long-term threats to the special relationship of trust between physicians and patients and to the physician's moral integrity. Deception may also have long-term negative effects on the patient's self-image. These are strong reasons for caution. Although it is sometimes acceptable to justify the use of deceptive means by the probable negative impact of truthful information on the patient's health, alternative non-deceptive means are usually more satisfactory.

A second reason for nondisclosure and deception is that health care professionals cannot know the "whole truth"—"you can never tell what will happen," "each patient is unique," etc. Even if professionals could know the whole truth, many patients and subjects would not be able to comprehend and understand the scope and implications of the information provided. This reason, however, does not undermine the obligation of veracity. Disclosure of the whole truth about a complex circumstance is an ideal against which health care professionals can measure their performance, but it can usually only be approximated, never fully realized. We can best use this ideal to help formulate a standard of *substantial* completeness that is realistic and appropriate for health care professionals (as discussed in Chapter 3).

A third argument is that some patients, particularly the very sick and the dying, do not want to know the truth about their condition. While proponents of this argument may be aware of surveys that almost universally indicate that the majority in the United States do want to know, they maintain that some patients indicate by signals, if not actual words, that they do not, in fact, want the truth. However, claims about what patients genuinely want are inherently dubious when they contradict the patients' own reports, and this third argument sets dangerous precedents for what are patently paternalistic actions, even though they masquerade as respect for autonomy. Nevertheless, more subtle versions of this third argument for incomplete disclosure point to a specific implicit request not to be informed. It is appropriate under these conditions, which are rare, for physicians to tailor their information to their patients' specific informational needs, interests, and wants. However, great sensitivity is needed in interpreting the patient's precise "request."

Subtleties in disclosing the whole truth. One Italian oncologist reports that she tries to tell her patients "the complete truth," but sometimes the patient's family asks her not to use the word "cancer."[16] She then relies on *nonverbal communication* to establish truthful therapeutic relationships with patients, listening to them and respecting their need for information. The emphasis placed on beneficence toward the patient in many Italian settings is not accompanied by quite the same cultural emphasis on autonomy that prevails in some other countries. Surveys show that Italians are divided, roughly 50:50, on whether they want truthful disclosures. In a study of 1171 breast cancer patients and their physicians and surgeons in general hospitals in Italy, only 47% of the women reported that they had been informed that they had cancer (by comparison, only 25% of their physicians indicated that they had not given accurate information).[17]

Although some of these social practices in Italy reflect different ideals than do practices in some other countries, they do not necessarily fail to respect individual autonomy. We can affirm the physician's obligation to respect the patient's autonomy, while recognizing that the ways in which patients exercise their autonomy will reflect their self-understandings, including socio-cultural expectations and their religious or other beliefs. A choice not to know can be as autonomous and as worthy of respect as a choice to know. Edmund Pellegrino rightly argues that "To thrust the truth or the decision on a patient who expects to be buffered against news of impending death is a gratuitous and harmful misinterpretation of the moral foundations for respect for autonomy."[18] Accordingly, care and sensitivity are required to respect a particular patient's autonomy by varying the information according to his or her actual preferences, not merely the physician's understanding of cultural ideals.

Attending to a particular patient's desires for information about prognosis is often very difficult. In one case, a 26-year-old woman, the mother of two young children, had an aggressive adenocarcinoma. Following radiation therapy and two different chemotherapeutic combinations, she was fragile but stable.[19] She was on oxygen continuously and took long-acting morphine (60 mg) three times a day. Yet she was energetic and life-affirming. She told the new hematology/oncology fellow that she had "a feeling" (based on her increased hip pain and enlarged nodules) that "things aren't going as well as people tell me they are" and hoped he had some new "tricks" up his sleeve. She eagerly and promptly consented to a new drug after he explained its administration, its potential adverse effects, and the ways they would try to prevent those effects, as well as his "hope that we would begin to see the long-sought-for response that might begin to heal her."

However, on the way to the chemotherapy unit, she turned to him to say that she had heard about a woman dying of leukemia who had written several stories for her children to remember her by. She continued: "My girlfriend said I should do the same thing for my kids, but I don't think I'm *that* far gone, am I, Doctor Dan?" Her physician reports his "stunned silence." He was unprepared for such a critical question, raised almost as afterthought, and unsure about how to respond there in the hall of a busy clinic, hardly the kind of setting in which to break bad news, according to the methods he had been taught. Faced with her radiant smile, he replied: "No, Lisa, I don't think you're at that point. I'm hopeful that this new treatment will work and that you will be able to spend a lot more time with your kids." "That's what I thought, Doctor Dan," she responded, "Thanks. Now on to round three." Fourteen days later, she died, without having written her stories for her children. Years later, the physician continues to hear the echo of his last words to her, wondering whether conveying a different message, with its bad news, would have allowed her to pen a few words of poems or to tape record thoughts or messages to provide her children a living memory of their dynamic, care-free mother.

Managing Negative Information Affecting Colleagues and Patients

Disclosure of medical malpractice and deficient health care professionals. Health care professionals often face quandaries about what to disclose about medical malpractice and about incompetent or unscrupulous colleagues. The AMA Principles of Medical Ethics require disclosure in certain contexts in order to preserve trust between the public and the medical profession: "A physician shall deal honestly with patients and colleagues, and strive to expose those physicians deficient in character or competence, or who engage in fraud or deception." Exposés by fellow physicians are, however, uncommon. Bonds of professional loyalty, accented in the Hippocratic and "gentlemanly" traditions of medical ethics, present a seemingly formidable barrier to many physicians. Yet this sociological fact does not excuse failures to expose serious deficiencies. Indeed, in some cases, the health professional has an obligation not only to investigate but also to ameliorate the problems.

Despite this obligation, a wall of silence frequently surrounds medical malpractice. In one case, a young boy's parents took him to a medical center for treatment of a respiratory problem. After being placed in the adult intensive care unit, he received ten times the normal dosage of muscle relaxant, and the respirator tube slipped and pumped oxygen into his stomach for several minutes. He suffered cardiac arrest and permanent brain damage. His parents accidentally

overheard a conversation that mentioned the overdose. While the physician involved explained that he had decided not to inform the parents of the mistake
because they "had enough on [their] minds already," the parents felt their tragedy
was compounded by the deception of the physician, whom they had previously
trusted.

Studies indicate that nondisclosure of malpractice—including a failure to accept responsibility and to apologize—threatens the relationship of trust between
professionals and patients and increases the risk of legal action.[20] A climate of
trust and moral seriousness among professionals is also needed to encourage disclosures of one's mistakes. For example, a promising young physician in Chicago
candidly reported that he had inadvertently used a swab on a patient that previously had been used on an HIV patient. Although this mistake apparently harmed
no one, the physician's honesty earned him dismissal along with collegial indifference to his plight.[21] The clear message imparted to younger physicians is that
nondisclosure and deception are more prudent than veracity.

Deception of third-party payers. In Chapter 3, we referred to a study in which
70% of the physicians responding to a scenario indicated that they would use the
words "rule out cancer" rather than "screening mammography" so that a patient's
insurance company would cover the costs. For the insurance company, the words
"rule out cancer" were to be used only if there was evidence of a breast mass or
objective clinical evidence of the possibility of breast cancer, neither of which
was present in this case. Surprisingly, 85% of these respondents did not think
that putting "rule out cancer" was deceiving the insurance company.[22]

Efforts to contain the costs of health care in the United States, particularly
through managed care organizations, have led some physicians to use deception
to secure third-party coverage. A physician in obstetrics and gynecology presented the following example: A 40-year-old woman underwent a diagnostic lap-
aroscopy for primary infertility. Because the woman's private insurance policy
did not cover this indication, the attending surgeon instructed the resident not to
put anything about infertility in the operative notes, but rather to stress the two
or three fine adhesions found in the pelvic area so that pelvic adhesions could
serve as the indication, and the patient's insurance would then cover the procedure. When the resident refused, the attending prepared the operative note.[23]

Several studies have attempted to determine the extent to which physicians use
or would be willing to use deception on behalf of their patients. According to
one study in 1999, close to 50% of the physicians surveyed admitted that they
had exaggerated the severity of their patients' medical condition so that those
patients would be covered for what the physicians believed they needed.[24] In
another survey in the late 1990s, 39% of physicians indicated that they had exaggerated the severity of patients' conditions, altered patients' filling diagnoses,
and/or reported signs or symptoms that patients did not have in order to help pa-

tients obtain coverage for needed care.[25] A third study attempted to determine the extent to which physicians were willing to deceive, or at least to sanction a colleague's deception of, a third-party payer in order to secure approval for patient procedures.[26] Using six vignettes of varying clinical severity, the researchers evaluated 169 randomly selected, board-certified internists from four high- and four low-managed-care penetration metropolitan markets in the United States: 57.7% sanctioned the use of deception for coronary bypass surgery, 56.2% for arterial revascularization, 47.5% for intravenous pain medication and nutrition, 34.8% for screening mammography, and 32.1% for emergent psychiatric referral in the vignettes presented. Only 2.5% were willing to use deception for cosmetic rhinoplasty. Not only were rates the highest for clinically severe vignettes, in which patients were at immediate risk, they were also the highest for physicians who practiced in predominantly managed-care markets.

A tension clearly exists between physicians' traditional conceptions of their moral role as patient advocates and their new roles within institutional structures that restrict both physician and patient choices about the use of financial resources to cover procedures. Without arguing that deception can never be justified, we believe that the current system needs other measures to deal with third-party–payer restrictions. The understandable temptations of deception in this system pose a significant threat to physician integrity and character as well as to fairness in the system.

Nondisclosure to third parties to protect patients. Health professionals can also experience a conflict between the obligation of veracity and the obligation of confidentiality when a third party enters the mix. For example, health care professionals in medical genetics sometimes discover nonpaternity. Consider a case in which, following the birth of a child with a genetic problem, a married couple seeks counseling about whether to have another child, and tests indicate that the husband is not the child's biological father. In a cross-cultural study of geneticists in 19 countries, 96% of respondents (and over 90% in all countries) indicated that they would not disclose false paternity to the husband. Eighty-one percent of respondents said they would tell the mother in private, away from the husband, and let her decide what to tell him, 13% would lie to the couple (e.g., by telling them that both are genetically responsible), and 2% would indicate that the child's disorder is the result of a new mutation. Only 4% of respondents would tell both the wife and the husband. The reasons for nondisclosure to the husband include preserving the family unit (58%), honoring the mother's right to decide (30%), and respecting the mother's right to privacy (13%). Although there were no gender differences in the response to the situation, female geneticists (75% of female respondents) were more likely than male counterparts (57% of male respondents) to use potential marital conflict as a reason for their decisions.[27]

A psychologically and ethically more complex case occurs when a physician has a patient, who, with her spouse, seeks help because she is infertile, and the counselor determines that she is an XY female—that is, genetically male but phenotypically female. One question is whether to provide the patient and the patient's husband with an accurate biological explanation of testicular feminization syndrome. In the cross-cultural study mentioned in the previous paragraph, the vast majority of counselors selected nondisclosure on grounds that they wanted to avoid causing psychological harm to the patient. However, at least three premises fuel an argument for disclosure: (1) the patient's infertility requires an explanation, and the genetic explanation may help relieve guilt; (2) surgical removal of the abdominal or inguinal testes is recommended to prevent cancer, but such surgery requires consent based on adequate information; and (3) the physician–patient relationship generally requires the disclosure of meaningful information to patients.[28]

What and how to disclose to the woman depend in part on the risks of disclosure (see our discussions of paternalism in Chapter 5 and informed consent in Chapter 3). Regarding disclosure to the husband, this case is analogous to the nonpaternity case and may be decided on similar grounds. Because no risk of physical harm exists for the husband, it is difficult to defend a breach of medical confidentiality against the wife's wishes. Nevertheless, the information will likely be important to the husband, and he too has come to the counsellor seeking help. Geneticists can encourage the wife to make disclosures to the husband, while offering assistance in counseling, and thus avoid a breach of confidentiality. In addition, we cannot rule out full disclosure to both parties *under some circumstances*, even if the wife resists disclosure to her husband and appeals to confidentiality. Indeed, in some cases, full disclosure to both parties may be the only responsible course of action.

Privacy

When syndicated columnist Jack Anderson reported that a well-known lawyer, Roy Cohn, was being treated for AIDS in an experimental trial of the drug AZT at the National Institutes of Health, critics charged that some health care professionals had violated Cohn's rights of privacy and confidentiality by releasing information to Anderson, who then violated Cohn's right of privacy by publishing the report.[29] Many such claims about obligations to protect privacy and confidentiality have affected controversies about policies to control the spread of HIV infection and AIDS. Various proposals to screen individuals to determine whether they are antibody-positive for HIV threaten a loss of privacy, and physicians question traditional obligations of confidentiality when patients with HIV infection refuse to inform or allow physicians to inform their spouses or lovers of their condition. Similar questions about privacy and confidentiality appear in several other areas of biomedicine.

Privacy in the Law and Legal Theory

Privacy received little explicit attention in the law or in legal theory until the late nineteenth century.[30] In the 1920s, the U.S. Supreme Court employed an expansive "liberty" interest to protect family decision-making about child rearing, education, and the like. It later adopted the term *privacy* and expanded the individual's and the family's protected interests in family life, child rearing, and other areas of personal choice. The Court's family-planning decisions most clearly articulate this privacy right. *Griswold v. Connecticut* (1965), a contraception case, was the first to construe the right to privacy not only as shielding information from others, but as protecting an area of individual and familial freedom from governmental interference. The Court's decision overturned state legislation that prohibited the use or dissemination of contraceptives. The right to privacy was said to protect liberty by demarcating a zone of private life that merits protection from state intrusion. In 1973, the Court expanded the scope of privacy rights by overturning restrictive abortion laws.[31]

It seems inapposite to make a right that protects individual or familial interests one of privacy rather than liberty or autonomy. However, the right to privacy encompasses both rights of limited physical and informational access, as well as rights of decisional freedom, and reducing this right to a right to be free to do something or a right to act autonomously creates confusion, for reasons we will now explore.

The Concept of Privacy

Some definitions of "privacy" focus on an agent's *control* over access to himself or herself, but these definitions confuse privacy, which is a state or condition of limited access, with an agent's control over privacy or a right to privacy, which involves the agent's right to control access. These definitions focus on powers or rights rather than privacy itself. A person can have privacy without having any *control* over access by others. Privacy exists, for example, in some long-term care facilities that render patients inaccessible.

Anita Allen has identified four forms of privacy that involve limited access to the person: *informational privacy*, which biomedical ethics often emphasizes; *physical privacy*, which focuses on persons and their personal spaces; *decisional privacy*, which concerns personal choices; and *proprietary privacy*, which highlights property interests in the human person.[32] Our discussion will emphasize informational, physical, and decisional privacy, but proprietary privacy also merits attention in biomedical ethics. The law extends property-like notions to individuals' interests in possessing and controlling aspects of their person. For example, laws and court decisions have imposed civil liability for the unauthorized appropriation of a person's name, portrait, or picture. Stored tissue samples may involve this kind of privacy interest, sometimes because one's genetic endowment is expressed in one's genes, but sometimes because of claims of ownership of the tissue sample and its products.[33]

A fifth form of privacy is *relational* or *associational*. It includes the family or other intimate relations, within which individuals in conjunction with others make decisions. This form of privacy recognizes that limited access to intimate relationships is central and that individuals, singly and jointly, make private decisions within these relationships.

As these different forms of privacy suggest, definitions of privacy are too narrow if presented solely in terms of limited access to *information* about a person. A loss of privacy occurs if others use any of several forms of access, including intervening in zones of secrecy, anonymity, seclusion, or solitude.[34] Privacy as limited access also extends to bodily products and objects intimately associated with the person, as well as to the person's intimate relationships with friends, lovers, spouses, physicians, and others.

It is sometimes desirable to provide a tighter definition of "privacy" because of the breadth of the concept. This objective may be imperative when developing policies regarding which forms of access to which aspects of persons will constitute losses and violations of privacy. We are, however, reluctant to castrate the concept to make it more serviceable for certain types of policy.[35] Instead, we recommend that those who propose policies carefully specify the conditions of access that will and will not count as a loss of privacy or a violation of the right to privacy. The policy should accurately define the zones that are considered private and not to be invaded, and should also identify interests that legitimately may be balanced against privacy interests. Often, the focus will be informational privacy and restricting modes of access to information about persons; but the strategy we have just suggested would also apply to policies that govern privacy in making decisions, in intimate relationships, and the like.

Finally, the value we place on a condition of limited access or nonaccess explains how it comes to be categorized as private. A loss of privacy may depend not only on the kind or amount of access but also on who has access through what means to which aspect of the person. As Charles Fried notes, "We may not mind that a person knows a general fact about us, and yet feel our privacy invaded if he knows the details. For instance, a casual acquaintance may comfortably know that I am sick, but it would violate my privacy if he knew the nature of the illness."[36]

Justifications of the Right to Privacy

In their celebrated 1890 article "The Right to Privacy," Warren and Brandeis argued that a legal right to privacy flows from fundamental rights to life, liberty, and property. They derived it largely from "the right to enjoy life—the right to be let alone." However, it is confusing to think of the right of privacy as nothing more than a right to be free to do something or a right to act autonomously. In addition, agents have to be able to act freely in the absence, for example, of certain forms of scrutiny by others. In recent discussions, several alternative justifications of the right to privacy have been proposed, three of which deserve attention.

One approach reduces the right to privacy to a cluster of other rights from which this right is derivative. According to Judith Thomson, this cluster of personal and property rights includes rights not to be looked at, not to be listened to, not to be caused distress (e.g., by the publication of certain information), not to be harmed, hurt, or tortured (in an effort to obtain certain information, say), and so on. However, Thomson's argument relies on several allegedly foundational rights that themselves have an uncertain status, such as the right not to be looked at. We are not convinced that each of these alleged rights is a right, and, more importantly, some of these rights may have the right to privacy as their basis, rather than the converse.[37] Indeed, one might plausibly argue that each violation of these "basic" rights is wrong because it involves wrongfully gaining access to a person—that is, because it violates a right to privacy.

Another approach emphasizes the instrumental value of privacy and the right to privacy by identifying various ends that rules of privacy promote. More specifically, different consequentialist theories, including utilitarianism, justify rules of privacy according to their instrumental value for such ends as personal development, creating and maintaining intimate social relations, and expressing personal freedom.[38] Fried, for example, argues that privacy is a necessary condition for maintaining intimate relationships of respect, love, friendship, and trust.[39] We do not deny that privacy has such instrumental value; we build and maintain various relationships by granting some and denying others certain kinds of access to ourselves. However, we question whether the instrumental value of privacy is the primary justification of rights to privacy.

The primary justification, we suggest, resides in a third rationale, based on the principle of respect for autonomy. We often respect persons by respecting their autonomous wishes not to be observed, touched, or intruded upon. On this account, rights of privacy are valid claims against unauthorized access that have their basis in *the right to authorize or decline access*. These rights are justified by rights of autonomous choice that are correlative to the obligations expressed in the principle of respect for autonomy. In this respect, the justification of the right to privacy parallels the justification of the right to give an informed consent that we developed in Chapter 3.

Joel Feinberg has observed that, historically, the language of autonomy has functioned as a political metaphor for a domain or territory in which a state is sovereign. Personal autonomy carries over the idea of a region of sovereignty for the self and a right to protect it by restricting access, an idea closely linked to the concepts of privacy and the right to privacy. Using the spatial and territorial model, Feinberg interprets the personal domain to include "a certain amount of 'breathing space' around one's body."[40] Other metaphors expressing privacy in the personal domain include zones and spheres of privacy that protect autonomy. The principle of respect for autonomy, therefore, includes the right to decide as far as possible what will happen to one's person—to one's body, to information about one's life, to one's secrets, and the like.

When individuals voluntarily grant others some form of access to themselves, their act is an *exercise* of the right to privacy, not a *waiver* of that right. For example, our decision to grant a physician access for diagnostic, prognostic, and therapeutic procedures is an exercise of our right to control access that includes the right to grant as well as to exclude access. The different kinds of access do not alter this conclusion. For example, a physician may need to take a personal history of certain private activities, touch our bodies, observe or listen to our bodies directly or through various instruments, run tests on our blood, and so on. With a psychotherapist, we expose our innermost thoughts, emotions, dreams, and fantasies. In these instances, we exercise the right to privacy by reducing privacy in order to achieve other goals.

Specifying and Balancing Rules of Privacy for Public Policy

Three examples will indicate how we propose to specify rules and rights of privacy, while allowing for justified intrusions on privacy that involve balancing privacy interests against other interests. These examples concern privacy in (1) screening and testing for HIV infection, (2) ensuring effective treatment for patients with active tuberculosis, and (3) applied human genetics.

Compulsory and voluntary screening for HIV. The HIV/AIDS epidemic has caused millions of deaths and vast suffering around the world. By June 30, 1999, more than 420,000 deaths from AIDS in the United States had been reported to the Centers for Disease Control, which estimates that 650,000 to 900,000 U.S. residents currently live with the HIV infection and that more than 200,000 of those residents are unaware of their infection. At first glance, screening appears to be a good public health strategy.[41] However, we need to ask what society plans to do with information about a person who is antibody-positive for HIV infection. No evidence exists that the virus is spread through casual contact, and most transmission occurs between parties in consensual, intimate relations under protected privacy. It is customary to distinguish between testing individuals and screening groups for antibodies to HIV, but we will use the term *screening* to cover both. Screening that identifies the individual screened necessarily involves some loss of privacy, because some persons gain access to private information. If testing is anonymous, no loss of privacy occurs, and the moral and policy issues are less complex. The following chart depicts possible policies toward screening (with identifiers) for exposure to HIV.

| | | Form of Authorization | |
		Voluntary	*Compulsory*
	Universal	1	2
Scope of Screening			
	Selective	3	4

No adequate justification has emerged for requiring either of the first two types of screening in public policy. Voluntary-universal screening rests on encouragement rather than coercion and consequently does not violate any moral rights of privacy and autonomy. However, neither voluntary nor compulsory universal screening is justified by current evidence. Universal screening is not necessary to protect the public health; HIV infection is not widespread outside groups engaging in high-risk activities; screening in groups or areas with low prevalence of HIV infection produces a high rate of false positives; and universal screening would be very costly and not cost-effective.

However, rejection of (1) and (2) is subject to reversal if various conditions change—for example, were the disease to spread so that it was far more difficult to identify persons at risk; were many people harmed by the failure of their partners to inform them of their infection; were improved techniques to emerge that could substantially reduce the false-positive and false-negative rates in testing without excessive costs; were increasingly effective anti-AIDS drugs to be developed; were the cost-effectiveness of screening programs to improve substantially; and were social policies to reduce the psychosocial risks to those identified as HIV-positive. Hence, our position does not oppose universal testing in principle, but universal testing cannot currently be justified for HIV infection.

Policy 3, voluntary-selective screening, can be justified, especially for people engaging in unsafe sexual practices and sharing needles in intravenous drug use. However, unresolved questions remain, including who should be encouraged to be tested, who should bear the costs, what sort of pre- and post-test counseling should be provided, and what conditions make the decision to undergo the test reasonable. Reasoned choice is particularly important because HIV screening presents major benefits and risks that need to understood and balanced.[42] If we assume the accuracy of the test results, the possible benefits of testing to those who test negative (seronegative) include reassurance, the opportunity to make future plans, and the motivation to make behavioral changes to prevent infection. Possible benefits to those who test positive (seropositive) include closer medical follow-up, earlier use of antiretroviral agents, prophylaxis or other treatment of associated diseases, protection of loved ones, and a clearer sense of the future.

No significant risks of HIV testing exist for seronegative individuals, but major risks are presented to seropositive individuals. These risks are both psychological and social, with interaction between the two. The psychological risks include anxiety and depression, followed by a higher rate of suicide than for the population at large. Social risks include stigmatization, discrimination, and breaches of confidentiality. Society can substantially reduce these risks by establishing firm rules to protect individuals against breaches of confidentiality and against discrimination in housing, employment, and insurance.

Finally, under option 4, several policies of compulsory-selective screening are justifiable. It is inappropriate to refer to some of these practices as compulsory in the strictest sense, because individuals often can choose whether to enter situations or institutions in which screening is mandatory, such as voluntary military service. Conditionally mandatory screening is justifiable whenever persons engage in actions or are involved in procedures that impose risks on others who cannot avoid those risks. Examples include blood donation, sperm donation, and organ donation.

Policies of screening pregnant women and newborns also raise ethical questions. The justification for mandatory HIV screening of newborns parallels the justification for mandatory newborn screening policies that are already in place in all U.S. states for several genetic diseases. States introduced the latter policies for serious genetic conditions for which presymptomatic interventions can prevent harms at acceptable cost–benefit trade-offs.[43] Neonatal screening for HIV could be justified by a similar rationale since more can now be done for infected newborns to extend their life expectancy at a higher quality.

For years, the risk of transmission of HIV infection from mother to offspring appeared to range from 25% to 30%, and debates occurred about whether it was morally responsible for HIV-infected women to continue pregnancy and about what counselors should recommend. Even if society could agree on the morally responsible choice in such a case, the legal enforcement of obligations presents additional problems because of moral constraints of privacy. For example, researchers undertook a clinical trial to determine whether azidothymidine (AZT) could reduce the rate of perinatal transmission of HIV infection. It became clear that AZT administered during the pregnancy and after delivery reduced the rate of transmission by two-thirds—from 25–30% to 8%.[44] The terms of the policy debate changed because it was now possible for pregnant women to greatly reduce the risk of transmitting HIV infection to their children, if they knew that they were HIV-infected and if they took AZT.[45] However, efforts to *mandate* prenatal testing would probably be ineffective, and perhaps counterproductive. For example, mandatory screening of all pregnant women who appear at clinics in areas with a high rate of HIV infection would put the women at social risk.[46] The policy most respectful of pregnant women's autonomy and privacy, and also the most likely to produce desirable consequences, is to offer pregnant women testing for HIV while providing them with information and appropriate counseling and support services, including, most importantly, access to AZT.

Related issues arise in institutional settings, which vary in the extent to which individuals are free to enter and leave and to control risky contacts within those settings. For example, it is doubtful that current policies of mandatory screening can be morally justified for foreign service applicants, officers, and their dependents, or for young people entering the U.S. Job Corps. Mandatory screening in the workplace is also inappropriate, except where exposure to bodily fluids could transmit the virus.

Mandatory treatment and detention of patients with tuberculosis. By contrast to HIV infection, tuberculosis (TB) is spread by airborne transmission. In the 1980s, public health officials predicted that tuberculosis could be eliminated in the United States within 25 years. Despite those predictions, the incidence of TB increased each year for a number of years (before again starting to decline), and a greater proportion of the cases involved multidrug-resistant, often fatal forms of TB. These forms of TB are difficult and costly to treat, requiring more than $200,000 in some cases, with limited success. Poverty, homelessness, inadequate and crowded housing, and substance abuse have long been associated with the spread of TB, but new problems include the susceptibility to TB infection among those who are HIV-infected.

A perennial moral problem concerns how to handle noncompliant patients who lack either the capacity or the will to complete the recommended treatments. Although treatment regimens for TB vary, the initial phase often requires daily medications for one to two months, followed by twice-weekly medications for several months (a total of six to nine months). The incidence of multidrug-resistant TB is much higher among previous recipients of anti-TB therapy, mainly because of their failure to continue the prescribed treatment until cured. In fact, their noncompliance or partial compliance with prescribed treatment regimens is the major cause of multidrug-resistant TB.

Obligations to respect privacy and autonomy dictate a priority for policies of voluntary compliance to control the TB epidemic, as in the AIDS epidemic. However, TB's different mode of transmission makes it easier to justify infringements of both autonomy and privacy. Mandatory TB screening is readily justifiable if substantial risk of transmission exists—for example, in crowded workplaces and prisons—and coercive police powers are justified to protect the public from persons identified to have active TB. Quarantine, isolation, and mandatory, directly observed treatment (DOT, which entails directly observing patients take their medication) are all justified in some circumstances. DOT has been used until patients with active TB become *noncontagious*, but many now argue that it should be used until such patients are *cured*. The rationale is not primarily paternalistic—to benefit the patient—but to protect others over time from exposure to TB.

If patients with TB do not continue their treatments until cured, they run the risk of developing multidrug-resistant forms that pose serious threats to those they infect, as well as to themselves.

According to some studies, about one-third of patients with TB fail to adhere to treatment. Their noncompliance stems from the conditions that foster TB, as well as from other social and psychological factors. Furthermore, professionals lack clear ways to identify noncompliant patients in advance. Those critical or suspicious of mandatory DOT contend that, because the majority of TB patients comply, it would be "wasteful, inefficient, and gratuitously annoying" to mandate DOT for all patients with TB. Moreover, to opt for DOT would be to fail to select the least restrictive and intrusive intervention for particular patients.[47] However, the risks of not implementing DOT include the further spread of TB, particularly its multidrug-resistant forms, and the escalation of treatment costs.[48] Several jurisdictions now invoke police powers to mandate DOT. While forcible detention is justified under some circumstances, respect for privacy and autonomy dictates giving primacy to various inducements and incentives, such as food and travel vouchers, to secure compliance with DOT.

An effective public health strategy in response to the TB epidemic should pay primary attention to conditions that cause TB and should give priority to policies that emphasize privacy and freedom of choice. However, coercive measures are justified when necessary to protect the public health, if priority is assigned to the least restrictive and least intrusive measures—first, induced DOT, then mandatory DOT. Both of these measures should have priority over detention.

Genetic privacy. Over the last decade, as mapping the human genome has progressed, concerns about "genetic privacy" have arisen. Of particular concern is the scope of rights of ownership to genetic information and the way this information can be joined with new information technologies to create threats to individual and familial privacy.[49]

One issue centers on whether genetic information is so different from other medical information that it merits separate protection. Some features of genetic information do provide plausible grounds for giving it special attention. For example, individuals and families often worry about genetic conditions that are *stigmatizing* more than they worry about other health problems. As in screening for HIV infection, the risks of genetic screening and testing are primarily psychosocial. Because of these risks, genetic screening and testing require justification in terms of their probable benefits, which vary from genetic condition to condition, depending on whether the screening and testing are for disease, disposing condition, or carrier status, whether preventive or treatment measures are available, whether the information is important for reproductive decisions, and the like. For any genetic screening or testing, fundamental questions concern who will use the resulting information, how they will use it, and for what purposes.[50]

Discriminatory uses of information are a major concern. Genetic testing has the potential to facilitate the exclusion of the genetically vulnerable from life and health insurance coverage, and potentially from employment. Many recognized from the beginning of the human genome project that genetic screening (that is, sorting an asymptomatic population to locate persons at elevated risk of genetic problems) would present issues of privacy and confidentiality involving employers, insurers, bankers, credit raters, and many others. Predictive uses of genetic information are not now sufficiently developed to affect a large number of underwriting decisions—and they are not cost-effective—but the human genome initiative will increasingly create a larger volume of predictive information to be added to the genetic information already available. If this information is obtainable, it will encourage insurance companies to make genetic tests cost effective. Companies can then deny coverage, increase charges, initiate exclusions, and the like. Such information also would be obtainable by persons at risk of disease, and they are more likely than others to purchase the relevant type of insurance in maximal amounts because they are more likely to experience claims in excess of premiums.

The costs of health care give employers a reason to avoid hiring persons who may get sick and file claims. Many companies already carry limited coverage in the case of diseases such as AIDS. At the present time, corporate policy often restricts so-called *group* insurance to ever-smaller subgroups, eliminating from the larger group persons who potentially will be most costly. The private health insurance industry views these strategies and adjustments as justifiable, because insurance policies are designed to limit risk as well as to protect the healthy, but a morally unsatisfactory feature marks the current American insurance scheme: Insurers want to avoid those most in need of insurance; the more insurance you need, the less you can obtain, or the more you pay. The situation will worsen as genetic information accumulates unless the information remains private. Lost in this upheaval is the moral goal of blindly pooling risks for groups in the face of the unknown lotteries of life.[51]

A basic question about a system of access to health care is whether it is ethical even to allow second parties to obtain information about genetic risks in the context of contracting for insurance policies, or whether health insurance should instead be distributed in accordance with the luck of the natural lottery, totally blinded from genetic information. It seems morally unjustified—a clear act of discrimination—to exclude persons from a health insurance pool merely because they were unlucky in the genetic or any other natural lottery. So-called "fair discrimination" in access to health insurance diminishes access to desperately needed health care, and rules of privacy may provide the best protection against such discrimination, unless the United States deeply reforms access to health care.

Employment discrimination is closely linked to these problems. Some employers find it advantageous to exclude potentially costly employees. Although relatively few employers currently use genetic testing, this situation will change as the benefits of testing shift and as the market fosters incentives to engage in testing. Worries about genetic discrimination led to a study by Paul Billings and associates of access to genetic information in the United States. He considered (1) whether incidents involving genetic discrimination are already common in the workplace, (2) access to social services, (3) insurance underwriting, and (4) the delivery of health care. The study described many difficulties that respondents had encountered in obtaining insurance coverage, finding or retaining employment, and the like. Here is a typical example involving the "asymptomatic ill," reported by a clinical geneticist treating individuals with PKU:

[Name withheld] is an eight-year-old girl who was diagnosed as having PKU at 14 days of age through the newborn screening program. . . . Growth and development have been completely normal. . . . The circumstances of the discrimination that this child has experienced involve rejection for medical insurance. She was covered by the company that provided group insurance for her father's previous employer. However, when he changed jobs recently, he was told that his daughter was considered to be a high risk patient because of her diagnosis and, therefore, ineligible for insurance coverage under their group plan.[52]

This and many other cases reported in the Billings study illustrate discrimination against persons who are completely asymptomatic; their only "abnormality" lies in their genotypes. Though healthy, these persons are treated as if disabled or chronically ill. If this information were protected as private (allowing an exception in the case of individuals who apply to increase or purchase extra coverage), such discrimination could not occur.

If we could protect privacy and confidentiality so that we could reduce the level of discrimination, or prevention information from being used for discriminatory purposes altogether, then individuals and families might find it more reasonable, on a risk–benefit calculation, to undergo genetic testing. As matters now stand, women with a family history of breast cancer sometimes refrain from undergoing genetic testing out of fear that the information, even if presented as private and confidential, will be used to discriminate against them in employment or health insurance.

The differences between genetic and other medical information are matters of degree rather than kind. Public policies therefore should address the privacy (and confidentiality) of medical information, in general, and then add special, additional protections for genetic information, if needed.[53]

Confidentiality

We necessarily surrender some of our privacy when we grant others access to our personal histories or bodies, but we also retain some control over information generated about us, at least in diagnostic and therapeutic contexts and in research. For example, physicians are obligated not to grant an insurance company or a prospective employer access to information about patients unless the patients authorize its release. When others gain access to protected information without our consent, we sometimes say that their access infringes our right to confidentiality and at other times say that it infringes our right to privacy.

From one standpoint, confidentiality is a branch or subset of informational privacy—it prevents *redisclosure* of information that was originally disclosed within a confidential relationship.[54] The basic difference between the concepts is this: An infringement of a person's right to confidentiality occurs only if the person (or institution) to whom the information was disclosed in confidence fails to protect the information or deliberately discloses it to someone without first-party consent. By contrast, a person who without authorization enters a hospital record room or computer data-bank violates rights of privacy rather than rights of confidentiality. Only the person (or institution) who receives information in a confidential relationship can be charged with violating rights of confidentiality.

Traditional Rules and Contemporary Practices

Rules of confidentiality have long been common in codes of medical ethics. Requirements of confidentiality appear as early as the Hippocratic Oath and continue in, for example, the World Medical Association's Declaration of Geneva, which asserts an obligation of "absolute secrecy" and includes the following pledge: "I will respect the secrets which are confided in me, even after the patient has died." The World Medical Association's International Code of Medical Ethics states the most stringent requirement of all: "A doctor shall preserve absolute secrecy on all he knows about his patient because of the confidence entrusted to him."

Some commentators ridicule such official rules as little more than a ritualistic formula or convenient fiction, publicly acknowledged by professionals but widely ignored and violated in practice. Mark Siegler has argued that "confidentiality in medicine" is a "decrepit concept," because what both physicians and patients have traditionally understood as medical confidentiality no longer exists. Rather, it is "compromised systematically in the course of routine medical care." To make his point graphic, Siegler presents the case of a patient who became concerned about the number of people in the hospital with apparent access to his record and threatened to leave prematurely unless the hospital would guarantee confidentiality. Upon inquiry, Siegler discovered that many more people than he had suspected had needs and responsibilities to examine the patient's chart. When he informed the patient of the number, approximately 75, he assured the patient that "these people were all involved in providing or supporting his health care services." The patient retorted, "I always believed that medical confidentiality was part of doctors' code of ethics. Perhaps you should tell me just what you people mean by 'confidentiality.' "[55]

This reaction is reasonable in contemporary health care. When William Behringer tested positive for HIV at the medical center in New Jersey where he worked as an otolaryngologist and plastic surgeon, he received numerous phone calls of sympathy within a few hours from members of the medical staff. Within a few days, he received similar calls from his patients, and shortly thereafter, his surgical privileges at the medical center were suspended and his practice ruined. Despite his expectation of and request for confidentiality, the medical center took no serious precautions to protect his medical records.[56] If physicians as patients cannot protect themselves in the system, it is unlikely that the system will adequately protect other patients.

According to one survey of patients, medical students, and house staff about expectations and practices of confidentiality, "patients expect a more rigorous standard of confidentiality than actually exists." Virtually all patients (96%) recognized the common practice of informally discussing patients' cases for second opinions; most (69%) expected cases to be discussed openly in professional settings in order to receive other opinions; a majority (51%) expected cases to be discussed in professional settings simply because they were medically interesting, and half of the patients expected cases to be discussed with office nursing staff. However, they generally did not expect cases to be discussed in other settings, such as in medical journals, at parties, or with spouses or friends. Yet, to take two examples, house staff and medical students reported that cases were frequently discussed with physicians' spouses (57%) and at parties (70%).[57]

Threats to confidentiality also emerge in many institutions with a capacity to store and disseminate confidential medical information, such as medical records on file, drugs prescribed, medical tests administered, and reimbursement records. In occupational medicine, for example, computerized records in corporations are growing rapidly, and data in these records can be searched quickly and thoroughly. If the company routinely offers medical examinations by a corporate physician, records can be computerized and merged with all claims filed by an employee's private physician for reimbursement under corporate insurance policies. Many employees (especially in industries with hazardous work environments) are concerned that this extensive, two-track medical history will be used against them if a question of continued employment arises. Companies can reduce this risk by severely limiting access to computerized information, but generally at least one physician and at least one employee in data-processing will have access to the full set of records, and access may also be granted to company epidemiologists, union officials, and the like.

It may be possible to alter current practices in the delivery of care to approximate more closely the traditional ideal of confidentiality, but a gulf will always remain because of the need for access to information in medicine.

The Nature of Medical Confidentiality

Confidentiality is present when one person discloses information to another, whether through words or an examination, and the person to whom the information is disclosed pledges not to divulge that information to a third party without the confider's permission. By definition, confidential information is both private and voluntarily imparted in confidence and trust. If a patient or research subject authorizes release of the information to others, then *no violation* of rights of confidentiality occurs, although a *loss* of both confidentiality and privacy may occur.

Acknowledged and justifiable exceptions exist to the kind of information that can be considered confidential in policy and practice. For example, legal rules may set external limits to confidentiality, as when they require practitioners to report gunshot wounds and venereal diseases. Some unwanted disclosures of information to third parties may not breach confidentiality because of the context in which the information was originally gathered. For example, IBM-physician Martha Nugent informed her employer about her belief that an employee, Robert Bratt, had a problem of paranoia relevant to behavior on the job.[58] Bratt knew that Nugent had been retained by IBM to examine him, but expected conventional medical confidentiality. The company held that the facts disclosed by Nugent were necessary for evaluating Bratt's request for transfer and, under law, were a legitimate business communication. In our view, it is a reasonable conclusion that such information is not confidential by the standards of medical confidentiality and that Nugent was not bound by obligations of confidentiality in the same way as a private physician.

This is not to say, however, that a physician employed by a corporation is free to disclose everything to the corporation. The point is that contracts for at least limited disclosures are not illegitimate as long as employees are aware of provisions in the contract. A similar point applies to military physicians who have a dual responsibility—to the soldier as patient and to the military. Nevertheless, the company and the military, along with the physicians in each context, do have a moral responsibility to ensure that employee-patients and soldier-patients understand at the outset the extent to which traditional rules of confidentiality do not apply.

The Justification of Obligations of Confidentiality

We can easily imagine a society that does not recognize any obligations of confidentiality. Indeed, many of the goods of medicine and research could be realized without rules of confidentiality. On what basis, then, can we justify a system of extensive protections of confidentiality? We believe that three types of argument justify (prima facie) rules to protect confidentiality: (1) consequence-based arguments, (2) rights-based autonomy and privacy arguments, and (3) fidelity-based arguments. These arguments also address legitimate exceptions to rules of confidentiality.

Consequentialist arguments. If patients could not trust physicians to conceal some information from third parties, patients would be reluctant to disclose full and forthright information or to authorize a complete examination and a full battery of tests. Without such information, physicians would not be able to make accurate diagnoses and prognoses or to recommend the best course of treatment. Although such consequentialist arguments establish a need for some rule of confidentiality, consequentialists disagree among themselves about which rule should be adopted, and about the rule's scope and weight.

Consequentialist arguments also support exceptions to the rule of confidentiality. In *Tarasoff* (Case 1), both the majority opinion, which affirmed that therapists have an obligation to warn third parties of their patients' threatened violence, and the dissenting opinion, which denied such an obligation, used consequentialist arguments. Their debate hinged on different predictions and assessments of the consequences of (1) a rule that *required* therapists to breach confidentiality by warning intended victims of a client's threatened violence, and (2) a rule that *allowed* therapists to breach confidentiality in the face of some peril to a member of the public. The majority opinion pointed to the victims who would be saved, such as the young woman who had been killed in this case, and contended that a professional's obligation to disclose information to third parties could be justified by the need to protect such potential victims. By contrast, the minority opinion contended that if it were common practice to override obligations of confidentiality, the fiduciary relation between the patient and the doctor would soon erode and collapse. Patients would lose confidence in psychotherapists and would refrain from disclosing information crucial to effective therapy. As a result, violent assaults would increase because dangerous persons would refuse to seek psychiatric aid or to disclose relevant information, such as their violent fantasies. Hence, the debate about different rules of confidentiality hinges in part on empirical claims about which rule more effectively protects the interests of other persons.

In the case of other legally accepted and mandated exceptions to confidentiality—such as requirements to report contagious diseases, child abuse, and gunshot wounds—no substantial evidence exists that these requirements have either reduced prospective patients' willingness to seek treatment and to cooperate with physicians or significantly impaired the physician–patient relationship.[59] Even in the aggregate, such reports are relatively isolated events with little effect on others' conduct.

A consequentialist justification for *nonabsolute* rules of confidentiality therefore has strong support. However, to accept this justification is not to overlook the fact that, when physicians breach medical confidentiality, they infringe their patients' rights whenever they have made a promise to keep confidentiality and their relationship was cemented by trust. Such an infringement has negative effects for confiders, and those effects can be outweighed only by substantial threats to others, to the public interest, or to the patient. A physician who breaks confidence cannot ignore the potential for eroding the system of medical confidentiality, trust, and fidelity. A consequentialist justification for breaching confidentiality can thus meet its own high standards only if it considers all such consequences.

Arguments from autonomy and privacy rights. A second approach to the justification of rules and rights of confidentiality looks to respect for autonomy and privacy. The argument for privacy in the previous section can here be extended to confidentiality, breaches of which have often been viewed primarily as violations of privacy and personal autonomy. It is true that such breaches acquire a special importance when disclosures of information subject a patient to legal jeopardy, loss of friends and lovers, emotional devastation, discrimination, loss of employment, and the like. However, an argument that uses an autonomy or privacy rationale does not appeal to these consequences. The thesis is that the values of the exercise of autonomy and privacy themselves support the rules of confidentiality.

Fidelity-based arguments. Another obligation explored later in this chapter is fidelity in the physician–patient relationship. The physician's obligation to live up to the patient's reasonable expectations of privacy and confidentiality is one way to specify the general obligation of fidelity. Medical practice requires the patient to disclose private and sensitive information to the physician, and a failure of fidelity thus tears at a significant dimension of the patient–physician relationship. Part of the binding force of confidentiality derives from the health care professional's implicit or explicit promise to the person seeking help. For example, if the professional's public oath or the accepted code of professional ethics pledges confidentiality, and if the professional does not expressly disavow confidentiality to the patient, the patient has a right to expect it.

Like the first argument, the second and third arguments do not support absolute rules of confidentiality. When rules of confidentiality are used as absolute shields, they can eventuate in outrageous and preventable injuries and losses. The best approach is to treat rules of confidentiality as prima facie in ethics as in law.[60] However, we will need a proper understanding of the circumstances under which other obligations validly override obligations of confidentiality—our next topic.

Justified Infringements of Rules of Confidentiality

When, all things considered, a person is not entitled to confidentiality, disclosure is sometimes *permissible* and at other times even *obligatory*. Obligations to divulge confidential information most commonly emerge when third parties face serious dangers.

Assessing and reducing risks to others. In assessing which risks to others, if any, outweigh the rule of confidentiality, we must balance both the probability that a harm will materialize and the magnitude of that harm against the obligation of confidentiality. The chart of risk assessment introduced in Chapter 5 supplies the basic categories:

		Magnitude of Harm	
		Major	*Minor*
Proba- bility of Harm	*High*	1	2
	Low	3	4

As health professionals' assessments of a situation approach a high probability of a major harm (1 above), the weight of the obligation to breach confidentiality increases. As the situation approaches 4, the weight decreases and it would usually be wrong to breach confidentiality. Many particularities of the case will determine whether the professional is justified in breaching confidentiality in 2 and 3, which are complicated borderline categories. These particularities include the foreseeability of a harm, the preventability of the harm through a health professional's intervention, and the potential impact of disclosure on policies and laws regarding confidentiality.

These abstractions are often difficult to put into practice. Our attempts to measure probability and magnitude of harm are imprecise in many cases, and uncertainty will be present.

Disclosure of HIV infection to third parties. Controversy surrounds the question whether physicians and other health care professionals should notify spouses and lovers that a patient has tested positive for HIV infection and, consequently, has the potential to infect others through sexual intercourse or other exchanges of body fluids, particularly through sharing needles in intravenous drug use.[61] In one case, after several weeks of dry persistent coughing and night sweats, a bisexual man visited his family physician, who arranged for a test to determine whether he had antibodies to HIV. The physician informed the patient of a positive test, of the risk of infection for his wife, and of the risk that their children might lose both parents. The patient refused to tell his wife and insisted that the physician maintain absolute confidentiality. The physician reluctantly yielded to this demand. Only in the last few weeks of his life did the patient allow the physician to inform his wife of the nature of her husband's illness, and a test then showed that she too was antibody-positive for HIV. When symptoms appeared a year later, she angrily, and we think appropriately, accused the physician of violating his moral responsibilities to her and to her children.[62] This case presents a high probability (if we assume unprotected sexual intercourse) of a major harm to an identifiable individual—the paradigm case of a justified breach of confidentiality.

Legal and moral rules of confidentiality are still evolving in response to the AIDS epidemic, based in part on how relevantly similar cases were handled previously. Many well-grounded reasons support informing spouses and sexual partners that a particular person has tested positive for exposure to the AIDS virus. For example, if people are at risk of serious harms, and the disclosure is necessary to prevent—and probably would prevent—the harms (to their spouses or lovers), disclosure is usually justified.

Variations on these conditions appear in several statements of professional ethics by medical associations. According to a committee of the American Psychiatric Association (APA), for example, if the physician has "convincing clinical information" that a patient is infected with HIV and also has "good reason to believe" that the patient's actions will place others at ongoing risk of exposure, then "it is ethically permissible for the physician to notify an identifiable person who the physician believes is in danger of contracting the virus." However, a breach of confidentiality is categorized as a "last resort," to be used only following "scrupulous attention . . . to all other alternatives," which include "the patient's agreement to terminate behavior that places other persons at risk of infection or to notify identifiable individuals who may be at continuing risk of exposure."[63]

Various ambiguities and gaps in this statement can serve as a case study to point to broader difficulties in specifying the nature and scope of the clinician's ethical obligation to protect third parties. First, which actions will discharge the physician's moral obligation to protect third parties? The guidelines do not hold that the physician has an obligation to determine whether the patient has, in fact, carried out the "agreement" to terminate the risky conduct or to warn those endangered, and it is not clear how far the physician should go in monitoring compliance, particularly without the patient's consent. One study concludes that it is very ineffective to leave partner-notification to patients.[64] Perhaps the only responsible strategy is the one proposed by the AMA's Council on Ethical and Judicial Affairs: A physician who "knows that a seropositive individual is endangering a third party . . . should (1) attempt to persuade the infected patient to cease endangering the third party; (2) if persuasion fails, notify authorities; and (3) if the authorities take no action, notify the endangered third parties."[65]

Second, how are we to interpret the patient's "agreement to terminate behavior that places others at risk of infection or to notify [them]"? In particular, how far must the patient go to reduce the risk of HIV transmission? Suppose the patient refuses to notify his or her sexual partner and refuses to abstain completely from sexual intercourse, but indicates that he or she will insist on the use of a condom. This promise is usually not sufficient to release the physician from an obligation of disclosure.

Third, the APA guidelines propose that physicians inform their patients in advance of the limits placed on confidentiality in their relationship. If the patient has understood in advance that certain information will not be kept confidential and the physician then discloses that information to a third party, no breach of confidentiality occurs. However, the guidelines are unclear regarding whether doctors can disclose the patient's HIV-positive status if the patient informed the doctor about his status prior to the physician's disclosure of the limits of confidentiality. While a physician need not have given prior notification that the HIV status would be disclosed to parties at risk, the physician should seek the patient's permission to warn a third party if the patient is unwilling to do so.

Fourth, the APA guidelines stress the ethical *permissibility* of the physician's disclosure, rather than its *obligatoriness*, whereas the Council on Ethical and Judicial Affairs of the American Medical Association (AMA) focuses on the physician's obligation. The primary justification for disclosure is that health professionals are *obligated* to reduce the risk of death. Public officials, on the other hand, need to consider carefully which societal rule of confidentiality would save more lives in the long run: One that permits or perhaps requires notification of sexual or needle-sharing partners or one that guarantees confidentiality.

Answers to this question hinge, in part, on disputed claims about the importance of voluntary testing in changing behavior and reducing risky conduct over time. One consequentialist argument is that people who have been exposed to the AIDS virus but do not yet have symptoms will be reluctant to seek testing unless confidentiality is protected. As a result, they will fail to obtain valuable information that could lead them to reduce risks to others. A counterargument holds that carefully limited breaches of confidentiality—namely, disclosure only to sexual partners or needle-sharing partners who are at risk of harm—would not deter people from seeking testing and medical attention. According to this argument, people would still seek testing if they were informed that confidentiality would be breached only under strictly limited conditions and then only to parties at risk of harm.[66]

We lack sufficient evidence regarding the effects of breaches of confidentiality or willingness to be tested to resolve this debate. However, successful notification of partners, whether by physicians to identifiable third parties or by public health officials, depends largely on patients' cooperation in providing information. A policy should be carefully hedged to gain such cooperation.[67]

Disclosure of genetic information to third parties. Genetic information about a particular individual may also reveal information about particular family members. Those who learn that they have a genetic condition have a moral obligation to share that information with relatives who may be able to take actions to reduce their risks or to seek treatment. Health care providers should underline this obligation. Genetic counselors in particular may have to overcome their proclivity for nondirective counseling and seek to persuade counselees to disclose this information, or, preferably, to allow the counselors to do so in order to ensure adequate information about risks and preventive or therapeutic options. However, directive counseling is different from actually disclosing the information to relatives against the counselee's explicit directives. We concur with the recommendation of the Institute of Medicine Committee on Assessing Genetic Risks that "confidentiality be breached and relatives informed about genetic risks only when (1) attempts to elicit voluntary disclosure fail, (2) there is a high probability of irreversible or fatal harm to the relative, (3) the disclosure of the information will prevent harm, (4) the disclosure is limited to the information necessary for diagnosis or treatment of the relative, and (5) there is no other reasonable way to avert the harm."[68]

In conclusion, we have argued that obligations of medical confidentiality are not, at present, well-delineated and need restructuring. On the one hand, if we are to honor obligations of respect for autonomy, institutions and professionals generally should tell patients more about practices of confidentiality and threats to confidentiality, such as computerized record keeping. Patients should be able to consent to the inclusion of information in their records, should have access to those records, and should be able to retain considerable control over others' access to those records. On the other hand, moral obligations to protect confidentiality sometimes must yield to other moral demands, such as protection of the rights and interests of third parties.

Fidelity

The late Paul Ramsey argued that the fundamental ethical question in research, medicine, and health care is, "What is the meaning of the faithfulness of one human being to another?"[69] Few today would agree that fidelity is the fundamental moral norm in health care and research, but many accept it as an essential norm.

The Nature and Place of Fidelity

Obligations of fidelity are best understood as norms that specify the moral principles discussed in previous chapters, especially respect for autonomy, justice, and utility. These principles justify the obligation to act in good faith to keep vows and promises, fulfill agreements, maintain relationships, and discharge fiduciary responsibilities. Both law and medical tradition distinguish the practice of medicine from business practices that rest on contracts and marketplace relationships. The patient–physician relationship is founded on trust and confidence; and the physician is therefore necessarily a trustee for the patient's medical welfare. This model of fidelity relies more on values of loyalty and trust than merely on being true to one's word. Whether or not the physician makes a pledge or takes an oath upon entry into the profession, obligations of fidelity arise in this model whenever the physician establishes a relationship with a patient. Similarly, abandonment is a breach of fidelity, an infidelity amounting to disloyalty.

Fiduciary relationships sometimes encounter competing moral obligations that limit and override obligations of fidelity. Determining obligations may require a discerning interpretation of the weight of special relationships and explicit or implicit promises. For example, in an epidemiological study of what happens to people who are antibody-positive for HIV but do not yet have signs of AIDS, some investigators indicated that they would treat the information gathered confidentially and use it exclusively for epidemiological purposes. But this assurance came into question when a researcher discovered that an antibody-positive subject had not informed his lover and continued to practice unprotected sex. In considering whether to warn the lover, this researcher had to weigh his specific promise of confidentiality against the obligation to prevent harm.[70]

Conflicts of Fidelity and Divided Loyalties

Several problems about the meaning and strength of obligations of fidelity arise because of conflicts of fidelity, which often produce divided loyalties. The phrase "conflicts of fidelity" is less familiar than "conflicts of loyalty" and "conflicts of interest," and we need first to analyze the meaning of each of these terms.

Professional fidelity or loyalty has been traditionally conceived as giving the patient's interests priority in two respects: (1) the professional effaces self-interest in any situation that may conflict with the patient's interests, and (2) the professional favors the patient's interests over others' interests.[71] In practice, of course, fidelity has never been so unadulterated. For instance, caring for patients in epidemics has often been considered praiseworthy and virtuous rather than an obligatory instance of fidelity, and physicians have never been expected to care for all patients free of charge.

Health care professionals regularly use their clinical skills to serve social purposes beyond the individual patient's interests. More specifically, physicians often incorporate public health concerns into caring for their patients. For instance, they may recommend vaccination when, in a context of high rates of immunization, its risks would outweigh its benefits to certain patients. Or physicians may select antibiotics in light of a concern about the development of antibiotic-resistant bacteria. Second, clinical skills serve various non-health–related social activities, such as criminal justice and war, as well as religious and cultural practices, such as male circumcision. Finally, physicians serve as gatekeepers for society's ascription of rights, responsibility, and opportunity by examining and assessing particular patients. Examples include providing psychiatric evaluation as part of a person's insanity defense in a criminal trial or conducting a medical review of a person's disability insurance claims.[72]

The rhetoric of the primacy of the patient's interests was once more plausible than it is now, because major changes in the structure, delivery, and financing of health care and its social context have produced divided loyalties in many areas of medical practice, nursing, and clinical research. Issuing orders and assigning duties create some forms of divided loyalty, but divided loyalty also occurs when fidelity to patients, subjects, or clients conflicts with allegiance to colleagues, institutions, funding agencies, corporations, or the state. In these cases, two or more roles and associated loyalties and their obligations become incompatible and irreconcilable, forcing a moral choice between them. This choice may alter the landscape of one's commitments.[73] A divided loyalty can be reconciled only by giving up or seriously modifying one or more of the conflicting loyalties. In extreme cases of divided loyalty, the professional faces conflicting moral obligations.

Third-party interests. Physicians, nurses, and hospital administrators sometimes find aspects of their role obligations in conflict with obligations to patients. For example, they may have a therapeutic contract with a party other than the patient. When parents bring a child to a physician for treatment, for instance, the physician's primary responsibility is to serve the child's interests, although the parents made the contract and the physician has obligations of fidelity to the parents. The latter obligations are sometimes easily and validly overridden, as occurs when physicians go to court to oppose parental decisions that seriously threaten children. For example, courts have often allowed adult Jehovah's Witnesses to reject blood transfusions for themselves, while rightly refusing to allow them to reject medically necessary blood transfusions for their children. Parents are also sometimes charged with child neglect when they fail to seek or permit potentially beneficial medical treatment recommended by physicians.[74]

Maternal–fetal relations have likewise become more complex and open to conflicts. The fetus typically becomes a patient because of the pregnant woman's decision to enter the health care system. Once both patients, the pregnant woman and the fetus, are under care, conflicting obligations of fidelity and divided loyalties may develop. For example, the possibility of cesarean sections late in pregnancy sometimes presents a conflict between the survival and health of the fetus and the wishes of the pregnant woman. The diagnosis and treatment of some fetal maladies in utero, such as the treatment of hydrocephalus through intrauterine surgery, can engender similar conflicts. Rules of privacy and informed consent usually allow the pregnant woman's interests to prevail in the legal arena in cases of conflict.

The sensational case of Angela Carder illustrates some of these contentious issues. This 27-year-old patient—referred to as "A. C."—was terminally ill with cancer and 26 weeks pregnant. A court ordered a cesarean section against her wishes, in part because doubt existed about her competence and the stability of her preferences. Attorneys for the hospital had sought a declaratory judgment to determine whether the hospital had a duty to attempt to save the baby's life through a cesarean section when it appeared that the woman's death was imminent. A superior court judge held a three-hour emergency hearing at the hospital, but never entered A. C.'s room, and ordered the cesarean section after a neonatologist estimated that the baby had perhaps a 50 to 60 percent chance of surviving the operation but that the operation could hasten the woman's death, which was already considered imminent. A three-judge panel of the District of Columbia Court of Appeals denied the request by A. C.'s counsel for a stay of the order. After the cesarean section was performed, the baby was named and a birth certificate issued; but the baby died within two and one-half hours, and the mother died two days later. They were buried together. The panel's opinion, filed five months later, noted that the pregnant woman was predicted, at best, to have only two days left of sedated life. The panel relied on previous court holdings that the state's interest in protecting innocent third parties from an adult's decision to refuse medical treatment may validly override the patient's interest in bodily integrity.[75]

Following major public controversy over this opinion, the full District of Columbia Court of Appeals reheard the case.[76] The majority opinion focused on the right of competent adults to make an informed choice to accept or forgo medical treatment. It noted that courts have consistently refused to compel someone to donate bodily tissue to benefit someone else through transplantation. According to this opinion, the trial court erred in balancing A. C.'s rights against the interests of the fetus without a prior effort to determine her informed choices—or, if she were incompetent, through substituted judgment (that is, ascertainment of "what the patient would do if faced with the particular treatment question"). The court held that the pregnant woman's wishes "will control in virtually all cases." Viewing the cesarean section as a "massive intrusion" comparable to organ and tissue removal, the court established a strong presumption against court-ordered cesarean sections.

Institutional interests. In some types of conflict that arise in institutions, it is also unclear what the health care professional owes the "patient." Often the institutions involved are not health care institutions, but, in order to discharge their functions, they may need medical information about individuals and may provide some care for those individuals. Examples include a physician's contract to provide medical examinations for applicants for positions in a company or to determine whether applicants for insurance policies are safe risks. The health care professional may rightly not regard the person examined as his or her patient, but the professional still has certain responsibilities of due care—for example, care in examinations so as not to injure the individual.

In some jurisdictions, the health care professional does not have a legal obligation to disclose the discovery of a disease to the examinee, although nondisclosure is a morally dubious practice. At a minimum, health care professionals have a moral responsibility to oppose, avoid, and withdraw from contracts that would require them to withhold information of significant potential benefit to examinees. Physicians similarly owe "due care" to individuals who become their patients under a third-party contract in an institutional arrangement. Examples include health care professionals in industries, prisons, and the armed services.

However, care of the patient occasionally conflicts with institutional objectives and policies, and the patient's needs may or may not take precedence, even when they are owed due care. For example, the military physician must accept a different set of obligations than the nonmilitary physician, in particular, to place the military's interests above both the patient's and the physician's interests. However, even in such a context, some actions so grossly violate canons of medical ethics that they warrant disobedience of orders and defiance of superiors, rather than loyalty and compliance. An example is a commander's order for a physician to help torture a prisoner of war in order to gain information or to verify the efficacy of the techniques being used.[77]

Medical assistance in prisons also presents explosive moral problems, in part because the institutional mandate to punish limits obligations of fidelity to the patient. Medical values are sometimes subordinated to the correctional institution's functions, and yet the physician is expected to be loyal to both. The correctional institution may expect physicians and other health care professionals to participate in the administration of justice and of punishment. Examples include surgical removal of a bullet for evidence when the bullet is not a hazard to the inmate and can be safely left in place, forced examinations of inmates' body cavities for evidence of contraband drugs, and participation in corporal or capital punishment—for example, by administering a lethal injection.[78]

Moral questions arise about medical assessments of prisoners' physical conditions to determine whether they can endure punishments, and about medical monitoring of these prisoners during punishment. Medical supervision can prevent extreme or unintended injury or harm, but participation in the administration of punishment, whether corporal or capital, represents a compromise of the profession's commitments of fidelity.[79] For similar reasons, the Council on Ethical and Judicial Affairs of the AMA has held for several years that physician participation in capital punishment through administration of a lethal injection is unethical. In 1992, it enlarged unethical participation to include administering tranquilizers or other medications as part of an execution, monitoring a condemned prisoner's vital signs, witnessing an execution in a professional capacity, or rendering technical advice for an execution.[80] The reason, we suggest, is that in these acts, a physician's conflicts of fidelity are unjustifiably resolved in favor of institutional needs that could be satisfied without the participation of physicians.

Nursing. Perhaps in no area of health care are conflicts among obligations of fidelity more pervasive and morally troubling than in nursing: "Traditionally, nurses have been discouraged from developing and acting on their own ethical judgments. Although the institutions of nursing and medicine developed separately until the late eighteenth century, the increasing importance of the hospital in health care brought nursing under the dual command of physicians and hospital administrators."[81] Codes of nursing ethics in the latter part of the twentieth century defined the moral responsibility of nurses in sharply different ways from earlier codes. For example, in 1950, the first code of the American Nurses' Association stressed the nurse's obligation to carry out the physician's orders, whereas the 1976 revision stressed the nurse's obligation to the client and the obligation to safeguard both the client and the public from the "incompetent, unethical or illegal" practices of any person.

Political as well as moral problems will persist in nursing as long as some professionals make the decisions and order their implementation by other professionals who have not participated in the decision-making. For example, in a study of relationships in health care, investigators examined different perceptions of ethical problems by nurses and doctors in acute care units. In structured interviews, both nurses and physicians said they frequently encountered ethical problems. Most of the physicians (21 of 24) and most of the nurses (25 of 26) recognized differences of opinion or ethical conflicts within the health care team. However, in 21 of the 25 cases reported by nurses, the ethical conflict was between a nurse and a physician, whereas only one physician reported a conflict with a nurse rather than with another physician. The authors of the study believe it is likely that conflicts with nurses occurred, but that the physicians "were not aware of them, or did not see conflict with a nurse as forming an *ethical* problem."[82]

Several features of the working relationship between physicians and nurses may explain these findings. Physicians write orders and nurses carry them out. By virtue of their close, sustained relationships with patients, nurses often experience the problems that arise from medical decisions more immediately than physicians. These common features of nursing roles sharpen obligations of fidelity to patients but also open avenues of conflict with colleagues.

Conflicts of Interest

Over the last several years, new, or at least more serious, conflicts have weakened traditional rules of fidelity. In particular, third-party payers and institutional providers increasingly impose constraints on medical decisions about diagnostic and therapeutic procedures, and many physicians rely on other funding sources for additional income. These economic interests form loyalties to these parties in addition to loyalties to patients.[83] Various mechanisms have emerged in efforts to control the escalating costs of health care, including utilization review, preferred provider arrangements, and sundry forms of managed care. These mechanisms often function to limit and constrict the physician's fidelity to the patient through a mixture of incentives and disincentives, some of which place the physician's self-interest in conflict with the patient's best medical interest, thereby producing serious conflicts of interest in addition to conflicts of fidelity.

Conflicts of interest emerge in medicine when, in addition to their obligations to protect and promote their patients' interests, physicians have a personal, often financial, interest at odds with fidelity or loyalty to their patients.[84] These conflicts of interest are common. They pervaded and continue to pervade fee-for-service medicine, which provides an incentive for physicians to use additional diagnostic and therapeutic procedures, even when they would not serve the patient's interests. On the whole, the medical profession has attempted to address specific conflicts of interest in financial arrangements, such as fee splitting, without attending to general and systemic issues of conflicts of interest.[85]

Society and the health professions need to address conflicts of interest in a more systematic way by *eliminating* some conflicts as well as by requiring *disclosure* of conflicts to alert parties at risk. At a minimum, laws (buttressed by professional sanctions) should ban or decline to enforce "gag clauses," which in some managed care contracts, prohibit clinicians from disclosing *conflicts of interest* (e.g., economic incentives for physicians to provide fewer or less expensive diagnostic and therapeutic procedures) and *conflicts of obligations* (e.g., the managed care organization's rationing strategy or clinical guidelines).

Financial and other incentives that motivate the clinician to consider the economic effects of particular clinical decisions are ubiquitous in modern medicine. For example, the majority of Health Maintenance Organizations (HMOs) retain part of the primary physician's income—10% to 30% (the higher figures appearing in for-profit HMOs). They return part or all at the end of the year, depending on the overall financial condition of the HMO and, in some cases, the physician's productivity and frugality. Such an arrangement creates an incentive for physicians to severely limit expensive procedures, a worrisome conflict of interest. The patient is in a different position when the physician has incentives to *restrict* needed treatment than when the physician has incentives to provide *unnecessary* treatment. In the latter situation, patients can obtain another opinion. In the former situation, patients may not be aware of a needed treatment.[86]

Widespread self-referral—that is, referral of patients to medical facilities or services that physicians own or in which they have some financial investment—also threatens fidelity to patients' interests by extending the temptation inherent in fee-for-service to provide unnecessary care or unnecessarily expensive care. Physicians create these economic conflicts of interest by owning or investing in medical facilities or services, such as diagnostic imaging centers, laboratories, or physical therapy services to which they refer patients. Evidence indicates that physician ownership of radiation therapy and physical therapy services, for instance, substantially increases both use and costs, without compensatory benefits, such as increased access.[87]

Fee-for-service is generally less problematic than self-referral, because the patient can more easily recognize the physician's economic gain in providing additional procedures and can exercise caution accordingly—for example, by seeking a second opinion. For this reason, some contend that the physician has an obligation to disclose economic conflicts of interest in instances of self-referral. Though such disclosure seems an ethical minimum of fidelity and honesty, it rarely occurs, and sometimes it occurs only in a manner calculated to protect physicians by reducing their risk of liability.[88] A strong case can be made that fidelity to patients requires a strict rule prohibiting "self-referral" (as the AMA has finally recognized, following years of vacillation). This prohibition of self-referral, allowing carefully circumscribed exceptions for disclosure when self-referral is necessary because of a lack of other facilities or services, is an essential expression of fidelity to patients. Numerous state statutes in the United States now appropriately prohibit forms of self-referral.[89]

Some relationships encountered in clinical research involve similar problems of conflict of interest. For example, many clinical trials are financially supported by companies willing to assume the financial risk because the returns from a successful trial can be extremely high. The financial advantages for physician-investigators and corporations promote a relationship with a consistent flow of funding. Such a relationship sometimes creates a subtle desire to arrange another and better contract or grant by producing research results that are favorable from a funding source's perspective. In some cases, the physician-investigator's personal financial interests are at stake. Medical centers, both inside and outside university research facilities, increasingly are staffed with physicians who have a financial interest in the drugs, medical devices, and technologies they prescribe or recommend to their patients. For example, some physicians have stock or stock options in companies that manufacture the products they recommend. In a few cases, investigators have advance knowledge of a medical device because of their research and they purchase stock in the belief its price will rise. Having clinician-investigators with an economic interest in products they are evaluating for safety and efficacy threatens both honesty and fidelity. Yet this arrangement is largely unchecked and growing.[90]

The Dual Roles of Physician and Investigator

The Declaration of Geneva of the World Medical Association affirms that "the health of my patient will be my first consideration," and the Physician's Oath of this same association demands that "Concern for the interests of the subject [of research] must always prevail over the interests of science and society." But can research involving patients and other subjects consistently honor these obligations? The dual roles of research scientist and clinical practitioner pull in different directions and present both conflicting obligations and conflicting interests. As an investigator, the physician acts to generate scientific knowledge to benefit individual patients in the future. As a clinician, responsibilities for care require acting in the best interests of present patients. Both roles are intended to benefit the sick, but the scientific role is directed at unknown, future patients, whereas the clinical role is aimed at known, current patients. Accordingly, responsibility to future generations may conflict with due care for particular current patients.

Research involving human subjects is socially important, but morally perilous because it exposes subjects to risk for the advancement of science. Ethically justified research must satisfy several conditions, including (1) a reasonable prospect that the research will generate the knowledge that is sought, (2) the necessity of using human subjects, (3) a favorable balance of potential benefits over risks to the subjects, and (4) fair selection of subjects.[91] Only after these conditions have been met, is it appropriate to ask potential subjects to participate.

Because society encourages and supports extensive research and because investigators and subjects are unequal in knowledge and vulnerability, public policy and review committees must act to prevent potentially exploitative contracts, to protect privacy and confidentiality, and the like. Some cases warrant a straightforward paternalistic decision. For example, if healthy persons with no heart disease volunteer as subjects in a protocol to have an artificial heart transplanted, as occurred at the University of Utah,[92] an IRB should declare that the risk relative to benefit for a healthy subject is too substantial to permit the research, although the risk relative to benefit for a patient with a seriously diseased heart may be acceptable.

These observations apply to both *nontherapeutic* research, which offers no prospect of medical benefit to the subject, and *therapeutic* research, which offers some prospect of medical benefit to the patient-subject and is usually conducted as a part of the care of the patient. We should use these terms with caution, because the term "therapeutic" can deflect attention from the fact that *research* is being conducted. As a scientific effort, therapeutic research is distinguishable from both routine therapy and experimental or innovative therapy, which are directed at particular patients. Attaching the favorable term "therapeutic" to research can be dangerous, because it suggests "justified intervention" in the care of particular patients and may create a misconception. Sick patients, who may be heavily dependent on a physician, may believe that anything the physician recommends will be beneficial. Therapeutic research must satisfy the conditions of justified research, just as much as nontherapeutic research.

Conflicts in Clinical Trials

Controlled clinical trials are sometimes needed to confirm that an observed effect, such as reduced mortality from a disease, results from a particular intervention rather than from an unknown variable in the patient population. The evidence supporting many available treatments is tenuous and needs validation, and some procedures have never been adequately tested for either safety or efficacy. If doubt surrounds the efficacy or safety of a treatment, or its relative merits in comparison to another treatment, scientific research that can resolve the doubt is in order. Controlled trials are scientific instruments intended to protect current and future patients against medical enthusiasm and hunches. In such research, one group receives the experimental therapy, while a "control group" receives either a standard therapy or a placebo in order to allow investigators to determine whether an experimental therapy is more effective and safer than a standard therapy or a placebo. Usually, subjects are randomly arraigned to control and experimental groups to avoid intentional or unintentional bias. Randomization is designed to keep variables other than the particular treatments under examination from distorting study results. Most controlled trials are randomized clinical trials (RCTs), which are generally preferred to observational or retrospective studies on grounds that their results have a higher degree of validity.

Blinding certain persons to some information about the RCT provides an additional protection against bias. An RCT may be single-blind (the subject does not know whether he or she is in the control group or the experimental group), double-blind (neither the subject nor the investigator knows), or unblinded (all parties know). Double-blind studies are designed specifically to reduce bias in observations and interpretations by subjects, physicians, and investigators. Blinding the physician-investigator, according to some interpretations, also serves an ethical function, because it obviates any conflict of interest for those who both provide therapy and conduct research.

Problems of consent. Potential subjects in RCTs usually do not know which treatment or placebo they will receive. In the specific case of randomized clinical trials, no justification exists for failing to disclose to potential subjects the full set of methods, treatments, and placebos (if any) that will be used, their known risks and benefits, and any uncertainties. Likewise, no justification exists for failing to disclose the fact of randomization and the rationale for it. Any physician-researcher with dual responsibilities has a fiduciary obligation to inform patient-subjects of matters directly relevant to their decisions, including any conflicts of interest.[43] If this information is supplied, potential subjects should have an adequate informational base for deciding whether to participate, despite the fact that they do not know whether they will receive a particular treatment or placebo.

In conventional RCTs, investigators screen patients for eligibility and then inform them about the study, its different arms, the risks and benefits, and the use of randomization for assignment to the different arms. If a patient consents to participate, he or she is then randomized to one arm of the study. Preconsent randomization, often called "prerandomization," modifies the standard approach: Randomization occurs prior to consent to participate.

The National Surgical Adjuvant Project for Breast and Bowel Cancers designed a study of treatments of breast cancer to determine whether survival rates differed among patients randomly assigned to simple mastectomy versus lumpectomy, with or without radiation. This RCT had a low rate of patient participation, and researchers thought it might have to be discontinued because the small number of subjects threatened the canons of statistical significance. Many of the problems with both physician and patient participation centered on the random assignment to different arms of the study. Physicians had difficulty approaching patients about the fact that *chance* determined the treatment. They had difficulty with informed consent in such a context, because of the uncertainty about which patients would receive "treatments," because they perceived conflicts between the role of scientist and the role of clinician, and because they would experience feelings of personal responsibility if one treatment proved superior to the other.

For their part, patients had difficulty accepting surgery not knowing whether their breasts would be removed.[94] For this RCT to be ethically justified, it had to be reasonable to assume that neither treatment was superior in survival rates. But if such conditions of "clinical equipoise" (see below) regarding survival are satisfied, considerations of quality-of-life become central in decisions to participate, and in this case, many women preferred the less invasive and disfiguring surgery. However, after a policy of prerandomization was adopted, the accrual rate increased sixfold and the trial was salvaged, producing sound evidence that the survival rates are as good with the less disfiguring surgery for early breast cancer.[95]

Critics have raised several moral questions about the use of prerandomization in this research protocol. It remains unclear how the mere shift in time of randomization—from randomization after consent to preconsent randomization—could increase patient accrual unless some distortion occurred in the information patients received. Even if they had no preference for one treatment over the other, some patients may have refused conventional randomization because of its uncertainty. However, some critics suspect that disclosure of information became distorted, perhaps unconsciously, when the physician knew the assigned treatment in advance.[96] Clearly, the *process* of obtaining informed consent under prerandomization merits unusually careful scrutiny to ensure adequate disclosure.

Even in the face of objective scientific evidence that two proposed treatments are roughly equal in safety and efficacy, patients may have strong subjective preferences for one treatment over another. Suppose two surgical procedures for treating the same disease appear to have the same survival rate (say, an average of 15 years), and suppose we test their effectiveness by an RCT. The patient might have a preference if treatment A has little risk of death during the operation but a high rate of death after ten years, whereas treatment B has a high risk of death during the operation or postoperative recovery but a low rate of death after recovery (say, for 30 years). A patient's age, family responsibilities, and other circumstances might be other factors leading to a preference for one over the other. If no known difference exists in the rates of survival between two interventions, patients may have a strong preference for one of them—for example, high-risk surgery rather than high radiation dosage, or for a less invasive or less disfiguring procedure. Some patients will prefer the lowest risk procedure, whereas others will gamble on risk for a potentially greater benefit.

The problem of clinical equipoise. Serving the patient's best interests seems inconsistent with assigning a treatment randomly in order to promote social goals of accumulating knowledge and benefitting future patients. No two patients are alike, and a physician should be able to modify the course of therapy, as required by the patient's best interests. But is this axiom of medical ethics consistent with randomized controlled trials?

Proponents argue that RCTs do not violate moral obligations to patients because they are used only in circumstances in which justifiable doubt exists about the merits of existing, standard, or new therapies. No one knows prior to conducting the research whether it is more advantageous to be in the control group or in the experimental group. Reasonable physicians are therefore in a state of "clinical equipoise"[97]: On the basis of the available evidence, members of the relevant expert medical community are equally poised between the treatment strategies being tested in the RCT, because they are equally uncertain about, and equally comfortable with, the known advantages and disadvantages of the treatments to be tested (or the placebo being used). No patient, then, will receive a treatment known to be less effective or more dangerous than an available alternative. Because current patients are not asked to sacrifice a superior treatment and may benefit from the experiment, the use of RCTs seems justifiable, especially in light of the promise of benefit to future patients. No reasonable person could have objective grounds before the trial for preferring to be in one group rather than another, although he or she may prefer one over the other on the basis of hunches or intuitions about effectiveness and safety or on the basis of factors not being studied in the trial. For example, as we noted above, if two treatments for breast cancer are in veritable clinical equipoise, a woman may prefer the less disfiguring treatment.

Whether a particular trial satisfies these justifying conditions is often a central issue.[98] If some cooperating physicians believe prior to the trial that one therapy is more beneficial or safer, they should not simply suspend this belief in the interests of scientific objectivity. It is not sufficient to argue that the trial provides a corrective to the physician's hunches, because this claim evades questions about whether the *physician* has an obligation not to participate or to inform patients about his or her belief. Physicians are obligated to communicate their beliefs about risks and benefits, together with an overall assessment of what they believe is in the patient's best interest. An honest communication will not conceal any of the physician's relevant beliefs and will disclose what will happen as the trial proceeds if the physician forms new or altered opinions.

The physician has a strict therapeutic obligation to offer his or her best professional judgment, but also to obtain the patient's informed consent prior to initiating treatment. The latter obligation entails explaining the risks and benefits of all reasonable alternatives, including enrollment in an appropriate RCT to test one treatment against another. As Don Marquis has pointed out, "physicians have a greater duty to offer patients enrollment in trials than has previously been realized," and to do so in the very context of offering their best professional judgment.[99]

The use of placebo controls. Some examples illustrate these and other controversial aspects of RCTs, particularly the use of placebo controls when no acceptable treatments exist and the condition is fatal. In one classic case, a conflict erupted over placebo-controlled trials of AZT in the treatment of AIDS. Promising laboratory tests led to a trial (phase I) to determine the safety of AZT among patients with AIDS. Several patients showed clinical improvement during this trial. Because AIDS was considered invariably fatal, many people argued that compassion dictated making it immediately available to all patients with AIDS and, perhaps, to those who were antibody-positive to the AIDS virus. However, the company did not have an adequate supply of the drug, and, as required by federal regulations, it used a placebo-controlled trial of AZT to determine its effectiveness for certain groups of patients with AIDS. A computer randomly assigned some patients to AZT and others to a placebo. For several months, no major differences emerged in effectiveness, but then patients receiving the placebo began to die at a significantly higher rate. Of the 137 patients on the placebo, 16 died. Of the 145 patients on AZT, only one died. In view of these results, a data and safety monitoring board advised terminating the trial. Subjects who had received the placebo in the trial were, as promised, the first to receive the drug.

Beginning in early 1987, the drug was distributed according to strict criteria because the supply was inadequate for all AIDS patients, there was inadequate evidence about its effectiveness for some groups of patients, and there was uncertainty about whether the risks of the drug (e.g., its toxicity) would outweigh its benefits to patients at earlier stages of the disease. Proponents of compassion for present patients have raised questions about starting such a placebo-controlled trial when a disease appears to be universally fatal and no promising alternative to the new treatment exists. They have also raised questions about when to stop a trial, as well as how to distribute a new treatment.[100]

Although commonly used in the investigation of pharmaceutical agents, RCTs (particularly placebo-controlled) are rare in surgery. Some worry that surgical procedures are too easily introduced without sufficiently rigorous evidence of their efficacy or safety. In one case, surgical researchers wanted to set up a clinical trial to determine whether transplanting fetal neural tissue into the brains of patients with Parkinson's disease (a disorder of motor function, marked by tremor, rigidity, unsteady walking, and unstable posture) would be safe and effective. Standard medical treatment consists of levodopa, which may not restore lost motor function, may have adverse effects over a long period, and may not adequately control new manifestations of the disease. Researchers contended that surgical therapy using cells is more like administration of pharmaceutical agents than conventional surgical procedures. In order to have the most rigorous investigation, they proposed a randomized, double-blind, placebo-controlled trial. Because surgery itself may have some effects, researchers believed that a placebo control was preferable to the use of standard medical treatment as the control. The placebo consisted of sham surgery—that is, the administration of general anesthesia followed by bilateral surgery, a skin incision with a partial burr hole that does not penetrate the skull's inner cortex. This sham surgery would be compared to two other procedures that would differ from each other only in the amount of fetal tissue transplanted. The 36 subjects in this study knew that 12 of them would undergo sham surgery, but researchers also promised them free access to the real surgery if the trial demonstrated its net benefits.

The basic moral argument against the use of the sham surgery as a placebo control in this research is that risks from the procedure and the anesthesia are substantial. In this trial, the best research design (from the standpoints of both the researchers involved and future patients) unduly conflicted with researchers' obligations of beneficence and nonmaleficence to current patients who were invited to serve as research subjects. From this perspective, appeals to the patient-subjects' consent were inadequate to justify the research.[101]

Early Termination of and Withdrawal from Clinical Trials

Physician-researchers sometimes face difficult questions about whether to stop an experiment before its planned completion, occasionally before they have sufficient data to support final conclusions. Access to data is limited during clinical trials to protect the integrity of the research. Consequently, physicians are excluded from access to information about trends to use in treating their patients. If they were aware of trends prior to the point of statistical significance, they might pull their patients from the trial, thereby invalidating the research.

However, if a physician determines that a patient's condition is deteriorating and that the patient's interests dictate withdrawal from the research, the physician should be free to act on behalf of the patient, assuming the patient concurs. In an RCT, it may be difficult to determine whether the experiment, as a whole, should be stopped even if some physician-researchers insist that they are satisfied by the preliminary evidence regarding trends. One procedural way to handle this ethical conflict is to differentiate roles. We can distinguish between individual physicians who must make decisions regarding their own patients and a data and safety monitoring committee established to determine whether to continue or stop a trial. Unlike the physicians, such a committee is charged to consider the impact of its decision on treatments for future patients, as well as on current patient-subjects. A major function of such committees is to stop a trial if accumulated data indicate that the circumstance of equipoise has shifted and uncertainty no longer prevails. Accordingly, any RCT needs a well-functioning data and safety monitoring committee to determine when clinical equipoise no longer exists.

This differentiation of roles by using a monitoring committee, particularly in a double-blind RCT, is procedurally sound, but it relocates rather than resolves some central ethical questions. The committee still must determine when, if ever, it is legitimate to impose risks on current patients in order to benefit future ones by establishing with a high degree of certainty the superiority of one treatment over another or over a placebo. A committee will likely take the perspective that clinical equipoise must have been eliminated *from the perspective of the expert medical community*.[102] However, the individual physician and his or her patient may be concerned primarily with whether clinical uncertainty has been eliminated *for them*.

Consent forms typically disclose that subjects may withdraw at any time, without detriment to their care. Many questions are relevant to a patient-subject's decision to withdraw from an RCT, including questions about interim data and early trends. Trends are often misleading and are sometimes later shown to be temporary aberrations. However, they might be relevant at a given point to a patient-subject's decision about whether to continue to participate, despite the fact that the evidence would not satisfy statisticians on the project or the expert medical community. As a rule, information about trends is not released prior to the completion or early termination of the RCT. This rule is justifiable if and only if prospective subjects understand and accept it as a condition for participating in the RCT.[103]

Justifying Conditions for Randomized Clinical Trials

Despite problems with RCTs, we believe they are justified if they satisfy the following conditions:

1. True clinical equipoise exists in the group of relevant medical experts;
2. The trial is designed as a crucial experiment between therapeutic alternatives and shows scientific promise of achieving this result;
3. An IRB has approved the protocol and certified that no physician has a conflict of interest or incentive that would threaten the patient–physician relationship;

4. Patient-subjects give comprehensive informed consent (as specified in Chapter 3);

5. Placebos cannot be used if an effective treatment exists for the condition being studied, if that condition involves death or serious morbidity, and if a new treatment is promising;

6. A data and safety monitoring committee will either end the trial when statistically significant data displace clinical equipoise or will supply physicians and patients with significant safety and therapeutic information that is relevant to a reasonable person's decision to remain in or to withdraw from the trial; and

7. Physicians have the right to recommend withdrawal, and patients have the right to withdraw at any time.

The first condition is worth stressing. Equipoise is essential for justified clinical research, because, without it, the superior treatment must be provided. In trials with several arms, every arm must exhibit equipoise. A shift in data that disturbs equipoise destroys the rationale for using the patients involved, because a treatment preference has emerged. Equipoise is also a necessary condition of all justified clinical research, not only of randomized clinical trials.

Beyond these conditions, we take the view that medical knowledge and scientific progress are vital societal goals, but that particular research protocols are often optional. Our obligations to future patients are so strong that we should permit, encourage, and support research that can generate knowledge, but do so without violating the rights and interests of current patients. RCTs should not become indispensable rituals or necessary canons of valid research. Historical controls may be sufficient, and, in some cases, prospective studies can be conducted without randomization, with evaluations performed by parties not involved in the research in order to eliminate bias.

Scientific research in the last half century has transformed medicine from a caretaking role with little power to cure serious disease to a robust practice capable of remarkable forms of cure, palliation, and risk reduction. This transformation has been sufficiently complete that we forget how profoundly biomedical research has shaped the modern world. Nonetheless, this research can present serious risks to its subjects. It requires constant scrutiny in light of the demands of fidelity and other fundamental moral commitments of the medical enterprise.

Conclusion

In this chapter, we have further interpreted and specified principles of respect for autonomy, nonmaleficence, beneficence, and justice for relationships in research and health care. We have concentrated on obligations and virtues that express these principles—obligations of veracity, privacy, confidentiality, and fidelity—and their conflicts. In each instance, we have explored the basis, meaning, limits, and stringency of these obligations in the context of professional and patient or subject relationships.

Notes

1. *Current Opinions of the Judicial Council of the American Medical Association* (Chicago: AMA, 1981), p. ix.
2. Henry Sidgwick, *The Methods of Ethics*, 7th ed. (Indianapolis, IN: Hackett Publishing Company, 1907), pp. 315–16.
3. G. J. Warnock, *The Object of Morality* (London: Methuen, 1971), p. 85.
4. See W. D. Ross, *The Right and the Good* (Oxford: Clarendon Press, 1930), ch. 2.
5. See the treatment of problems in the obligation of veracity in Nancy Potter, "Discretionary Power, Lies, and Broken Trust: Justification and Discomfort," *Theoretical Medicine* 17 (1996): 329–52; Christopher James Ryan, et al., "Becoming None But Tradesmen: Lies, Deception and Psychotic Patients," *Journal of Medical Ethics* 21 (1995): 72–76; Roger Higgs, "Truth-Telling, Lying and the Doctor-Patient Relationship," in *Principles of Health Care Ethics,* ed. Raanan Gillon (London: Wiley, 1994), pp. 499–509.
6. For a sensitive analysis of the actual practices of American doctors in truth-telling with dying patients (an analysis based on semistructured interviews with 32 physicians in a teaching hospital), see Naoko T. Miyaji, "The Power of Compassion: Truth-Telling Among American Doctors in the Care of Dying Patients," *Social Science and Medicine* 36 (1993): 249–64.
7. For valuable overviews of sociocultural contexts of physician–patient communication about cancer and nondisclosure, with reports on a number of different countries, see Antonella Surbone and Matjaz Zwitter, eds., *Communication with the Cancer Patient: Information and Truth, Annals of the New York Academy of Sciences* 809 (February 20, 1997). See also Ole Thomsen, Henrik Wulff, Alessandro Martin, and Peter A. Singer, "What Do Gastroenterologists in Europe Tell Cancer Patients?" *Lancet* 341 (Feb. 20, 1993): 473–76.
8. This case is discussed in Bettina Schöne-Seifert and James F. Childress, "How Much Should the Cancer Patient Know and Decide?" *CA-A Cancer Journal for Physicians* 36 (1986): 85–94.
9. See Donald Oken, "What To Tell Cancer Patients: A Study of Medical Attitudes," *Journal of the American Medical Association* 175 (1961): 1120–28; Dennis H. Novack, et al., "Changes in Physicians' Attitudes Toward Telling the Cancer Patient," *Journal of the American Medical Association* 241 (March 2, 1979): 897–900; Saul S. Radovsky, "Bearing the News," *New England Journal of Medicine* 313 (August 29, 1985): 586–88.
10. Thurstan B. Brewin, "Telling the Truth" (Letter), *The Lancet* 343 (June 11, 1994): 1512. Several subsequent letters to the editor support the physician's response; see *The Lancet* 344 (July 16, 1994): 196.
11. Nicholas A. Christakis, *Death Foretold: Prophecy and Prognosis in Medical Care* (Chicago: University of Chicago Press, 1999), esp. ch. 5. See also Afaf Girgis and Rob Sanson-Fisher, "Breaking Bad News: Consensus Guidelines for Medical Practitioners," *Journal of Clinical Oncology* 13 (1995): 2449–56; J. T. Ptacek and Tara Eberhardt, "Breaking Bad News: A Review of the Literature," *Journal of the American Medical Association* 276 (August 14, 1996): 496–502; and George J. Annas,

"Informed Consent, Cancer, and Truth in Prognosis," *New England Journal of Medicine* 330 (January 20, 1994): 223–25.

12. See Naoko T. Miyaji, "The Power of Compassion: Truth-Telling Among American Doctors in the Care of Dying Patients," pp. 249–64, and Letter to the Editor, "Informed Consent, Cancer, and Truth in Prognosis," *New England Journal of Medicine* 331 (September 22, 1994): 810. In European countries, physicians also provide more information about diagnosis and treatment than they do about prognosis. See E. Espinosa, P. Zamora, and M. Gonzalez Baron, Letter to Editor, "Informed Consent, Cancer, and Truth in Prognosis," *New England Journal of Medicine* 331 (September 22, 1994): 811; and E. Espinosa, et al., "The Information Given to the Terminal Patient with Cancer," *European Journal of Cancer* 29A (1993): 1795–96.

13. Joel Stein, "A Fragile Commodity," *Journal of the American Medical Association* 283 (January 19, 2000): 305–06.

14. James Boswell, *Life of Johnson*, as quoted in Alan Donagan, *The Theory of Morality* (Chicago: University of Chicago Press, 1979), p. 89.

15. Leo Tolstoy, *The Death of Ivan Ilych,* trans. Aylmer Maude, in *The Death of Ivan Ilych and Other Stories* (New York: The New American Library, 1960), p. 137.

16. Antonella Surbone, "Truth Telling to the Patient," *Journal of the American Medical Association*, 268 (October 7, 1992): 1661–62; and Surbone, "Truth-Telling, Risk, and Hope," in *Communication with the Cancer Patient: Information and Truth, Annals of the New York Academy of Sciences* 809 (February 20, 1997): 72–79.

17. See P. Mosconi, B. E. Meyerowitz, M. C. Liberati, et al., "Disclosure of Breast Cancer Diagnosis," *Annuals of Oncology* 2 (1991): 273–80, as discussed in Surbone, "Truth Telling to the Patient."

18. Edmund D. Pellegrino, "Is Truth Telling to the Patient a Cultural Artifact?" *Journal of the American Medical Association* 268 (October 7, 1992): 1734–35.

19. Daniel Rayson, "Lisa's Stories," *Journal of the American Medical Association* 282 (November 3, 1999): 1605–06.

20. C. Vincent, M. Young, and A. Phillips, "Why Do People Sue Doctors? A Study Of Patients And Relatives Taking Legal Actions," *The Lancet* 343 (1994): 1609–13; Amy B. Witman, Deric M. Park, and Steven B. Hardin, "How Do Patients Want Physicians to Handle Mistakes? A Survey of Internal Medicine Patients in an Academic Setting," *Archives of Internal Medicine* 156 (December 9–23, 1996): 2565–69. For a discussion of ethical issues, see several articles in *Journal of Clinical Ethics* 8 (Winter 1997): 323–58.

21. See Michael A. Greenberg, "The Consequences of Truth Telling," *Journal of the American Medical Association* 266 (July 3, 1991): 66.

22. Dennis H. Novack, Barbara J. Detering, Robert Arnold, et al., "Physicians' Attitudes Toward Using Deception to Resolve Difficult Ethical Problems," *Journal of the American Medical Association* 261 (May 26, 1989): 2980–85.

23. Joanna M. Cain, "Is Deception for Reimbursement in Obstetrics and Gynecology Justified?" *Obstetrics & Gynecology* 82 (September 1993): 475–78.

24. Kaiser Family Foundation, "Survey of Physicians and Nurses," at http://www.kff.org/1999/1503.

25. M. K. Wynia, D. S. Cummins, J. B. VanGeest, and I. B. Wilson, "Physician Manipulation of Reimbursement Rules for Patient: Between a Rock and a Hard Place," *Journal of the American Medical Association* 283 (April 12, 2000): 1858–65, and the Commentary by M. Gregg Bloche, "Fidelity and Deceit at the Bedside" in the same issue, pp. 1881–84. Contrast the report (in a study conducted during the same

period) in James L. Bernat, et al., "Attitudes of U.S. Neurologists concerning the Ethical Dimensions of Managed Care," *Neurology* 49 (1997): 4–13.

26. Victor G. Freeman, Saif S. Rathore, Kevin P. Weinfurt, et al., "Lying for Patients: Physician Deception of Third-Party Payers," *Archives of Internal Medicine* 159 (October 25, 1999): 2263–70. For the ethical debate about such practices, see "Intentional Deception by Physicians," *Journal of the American Medical Association* 282 (November 3, 1999): 1674–79. See also Robert L. Prosser, Jr., "Alternation of Medical Records Submitted for Medicolegal Review," *Journal of the American Medical Association* 267 (May 20, 1992): 2630–31; Paul Jesilow, Gibert Geis, and Henry Pontell, "Fraud by Physicians Against Medicaid," *Journal of the American Medical Association* 266 (December 18, 1991): 3318–22; and Gail Sekas and William R. Hutson, "Misrepresentation of Academic Accomplishments by Applicants for Gastroenterology Fellowships," *Annals of Internal Medicine* 123 (July 1, 1995): 38–41.

27. Dorothy C. Wertz, "The 19-Nation Survey: Genetics and Ethics Around the World;" and John C. Fletcher, "Ethics and Human Genetics: A Cross-Cultural Perspective," in *Ethics and Human Genetics: A Cross-Cultural Perspective*, ed. Wertz and Fletcher (New York: Springer-Verlag, 1989), pp. 13–17.

28. See Fletcher, "Ethics and Human Genetics: A Cross-Cultural Perspective," p. 482.

29. See Jonathan Alter with Peter McKillop, "AIDS and the Right To Know: A Question of Privacy," *Newsweek*, August 18, 1986, pp. 46–47.

30. A useful history of privacy in American law, including original sources, appears in Richard C. Turkington, George B. Trubow, and Anita L. Allen, eds., *Privacy: Cases and Materials* (Houston, TX: John Marshall Publishing Co., 1992), ch. 1. See also Samuel Warren and Louis Brandeis, "The Right to Privacy," *Harvard Law Review* 4 (1890): 193–220; Lawrence O. Gostin, et al., "The Public Health Information Infrastructure: A National Review of the Law on Health Information Privacy," *Journal of the American Medical Association* 275 (June 26, 1996): 1921–27. Our analysis of privacy has benefited from an unpublished paper by and discussion with Michael Duffy.

31. *Griswold v. Connecticut* [381 U.S. 479 (1965), at 486]. Some subsequent Supreme Court decisions held that the right to privacy, although not explicitly enumerated in the Bill of Rights, emanates from the "penumbra" of the first, third, fourth, fifth, ninth, and fourteenth amendments to the Constitution. The thesis is that a personal right to privacy exists because these amendments imply it. See also *Roe v. Wade*, 410 U.S. 113 (1973); a critical intervening case is *Eisenstadt v. Baird*, 405 U.S. 438 (1972), esp. at 453, and *Planned Parenthood of Southeastern Pennsylvania v. Casey*, 112 S.Ct. 2791 (1992), esp. at 851. See also *Bowers v. Hardwick*, 478 U.S. 186 (1986). Many problems have beset privacy-rights doctrine in law, especially its extension to areas involving the right to die. See *Cruzan v. Director, Missouri Dept. of Health*, 110 S.Ct. 2841, at 2851; Carl E. Schneider, "*Cruzan* and the Constitutionalization of American Life," *The Journal of Medicine and Philosophy* 17 (1992): 589–604; and Thomas Halper, "Privacy and Autonomy: From Warren and Brandeis to *Roe* and *Cruzan*," *Journal of Medicine and Philosophy* 21 (1996): 121–35.

32. Anita L. Allen, "Genetic Privacy: Emerging Concepts and Values," in Mark A. Rothstein, ed., *Genetic Secrets: Protecting Privacy and Confidentiality in the Genetic Era* (New Haven, CT: Yale University Press, 1997), pp. 31–59. Judith Wagner DeCew characterizes privacy as "a complex of three related clusters of claims concerning information, access, and activities." In *Pursuit of Privacy: Law, Ethics, and the Rise of Technology* (Ithaca, NY: Cornell University Press, 1997).

33. See the discussion and recommendations in *Research Involving Human Biological Materials: Ethical Issues and Policy Guidance*, Vol. I: Report and Recommendations of the National Bioethics Advisory Commission (Rockville, MD: NBAC, August 1999).

34. Ruth Gavison, "Privacy and the Limits of Law," *The Yale Law Journal* 89 (1980): 428.

35. Some definitions center on a narrow range of conditions, under which intrusions constitute losses of privacy, whereas other definitions center on a broader range of conditions. Some definitions view privacy as a condition of the person, others as a condition of control by the person over access to information. Some definitions place a value on privacy, others do not. See Madison Powers' survey of several definitions in "A Cognitive Access Definition of Privacy," *Law and Philosophy* 15 (1996): 369–86, and Anita L. Allen's examination of restricted-access definitions in *Uneasy Access: Privacy for Women in a Free Society* (Totowa, NJ: Rowman and Littlefield, 1988), esp. pp. 11–17.

36. Charles Fried, "Privacy: A Rational Context," *The Yale Law Journal* 77 (1968): 475–93.

37. Thomson, "The Right to Privacy," *Philosophy and Public Affairs* 4 (Summer 1975): 295–314, as reprinted in Schoeman, ed., *Philosophical Dimensions of Privacy* (New York: Cambridge University Press, 1984), pp. 272–89; esp. 280–87.

38. James Rachels, "Why Privacy Is Important," p. 292, and Edward Bloustein, "Privacy as an Aspect of Human Dignity," both as reprinted in Schoeman, ed., *Philosophical Dimensions of Privacy.*

39. Fried, "Privacy: A Rational Context."

40. Joel Feinberg, *Harm to Self,* Vol. III in *The Moral Limits of the Criminal Law* (New York: Oxford University Press, 1986), ch. 19.

41. National Institute of Allergy and Infectious Diseases, *National Institutes of Health, HIV/AIDS Statistics* (December 1999).

42. Bernard Lo, Robert L. Steinbrook, Moly Cooke, et al., "Voluntary Screening for Human Immunodeficiency Virus (HIV) Infection: Weighing the Benefits and Harms," *Annals of Internal Medicine* 110 (May 1989): 730. Our account of risks and benefits relies in part on this account. For a European perspective, with an emphasis on reciprocity of obligations, see Rebecca Bennett and Charles A. Erin, *HIV and AIDS: Testing, Screening, and Confidentiality* (Oxford: Oxford University Press, 1999).

43. See Kathleen Nolan, "Ethical Issues in Caring for Pregnant Women and Newborns at Risk for Human Immunodeficiency Virus Infection," *Seminars in Perinatology* 13 (February 1989): 55–65. See also Jeffrey T. Berger, Fred Rosner, and Peter Farnsworth, "The Ethics of Mandatory HIV Testing in Newborns," *Journal of Clinical Ethics* 7 (1996): 77–84; Carol Levine and Ronald Bayer, "The Ethics of Screening for Early Intervention in HIV Disease," *American Journal of Public Health* 79 (December 1989): 1661–67; and several essays in Ruth Faden, Gail Geller, and Madison Powers, eds., *AIDS, Women and the Next Generation* (New York: Oxford University Press, 1991).

44. See E. M. Connor, R. S. Sperling, R. Gelber, et al., "Reduction of Maternal-Infant Transmission of Human Immunodeficiency Virus Type 1 with Zidovudine Treatment," *New England Journal of Medicine* 331 (1994): 1173–80.

45. See, for example, Martha F. Rogers and Nathan Shaffer, "Reducing the Risk of Maternal-Infant Transmission of HIV by Attacking the Virus," *New England Journal of Medicine* 341 (August 5, 1999): 441–43.

46. Nolan, "Ethical Issues in Caring for Pregnant Women and Newborns," p. 64. See also LeRoy Walters, "Ethical Issues in HIV Testing During Pregnancy," in *AIDS, Women and the Next Generation*, ch. 4.
47. George J. Annas, "Control of Tuberculosis—The Law and the Public's Health," *New England Journal of Medicine* 328 (February 25, 1993): 585–88; see also M. Rose Gasner, et al., "The Use of Legal Action in New York City to Ensure Treatment of Tuberculosis," *New England Journal of Medicine* 340 (February 4, 1999): 359–66; Ronald Bayer and Laurence Dupuis, "Tuberculosis, Public Health, and Civil Liberties," *Annual Review of Public Health* 16 (1995): 307–26; and Lawrence O. Gostin, "Controlling the Resurgent Tuberculosis Epidemic," *Journal of the American Medical Association* 269 (January 13, 1993): 255–61.
48. Michael D. Iseman, David L. Cohn, and John A. Sbarbaro, "Directly Observed Treatment of Tuberculosis: We Can't Afford Not To Try It," *New England Journal of Medicine* 328 (February 25, 1993): 576–78; Tom Oscherwitz, et al., "Detention of Persistently Nonadherent Patients with Tuberculosis," *Journal of the American Medical Association* 278 (September 10, 1997): 843–46.
49. See Joke I. de Witte and Henk ten Have, "Ownership of Genetic Material and Information," *Social Science and Medicine* 45 (1997): 51–60; and Sonia M. Suter, "Whose Genes are They Anyway?: Familial Conflicts over Access to Genetic Information," *Michigan Law Review* 91 (1993): 1854–1908.
50. See Scott Burris and Lawrence O. Gostin, "Genetic Screening from a Public Health Perspective: Some Lessons from the HIV Experience," in Rothstein, ed., *Genetic Secrets*, pp. 137–58.
51. See Alexander M. Capron, "Which Ills to Bear?: Reevaluating the 'Threat' of Modern Genetics," *Emory Law Journal* 39 (1990): 678–96.
52. Paul R. Billings, Mel A. Kohn, Margaret de Cuevas, et al., "Discrimination as a Consequence of Genetic Testing," *American Journal of Human Genetics* 50 (1992): 476–82.
53. Lawrence O. Gostin, "Genetic Privacy," *Journal of Law, Medicine & Ethics* 23 (1995): 320–30. See also his "Health Information Privacy," *Cornell Law Review* 80 (1995): 101–84.
54. Mark A. Rothstein, "Genetic Secrets: A Policy Framework," in Rothstein, ed., *Genetic Secrets*, p. 453; and Rothstein, "Genetic Privacy and Confidentiality: Why They Are So Hard To Protect," *Journal of Law, Medicine and Ethics* 26 (1998): 198–204.
55. Mark Siegler, "Confidentiality in Medicine—A Decrepit Concept," *New England Journal of Medicine* 307 (1982): 1518–21; see further Bernard Friedland, "Physician–Patient Confidentiality: Time to Re-examine a Venerable Concept in Light of Contemporary Society and Advances in Medicine," *Journal of Legal Medicine* 15 (1994): 249–77.
56. Superior Court of New Jersey, Law Division, Mercer County, Docket No. L88-2550 (April 25, 1991).
57. Barry D. Weiss, "Confidentiality Expectations of Patients, Physicians, and Medical Students," *Journal of the American Medical Association* 247 (1982): 2695–97.
58. *Bratt v. IBM*, 467 N.E.2d 126 (1984).
59. See Kenneth Appelbaum and Paul S. Appelbaum, "The HIV Antibody-Positive Patient," in *Confidentiality Versus the Duty To Protect: Foreseeable Harm in the Practice of Psychiatry*, ed. James C. Beck (Washington, DC: American Psychiatry Press, Inc., 1990), pp. 127–28.
60. Cf. Gregory Larkin, John Moskop, Arthur Sanders, and Arthur Derse, "The Emer-

gency Physician and Patient Confidentiality: A Review," *Annals of Emergency Medicine* 24 (1994): 1161–67. For views to the contrary that propose absolute or near-absolute rules, see Michael H. Kottow, "Medical Confidentiality: An Intransigent and Absolute Obligation," *Journal of Medical Ethics* 12 (1986): 117–22; and H. T. Engelhardt, Jr., *The Foundations of Bioethics*, 2nd ed. (New York: Oxford University Press, 1996), pp. 336–40.

61. For empirical information about the extent of the problem of nondisclosure and unprotected sex, see Michael D. Stein, et al., "Sexual Ethics: Disclosure of HIV-Positive Status to Partners," *Archives of Internal Medicine* 158 (February 1998): 253–57. This study concludes that sexual partners of HIV-infected persons continue to be at significant risk for HIV transmission as a result of nondisclosure.

62. See Grant Gillett, "AIDS and Confidentiality," *Journal of Applied Philosophy* 4 (1987): 15–20, from which this case study has been adapted.

63. Ad Hoc Committee on AIDS Policy, subsequently approved by Board of Trustees, APA, "AIDS Policy: Confidentiality and Disclosure," *American Journal of Psychiatry* 145 (1988): 541. See also APA, "Guidelines on Confidentiality," *American Journal of Psychiatry* 144 (1987): 1522–26.

64. See Susanne E. Landis, Victor J. Schoenbach, David J. Weber, et al., "Results of a Randomized Trial of Partner Notification in Cases of HIV Infection in North Carolina," *New England Journal of Medicine* 326 (January 9, 1992): 101–06.

65. Council on Ethical and Judicial Affairs, "Ethical Issues Involved in the Growing AIDS Crisis," *Journal of the American Medical Association* 259 (March 4, 1988): 1360–61.

66. See Gillett, "AIDS and Confidentiality"; and Case Studies, "AIDS and a Duty to Protect," *Hastings Center Report* 17 (February 1987): 22–23, with commentaries by Morton Winston and Sheldon H. Landesman.

67. See Ronald Bayer and Kathleen E. Toomey, "HIV Prevention and the Two Faces of Partner Notification," *American Journal of Public Health* 82 (August 1992): 1158–64.

68. Lori B. Andrews, Jane E. Fullarton, Neil A. Holtzman, and Arno G. Motulsky, eds. for the Committee on Assessing Genetic Risks, Institute of Medicine, *Assessing Genetic Risks: Implications for Health and Social Policy* (Washington, DC: National Academy Press, 1994), pp. 264–73, 278. See also the guidelines for resolving issues of confidentiality, along with cases, in David H. Smith, Kimberly A. Quaid, Roger B. Dworkin, et al., *Early Warning: Cases and Ethical Guidance for Presymptomatic Testing in Genetic Diseases* (Bloomington, IN: Indiana University Press, 1998); and Ruth Macklin, "Privacy and Control of Genetic Information," in *Gene Mapping: Using Law and Ethics as Guides*, ed. George J. Annas and Sherman Elias (New York: Oxford University Press, 1992).

69. Paul Ramsey, *The Patient as Person* (New Haven, CT: Yale University Press, 1970), p. xii.

70. This case was prepared by John Fletcher.

71. On professional self-effacement, see Edmund Pellegrino, "Altruism, Self-Interest, and Medical Ethics," *Journal of the American Medical Association* 258 (October 9, 1987): 1939–40.

72. See M. Gregg Bloche, "Clinical Loyalties and the Social Purposes of Medicine," *Journal of the American Medical Association* 281 (January 20, 1999): 268–74.

73. Our formulation is indebted to Stephen Toulmin, "Divided Loyalties and Ambiguous Relationships," *Social Science and Medicine* 23 (1986): 784.

74. *In re Sampson*, 317 N.Y.S.2d (1970).

75. *In re A.C.*, 533 A.2d 611 (D.C. App. 1987), vacated and reh'g granted 539 A. 2d 203 (1988).

76. *In re A.C.*, 573 A.2d 1235 (D.C. App. 1990).

77. See Leonard A. Sagan and Albert Jonsen, "Medical Ethics and Torture," *New England Journal of Medicine* 294 (1976): 1428. See also *Medicine Betrayed: The Participation of Doctors in Human Rights Violations*, Report of a Working Party, British Medical Association (London: Zed Books, 1992).

78. See Curtis Prout and Robert N. Ross, *Care and Punishment: The Dilemmas of Prison Medicine* (Pittsburgh, PA: University of Pittsburgh Press, 1988).

79. Richard J. Bonnie, "The Death Penalty: When Doctors Must Say No," *British Medical Journal* 305 (August 15, 1992): 381–82; A. Sikora and Alan R. Fleischman, "Physician Participation in Capital Punishment: A Question of Professional Integrity," *Journal of Urban Health* 76 (1999): 400–08; and Michael Davis, "The State's Dr. Death: What's Unethical About Physicians Helping at Executions?" *Social Theory and Practice* 21 (1995): 31–60.

80. See Robert D. Truog and Troyen Brennan, "Participation of Physicians in Capital Punishment," *New England Journal of Medicine* 329 (October 28, 1993): 1346–50. See also Letters and Comments in *New England Journal of Medicine* 330 (March 31, 1994): 935–37.

81. Martin Benjamin and Joy Curtis, "Ethical Autonomy in Nursing," in *Health Care Ethics*, ed. Donald VanDeVeer and Tom Regan (Philadelphia, PA: Temple University Press, 1987), p. 394.

82. Gregory F. Gramelspacher, Joel D. Howell, and Mark J. Young, "Perceptions of Ethical Problems by Nurses and Doctors," *Archives of Internal Medicine* 146 (March 1986): 577–78.

83. See E. Haavi Morreim, *Balancing Act: The New Medical Ethics of Medicine's New Economics* (Boston: Kluwer Academic Publishers, 1991), which has influenced the following paragraphs.

84. Conflicts of interest may emerge from past actions, such as accepting gifts from corporations. Evidence indicates that some pharmaceutical manufacturers have been able to influence physicians' prescribing behavior through the estimated $8,000 to $10,000 spent each year on each physician. See Ashley Wazana, "Physicians and the Pharmaceutical Industry: Is a Gift Ever Just a Gift?" *Journal of the American Medical Association* 283 (January 19, 2000): 373–80; and Robert M. Tenery, Jr., "Interactions Between Physicians and the Health Care Technology Industry," in the same issue, pp. 391–93. See also Marc A. Rodwin, *Medicine, Money, and Morals: Physicians' Conflicts of Interest* (New York: Oxford University Press, 1993); and Edmund Erde, Roy G. Spece, Jr., David S. Shimm, and Allen E. Buchanan, eds., *Conflicts of Interest in Clinical Practice and Research* (New York: Oxford University Press, 1996), p. 33.

85. See George Khushf and Robert Gifford, "Understanding, Assessing, and Managing Conflicts of Interest," in *Surgical Ethics*, ed. Laurence B. McCullough, James W. Jones, and Baruch A. Brody (New York: Oxford University Press, 1998), pp. 342–66.

86. Morreim, *Balancing Act*, p. 37.

87. See Jean M. Mitchell and T. R. Sass, "Physician Ownership of Ancillary Services: Indirect Demand Inducement or Quality Assurance?" *Journal of Health Economics* 14 (August 1995): 263–89; L. Cohen, "Issue of Fraud Raised as MD Self-Referral Comes Under Spotlight in Ontario," *Canadian Medical Association Journal* 154

(June 1, 1996): 1744–46; Julie E. Mathews, "The Physician Self-Referral Dilemma: Enforcing Antitrust Law as a Solution," *American Journal of Law and Medicine* 19 (1993): 523–46; Jean M. Mitchell and Elton Scott, "Physician Ownership of Physical Therapy Services: Effects on Charges, Utilization, Profits, and Service Characteristics," *Journal of the American Medical Association* 268 (October 21, 1992): 2055–59; Jean M. Mitchell and Jonathan H. Sunshine, "Consequences of Physicians' Ownership of Health Care Facilities—Joint Ventures in Radiation Therapy," *New England Journal of Medicine* 327 (November 19, 1992): 1497–1501; Arnold S. Relman, " 'Self-Referral'—What's At Stake?" *New England Journal of Medicine* 327 (November 19, 1992): 1522–24.

88. Marc A. Rodwin, "Physicians' Conflicts of Interest: The Limitations of Disclosure," *New England Journal of Medicine* 321 (November 16, 1989): 1405–08.

89. See the discussion in Jean M. Mitchell, "Physician Joint Ventures and Self-Referral: An Empirical Perspective," pp. 314–315; and Paul E. Kalb, "Health Care Fraud and Abuse," *Journal of the American Medical Association* 282 (September 22–29, 1999): 1163–68.

90. See several chapters in Part IV, "Clinical Research," in Erde, Spece, Shimm, and Buchanan, eds., *Conflicts of Interest in Clinical Practice and Research*; see also William F. May, "Money and the Medical Profession," *Kennedy Institute of Ethics Journal* 7 (1997): 1–13.

91. See the Nuremberg Code and *The Belmont Report* of the National Commission for the Protection of Human Subjects. See also Alexander M. Capron, "Human Experimentation," in *Medical Ethics*, 2nd ed., ed. Robert M. Veatch (Boston: Jones and Bartlett Publishers, 1997), ch. 6.

92. Disclosed by surgeon William DeVries, as reported in Denise Grady, "Summary of Discussion on Ethical Perspectives," in *After Barney Clark: Reflections on the Utah Artificial Heart Program*, ed. Margery W. Shaw (Austin, TX: University of Texas Press, 1984), p. 49. DeVries and his colleagues at the University of Utah implanted the first artificial heart with the intention that it be permanent in December 1982; the patient, Barney Clark, survived 112 days.

93. See Gunnel Elander and Goran Hermeren, "Placebo Effect and Randomized Clinical Trials," *Theoretical Medicine* 16 (1995): 171–82; B. P. Minogue, et al., "Individual Autonomy and the Double-Blind Controlled Experiment: The Case of Desperate Volunteers," together with Gerald Logue and Stephen Wear, "A Desperate Solution: Autonomy and the Double-Blind Controlled Experiment," both in *Journal of Medicine and Philosophy* (1995): 43–64; and Fried, *Medical Experimentation*, p. 71.

94. C. Redmond and M. Bauer, "Statisticians' Report on Prerandomization," *NSABP Progress Report* (Pittsburgh, PA: National Surgical Adjuvant Project for Breast and Bowel Cancers, 1979), as quoted in Kenneth F. Schaffner, "Ethical Problems in Clinical Trials," *Journal of Medicine and Philosophy* 11 (November 1986): 306; and Kathryn M. Taylor, Richard Margolese, and Colin L. Soskolne, "Physicians' Reasons for not Entering Eligible Patients in a Randomized Clinical Trial of Surgery for Breast Cancer," *New England Journal of Medicine* 310 (May 4, 1984): 1363.

95. Bernard Fischer, et al., "Five-Year Results of a Randomized Clinical Trial Comparing Total Mastectomy and Segmental Mastectomy With or Without Radiation in the Treatment of Breast Cancer," *New England Journal of Medicine* 312 (1985): 665–73.

96. See Don Marquis, "An Argument that All Prerandomized Clinical Trials Are Unethical," *Journal of Medicine and Philosophy* 11 (November 1986): 377, 380; Mar-

cia Angell, "Patient Preferences in Randomized Clinical Trials," *New England Journal of Medicine* 310 (May 24, 1984): 1385–87; and Susan S. Ellenberg, "Randomization Designs in Comparative Clinical Trials," *New England Journal of Medicine* 310 (May 24, 1984): 1404–08. Contrast Kopelman, "Consent and Randomized Clinical Trials," pp. 334–36.

97. See the specific proposals by Benjamin Freedman, "Equipoise and the Ethics of Clinical Research," *New England Journal of Medicine* 317 (July 16, 1987): 141–45; and Eugene Passamani, "Clinical Trials—Are They Ethical?," *New England Journal of Medicine* 324 (May 30, 1991): 1590–91.

98. Fred Gifford, "Community-Equipoise and the Ethics of Randomized Clinical Trials," *Bioethics* 9 (1995): 127–48; and Ezekiel Emanuel, W. Bradford Patterson, and Samuel Hellman, "Ethics of Randomized Clinical Trials," *Journal of Clinical Oncology* 16 (1998): 365–71.

99. Don Marquis, "How to Resolve an Ethical Dilemma Concerning Randomized Clinical Trails," *New England Journal of Medicine* 341 (August 26, 1999): 691–93.

100. See M. A. Fischl, et al., "The Efficacy of Azidothymidine (AZT) in the Treatment of Patients with AIDS-Related Complex: A Double-Blind, Placebo-Controlled Trial," *New England Journal of Medicine* 317 (1987): 185–91; and D. D. Richman, et al., "The Toxicity of Azidothymidine (AZT) in the Treatment of Patients with AIDS and AIDS-Related Complex: A Double-Blind, Placebo-Controlled Trial," *New England Journal of Medicine* 317 (1987): 192–97.

101. For an unconvincing defense of this trial, see Thomas B. Freeman, Dorothy E. Vawter, Paul E. Leaverton, et al., "Use of Placebo Surgery in Controlled Trials of a Cellular-Based Therapy for Parkinson's Disease," *New England Journal of Medicine* 341 (September 23, 1999): 988–92; for an able critique, see Ruth Macklin, "The Ethical Problems with Sham Surgery in Clinical Research," *New England Journal of Medicine* 341 (September 23, 1999): 992–96.

102. This was Freedman's proposal in "Equipoise and the Ethics of Clinical Research."

103. See the sensitive treatments of issues of consent, data monitoring, and the control of information in Robert J. Levine and David K. Dennison, "Randomized Clinical Trials in Periodontology: Ethical Considerations," *Annals of Periodontology* 2 (1997): 83–94; and Valery M. Gordon, Jeremy Sugarman, and Nancy Kass, "Toward a More Comprehensive Approach to Protecting Human Subjects: The Interface of Data Safety Monitoring Boards and Institutional Review Boards in Randomized Clinical Trials," *IRB: A Review of Human Subjects Research* 20 (1998): 1–5.

PART III

8

Moral Theories

This chapter will examine several moral theories and approaches that we mentioned but did not pursue in Chapters 1 and 2. It treats five types of moral theory: utilitarianism, Kantianism, liberal individualism, communitarianism, and the ethics of care. Some knowledge of these general perspectives is indispensable for reflective study in biomedical ethics because much of the field's literature draws on their methods and conclusions.

A textbook approach to moral theory presents several competing theories and then proceeds to criticize each one. Typically, the criticisms are so harsh that each type of theory seems irreparably wounded. As a result, readers become skeptical about the value of ethical theory. This outcome is unfortunate and unnecessary. Defects and excesses appear in all general theories, but the theories discussed in this chapter all contain insights and arguments that deserve careful study. Our goal is to eliminate what is unacceptable in each type of theory and to appropriate what is relevant and acceptable.

We often refer to our own account of ethics as a *theory*, but a word of caution is in order about this term. It is commonly used to refer to each of the following: (1) abstract reflection and argument, (2) a systematic presentation of the basic components of ethics, (3) an integrated body of principles, and (4) a systematic justification of those principles. We have attempted in this book to construct a coherent account adequate for the subject of biomedical ethics. We do not claim to have developed or to presuppose a comprehensive ethical theory in ways suggested by the combination of (3) and (4). We engage *in theory* (e.g., in evaluating other ethical theories), and in doing so we engage in abstract reflection and argument (1). We also present an organized system of principles (3) and engage in systematic reflection and argument (2). But, at best, we present only some elements of a comprehensive *general* theory. Our own theory and method appear in Chapter 9.

Each section of this chapter, except the first and the last, is divided into subsections that are structured as follows: (1) an overview of the characteristic features of the theory being considered (introduced by examining how its proponents would approach a case); (2) a more detailed presentation of the salient features of the theory; (3) an examination of criticisms that point to the theory's limitations and problems; and (4) an indication of the theory's strengths and potential or actual contribution. This structure may seem to imply that we accept several moral theories. We do accept as legitimate various *aspects* of many theories advanced in the history of ethics.[1] However, we reject both the hypothesis that all leading principles in the different major moral theories can be assimilated into a coherent whole and the hypothesis that each of the theories offers an equally tenable moral framework.

Criteria for Theory Construction

We begin with eight conditions of adequacy for an ethical theory. These criteria for theory construction set forth exemplary or ideal conditions for theories, but not so exemplary or ideal that no theory could satisfy them. The fact that all available theories only partially satisfy these conditions does not concern us here. Our objective is to provide a basis from which to assess various theories.

Satisfying at least some of these conditions should protect a theory from criticism as a mere list of ad hoc or poorly assembled norms generated from pretheoretic beliefs. However, some philosophers attack even the criteria that we consider for presenting a distorted view of ethics or for improperly borrowing from scientific, legal, or political theory. We cannot fully engage this controversy, but we offer two observations: First, we have ourselves found these criteria useful guides in assessing general positions in ethics, including our own. Second, however effective these criteria are, we have also found that careful attention to actual moral practices often yields more insight into the moral life than general theories. Even illuminating theories cannot claim to be the only source of moral insight. These theories are usually more plausible if applied to some *limited range* of morality rather than to all of it. For example, utilitarianism seems a better theoretical model for public policy than for clinical medical ethics.

These problems, in part, reflect a conflict between a once-popular conception of ethical theory and a newer and less settled account. In the older conception, popular from the late eighteenth century to the late twentieth century, the task of moral theory is to prescribe and justify general norms as a system. In the newer and less determinate conception, the task of ethics is to reflect critically on actual moral norms and practices. Attitudes toward these criteria may co-travel with how we understand our own moral reflections and those of others we have found insightful.

Eight conditions express a more or less traditional understanding of criteria for ethical theories:[2]

1. *Clarity.* A theory should be as clear as possible, as a whole and in its parts. Although we can expect only as much precision of language as is appropriate, more obscurity and vagueness exist in the literature of ethical theory and biomedical ethics than is necessary or justified by the subject matter.

2. *Coherence.* An ethical theory should be internally coherent. There should be neither conceptual inconsistencies (e.g., "strong medical paternalism is justified only by consent of the patient") nor apparently contradictory statements or positions (e.g., "to be virtuous is a moral obligation, but virtuous conduct is not obligatory"). Ralph Waldo Emerson dismissed a foolish consistency as "the hobgoblin of little minds, adored by little statesmen and philosophers and divines." This obscure insight requires interpretation. Consistency should never be taken as a *sufficient* condition of a good theory, only a *necessary* condition. More importantly, if an account has implications that are incoherent with other parts of that account, some aspect of the theory needs to be changed in a way that does not produce further incoherence. As we indicate in Chapters 1 and 9, a major goal of a theory is to bring into coherence all its various normative elements (e.g., principles, rights, and considered judgments).

3. *Completeness and Comprehensiveness.* A theory should be as complete and comprehensive as possible. A theory would be fully comprehensive if it could account for all moral values and judgments. Any theory that includes fewer moral values will fall somewhere on a continuum, from partially complete to empty of important values. Although the principles presented in this book under the headings of respect for autonomy, nonmaleficence, beneficence, and justice are far from a complete system for general normative ethics, they do, when specified, provide a sufficiently comprehensive general framework for *biomedical ethics.* We do not need additional general principles, such as promise-keeping, avoiding killing, human dignity, keeping contracts, and the like. Instead, we draw on our basic principles to help justify rules, such as those of promise-keeping, truthfulness, privacy, and confidentiality (see especially Chapter 7). These rules increase the system's comprehensiveness by specifying the fundamental principles.

4. *Simplicity.* If a theory with a few basic norms generates sufficient moral content, then that theory is preferable to a theory with more norms but no additional content. A theory should have no more norms than are necessary, and no more than people can use without confusion. However, morality is complicated, and any comprehensive moral theory will be complex.

5. *Explanatory power*. A theory has explanatory power when it provides enough insight to help us understand the moral life: its purpose, its objective or subjective status, how rights are related to obligations, and the like.

6. *Justificatory power*. A theory should also give us grounds for *justified* belief, not merely a reformulation of beliefs we already possess. For example, the distinction between acts and omissions underlies many critical beliefs in biomedical ethics, such as the belief that killing is impermissible and allowing to die permissible. But a moral theory would be impoverished if it only incorporated this distinction without determining whether the distinction was itself justifiable. A good theory also should have the power to criticize defective beliefs, no matter how widely accepted those beliefs may be.

7. *Output power*. A theory has output power when it produces judgments that were not in the original data base of particular and general considered judgments on which the theory was constructed. If a normative theory did no more than repeat the list of judgments thought to be sound prior to the construction of the theory, it would have accomplished nothing. For example, if the parts of a theory pertaining to obligations of beneficence do not yield new judgments about role obligations of care in medicine beyond those assumed in constructing the theory, the theory will amount to no more than a classification scheme. A theory, then, must generate more than a list of the axioms already present in pretheoretic belief.

8. *Practicability*. A proposed moral theory is unacceptable if its requirements are so demanding that they probably cannot be satisfied or could be satisfied by only a few extraordinary persons or communities. A moral theory that presents utopian ideals or unfeasible recommendations fails the criterion of practicability. For example, if a theory proposed such high requirements for personal autonomy (see Chapter 3) or such lofty standards of social justice (see Chapter 6) that, realistically, no person could be autonomous and no society could be just, the proposed theory would be deeply problematic.

We could formulate other general criteria, but the eight sketched above are the most important for present purposes. A theory can receive a high score on the basis of one or more criteria and a low score on the basis of other criteria. For example, early in this chapter we depict utilitarianism as an internally coherent, simple, and comprehensive theory with exceptional output power, but it is not coherent with some of our vital considered judgments, especially with certain judgments about justice, human rights, and the importance of personal projects. By contrast, Kantian theories are consistent with many of our considered judgments, but their clarity, simplicity, and output power are limited.

Utilitarianism: Consequence-Based Theory

Consequentialism is a label affixed to theories holding that actions are right or wrong according to the balance of their good and bad consequences. The right act in any circumstance is the one that produces the best overall result, as determined from an impersonal perspective that gives equal weight to the interests of each affected party. The most prominent consequence-based theory, utilitarianism, accepts one and only one basic principle of ethics: the principle of utility. This principle asserts that we ought always to produce the maximal balance of positive value over disvalue (or the least possible disvalue, if only undesirable results can be achieved). The classical origins of this theory are found in the writings of Jeremy Bentham (1748–1832) and John Stuart Mill (1806–1873).

At first sight, utilitarianism seems entirely compelling. Who would deny that agents should minimize evil and increase positive value? Moreover, utilitarians offer many examples from everyday life to show that the theory is practicable and that we all engage in a utilitarian method of calculating what should be done by balancing goals and resources and considering the needs of everyone affected. Examples include designing a family budget and creating a new public park in a wilderness region. Utilitarians maintain that their theory simply renders explicit and systematic what is already implicit in everyday deliberation and justification.

The Concept of Utility

Although utilitarians share the conviction that we should morally assess human actions in terms of their production of maximal value, they disagree concerning which values should be maximized. Many utilitarians maintain that we ought to produce *agent-neutral* or *intrinsic* goods—that is, goods such as happiness, freedom, and health that every rational person values.[3] These goods are valuable in themselves, without reference to their further consequences or to the particular values held by individuals.

Bentham and Mill are *hedonistic* utilitarians because they conceive utility entirely in terms of happiness or pleasure, two broad terms that they treat as synonymous.[4] They appreciate that many human actions do not appear to be performed for the sake of happiness. For example, when highly motivated professionals, such as research scientists, work themselves to the point of exhaustion in search of new knowledge, they often do not appear to be seeking pleasure or personal happiness. Yet Mill proposes that such persons are initially motivated by success or money, both of which promise happiness. Along the way, either the pursuit of knowledge provides pleasure or such persons never stop associating their hard work with the success or money they hope to gain.

However, many recent utilitarian philosophers have argued that values other than happiness have intrinsic worth. Some list friendship, knowledge, health, and beauty among these intrinsic values, whereas others list personal autonomy, achievement and success, understanding, enjoyment, and deep personal relationships.[5] Even when their lists differ, these utilitarians concur that we should assess the greatest good in terms of the total intrinsic value produced by an action.

Still other utilitarians hold that the concept of utility does not refer to intrinsic goods, but to an individual's preferences; that is, we are to maximize the overall satisfaction of the preferences of the greatest numbers of individuals.

A Case of Risk and Truthfulness

To distinguish the major themes of each theory treated in this chapter, each section devoted to a theory explicates how its proponents might approach the same case, which centers on a five-year-old girl who has progressive renal failure and is not doing well on chronic renal dialysis. The medical staff is considering a renal transplant, but its effectiveness is "questionable" in her case. Nevertheless, a "clear possibility" exists that the transplanted kidney will not be affected by the disease process. The parents concur with the plan to try a transplant, but an additional obstacle emerges: The tissue typing indicates that it would be difficult to find a match for the girl. The staff excludes her two siblings, ages two and four, as too young to be donors. The mother is not histocompatible, but the father is compatible and has "anatomically favorable circulation for transplantation."

Meeting alone with the father, the nephrologist gives him the results and indicates that the prognosis for his daughter is "quite uncertain." After reflection, the father decides that he does not wish to donate a kidney to his daughter. His several reasons include his fear of the surgery, his lack of courage, the uncertain prognosis for his daughter even with a transplant, the slight prospect of a cadaver kidney, and the suffering his daughter has already sustained. The father then asks the physician "to tell everyone else in the family that he is not histocompatible." He is afraid that if family members know the truth, they will accuse him of intentionally allowing his daughter to die. He maintains that truth-telling would have the effect of "wrecking the family." The physician is uncomfortable with this request, but after further discussion he agrees to tell the man's wife that "for medical reasons, the father should not donate a kidney."[6]

Utilitarians evaluate this case in terms of the consequences of the different courses of action open to the father and the physician. The goal is to realize the greatest good by balancing the interests of all affected persons. This evaluation depends on judgments about probable outcomes. Whether the father ought to donate his kidney depends on the probability of successful transplantation as well as the risks and other costs to him (and indirectly to other dependent members of the family). The probability of success is not high. The effectiveness is questionable and the prognosis uncertain, although a possibility exists that a transplanted kidney would not undergo the same disease process, and there is a slight possibility that a cadaver kidney could be obtained.

The girl will probably die without a transplant from either a cadaveric or a living source, but the transplant also offers only a small chance of survival. The risk of death to the father from anesthesia in the kidney removal is 1 in 10,000 to

15,000; it is difficult to put an estimate on other possible long-term health effects. Nevertheless, because the chance of success is likely greater than the probability that the father will be harmed, many utilitarians would hold that the father or anyone else similarly situated is *obligated* to undertake what others would consider a heroic act that surpasses obligation. On a certain balance of probable benefits and risks, an uncompromising utilitarian would suggest tissue typing the patient's two siblings and then removing a kidney from one if there were a good match and parental approval. However, utilitarians differ among themselves in these various judgments because of their different theories of value and their different assessments of probable outcomes.

Probabilistic judgments would likewise play a role in the physician's utilitarian calculation of the right action in response to the father's request to camouflage why he will not donate a kidney. Primary questions include whether a full disclosure would wreck the family, whether lying to the family would have serious negative effects, and whether the father would subsequently experience serious guilt from his refusal to donate, thereby jeopardizing relations within the family. Studies indicate that families caring for chronically ill children break up at a higher rate than other families, and perhaps this family is already beyond repair. The utilitarian proposes that the physician is obligated to consider the whole range of facts and possible consequences in light of the best available information about their probability and magnitude.

So far we have taken primarily the perspective of a utilitarian who focuses on *particular acts*. Other utilitarians focus on the relevant *principles and rules* of parental obligation and professional practice that, over time, maximize overall welfare. We turn now to this distinction, which divides utilitarians into two major types.

Act and Rule Utilitarianism

The principle of utility is the ultimate standard of rightness and wrongness for all utilitarians. Controversy has arisen, however, over whether this principle pertains to particular acts in particular circumstances or instead to general rules that then determine which acts are right and wrong. Whereas the rule utilitarian considers the consequences of adopting certain rules, the act utilitarian skips the level of rules and justifies actions by appealing directly to the principle of utility, as the following chart indicates:

Rule Utilitarianism	*Act Utilitarianism*
Principle of Utility	Principle of Utility
↑	
Moral Rules	↑
↑	
Particular Judgments	Particular Judgments

The act utilitarian asks, "What good and bad consequences will result from *this action in this circumstance?*" For the act utilitarian, moral rules are useful in guiding human actions, but are also expendable if they do not promote utility in a particular context. For the rule utilitarian, by contrast, an act's conformity to a justified rule (that is, a rule justified by utility) makes the act right, and the rule is not expendable in a particular context, even if following the rule in that context does not maximize utility.[7]

Physician Worthington Hooker, a prominent nineteenth-century figure in academic medicine and medical ethics, was a rule utilitarian who attended to rules of truth-telling in medicine as follows:

> The good, which may be done by deception in a *few* cases, is almost as nothing, compared with the evil which it does in *many*, when the prospect of its doing good was just as promising as it was in those in which it succeeded. And when we add to this the evil which would result from a *general* adoption of a system of deception, the importance of a strict adherence to the truth in our intercourse with the sick, even on the ground of expediency, becomes incalculably great.[8]

Hooker agreed that a physician can sometimes best advance a patient's health through deception, but he argued that widespread deception in medicine will have an increasingly negative effect over time and will eventually produce more harm than good. He therefore defended the rule-utilitarian prohibition of deception in medicine.

Act utilitarians, by contrast, argue that observing a rule such as truth-telling does not always maximize the general good, and that such rules are properly understood as rough guidelines. They regard rule utilitarians as unfaithful to the fundamental demand of the principle of utility: Maximize value. In some circumstances, they argue, abiding by a generally beneficial rule will not prove most beneficial to the persons affected by the action, even in the long run. According to one act utilitarian, J. J. C. Smart, a third possibility exists between never adopting any rules and always obeying rules—namely, *sometimes* obeying rules.[9] From this perspective, physicians do not and should not always tell the truth to their patients or their families. Sometimes physicians should even lie to give hope. They do so justifiably if it is better for the patients and for all concerned and if their acts do not undermine general conformity to moral rules. According to Smart, selective obedience does not erode either moral rules or general respect for morality.

Because of the benefits to society of the general observance of moral rules, the rule utilitarian does not abandon rules, even in difficult situations (although the rule utilitarian may accept rules only as statements of prima facie obligation). Abandonment threatens the integrity and existence of both the particular rules and the whole system of rules.[10] The act utilitarian's reply is that although promises usually should be kept in order to maintain trust, this consideration should be set aside in cases in which breaking the promise would produce overall good. The act utilitarian might also argue that making exceptions to accepted rules is consistent with ordinary moral beliefs, because we often make exceptions to rules without acting wrongly. The act utilitarian further contends that when breaking rules justifiably clashes with our traditional moral convictions, we need to revise our convictions rather than discard act utilitarianism.

An example of the act utilitarian's point appears in a comment by former Colorado Governor Richard Lamm, who once observed that, in light of increasing financial costs of medical care, the terminally ill have "a duty to die and get out of the way with all of our machines and artificial hearts and everything else." This statement clearly conflicts with ordinary morality and provoked an outcry of indignation and shock that a public official would brush aside considered moral rules that protect our rights. Lamm chose an unfortunate word when he stated that the terminally ill have a "duty" to die, but in context he provided an act-utilitarian answer to what he correctly referred to as an "ethical question." His point was that we cannot continue public funding for medical technology without assessing costs and trade-offs, even if we must subsequently revise our traditional views and let some people die because a technology is not funded. The act utilitarian likewise believes that traditional moral rules cannot handle many other questions posed by technological developments.

An Absolute Principle with Derivative Contingent Rules

From the utilitarian's perspective, the principle of utility is the sole absolute principle. No derivative rule is absolute, and no rule is unrevisable. Even rules against killing in medicine may be overturned or substantially revised. For example, we had occasion in Chapter 4 to discuss current debates in biomedical ethics regarding whether seriously suffering patients should, at their request, be killed rather than "allowed to die," although such acts would revise traditional beliefs in medicine. The rule utilitarian argues that we should support rules permitting killing if and only if those rules would produce the most favorable consequences. Likewise, there should be rules against killing if and only if those rules would maximize good consequences. Utilitarians often point out that we do not presently permit physicians to kill patients because of the adverse social consequences that we believe would follow for those directly and indirectly affected. But if, under a different set of social conditions, legalization of mercy killing would maximize overall social welfare, the utilitarian would see no reason to prohibit such killing. Utilitarians thus regard their theory as responsive in constructive ways to changing social conditions.

A Critical Evaluation of Utilitarianism

Several problems suggest that utilitarianism is not a fully adequate moral theory.

Problems with immoral preferences and actions. Problems arise for utilitarians who are concerned about the maximization of individual preferences when some of these individuals have what our considered judgments tell us are morally unacceptable preferences. For example, if a researcher derived supreme satisfaction from inflicting pain on animals or on human subjects in experiments, we would condemn this preference and would seek to prevent it from being actualized. Utilitarianism based on subjective preferences is thus a defensible theory only if we can formulate a range of *acceptable* preferences and determine "acceptability" independently of agents' preferences. This task seems inconsistent with a pure preference approach.[11]

There is an additional problem of immoral actions. Suppose the only way to achieve the maximal utilitarian outcome is to perform an immoral act (as judged by the standards of the common morality). For example, suppose a country can end a devastating war only by using extremely painful methods of torturing captured children whose soldier fathers instructed them not to reveal their fathers' location. Utilitarianism seems to say not only that torturing the children is permissible, but that it is morally obligatory. Yet this requirement seems immoral. If so, utilitarianism permits or requires apparently immoral actions without giving sufficient reason to abandon our reigning restraints on utilitarian thinking.

Does utilitarianism demand too much? Some forms of utilitarianism seem to demand too much in the moral life, because the principle of utility requires *maximizing* value. Utilitarians have a difficult time maintaining a crucial distinction between (1) *morally obligatory actions*, and (2) *supererogatory actions* (those above the call of moral obligation and performed for the sake of personal ideals). Registering this objection, Alan Donagan describes situations in which utilitarian theory regards an action as obligatory against our firm moral conviction that the action is ideal and praiseworthy rather than obligatory.[12]

Donagan would regard the suicide of frail elderly and persons with severe disabilities who are no longer useful to society as an example of acts that could never rightly be considered obligatory, regardless of the consequences. Heroic donation of bodily parts such as kidneys and even hearts to save another person's life is another example. If utilitarianism makes such actions obligatory, then it is a defective theory. Donagan argues, and we agree, that all utilitarians face these problems, because none can rule out the ever-present possibility that what is today praiseworthy (but optional) will, through altered social circumstances, become obligatory by utilitarian standards. (At the same time, we should recognize that utilitarians are sometimes right in arguing that various moral conventions and beliefs are too weak or vague and need upgrading by more demanding requirements.)[13]

Bernard Williams and John Mackie offer extensions of the thesis that utilitarianism demands too much. Williams argues that utilitarianism abrades personal integrity by making persons as morally responsible for consequences that they *fail to prevent* as for those outcomes they *directly cause*, even when the consequences are not of their doing. Mackie similarly argues that a utilitarian "test of right actions" is so distant from our moral experience that it becomes "the ethics of fantasy," because it demands that people strip themselves of many goals and relationships they value in life in order to maximize outcomes for others. From this perspective, the utilitarian demands that we act like saints without personal interests and goals.[14] These criticisms also suggest that utilitarianism fails the test of *practicability* presented at the beginning of this chapter.

Problems of unjust distribution. A third problem is that utilitarianism, in principle, permits the interests of the majority to override the rights of minorities, and cannot adequately disavow unjust social distributions. The charge is that utilitarians assign no independent weight to justice and are indifferent to unjust distributions because they distribute value according to net aggregate satisfaction. If an already prosperous group of persons could have more value added to their lives than could be added to the lives of the indigent in society, the utilitarian must recommend that the added value go to the prosperous group.

An example of problematic (although not necessarily unjust) distribution appears in the following case. Two researchers wanted to determine the most cost-effective way to control hypertension in the American population. As they developed their research, they discovered that it is more cost-effective to target patients already being treated for hypertension than to identify new cases of hypertension among persons without regular access to medical care: younger men, older women, and patients with exceptionally high blood pressure. And they concluded that "a community with limited resources would probably do better to concentrate its efforts on improving adherence of known hypertensives (that is, those already identified as sufferers of hypertension), even at a sacrifice in terms of the numbers screened." If accepted by the government, this recommendation would exclude the poorest sector, which has the most pressing need for medical attention, from the benefits of high blood pressure education and management.

The investigators were concerned because of the apparent injustice in excluding the poor and minorities by a public health endeavor aimed at the economically advantaged sector of society. Yet their statistics were compelling. No matter how carefully planned the efforts, nothing worked efficiently (that is, nothing produced utilitarian results), except programs directed at known hypertensives already in contact with physicians. The investigators therefore recommended what they explicitly referred to as a utilitarian allocation.[15]

Medical research since this study has continued to support its findings. Nonadherence to treatment programs for hypertension is one of the most important antecedent conditions leading to serious hypertension-related medical problems. In poor sections of inner cities, nonadherence is much higher among patients who are screened and treated for hypertension in the emergency room than for those treated by their own primary-care physicians. This problem is significant because many poor people do not have primary-care physicians. Low economic status also correlates with fewer visits per year to physicians' offices. In addition, research indicates that the prevalence of hypertension is 50% higher among African Americans than among whites. Thus, the problems identified in the earlier study remain largely unchanged today: The society could probably achieve a greater net improvement in overall public health by targeting patients who have and who visit primary-care physicians, yet such a strategy is likely to underserve poor and minority populations who already suffer disproportionately from health problems.[16]

A Constructive Evaluation of Utilitarianism

Despite these criticisms, utilitarianism has many strengths, two of which we have appropriated in other chapters. The first is the acceptance of a significant role for the principle of utility in formulating public policy. The utilitarian's requirements of an objective assessment of everyone's interests and of an impartial choice to maximize good outcomes for all affected parties are acceptable norms of public policy. Second, when we formulated principles of beneficence in Chapter 5, utility played an important role. Although we have characterized utilitarianism as primarily a *consequence*-based theory, it is also *beneficence*-based. That is, the theory sees morality primarily in terms of the goal of promoting welfare.

A theory with a principle of beneficence that is balanced by other principles should eliminate all the problems with an unqualified use of the principle of utility that we encountered in the criticisms offered in the preceding section. This point holds even if beneficence is developed primarily in terms of producing good consequences. As political economist Amartya Sen notes, "Consequentialist reasoning may be fruitfully used even when consequentialism as such is not accepted. To ignore consequences is to leave an ethical story half told."[17]

A *strict* or *pure* utilitarianism also has strengths, as we can see by reconsidering the objection that utilitarianism is overdemanding. Utilitarianism often demands more than the rules of the common morality do, but this apparent weakness can be a hidden strength. For example, morality generally demands that we not override individuals' rights to maximize social consequences. But if we can more effectively protect almost everyone's interests by overriding some property rights or autonomy rights, this course of action might not be wrong merely because it contravenes conventional morality and pursues the goal of social utility. In many circumstances, then, utilitarians make a compelling case in advising us to rely less on traditional convictions and more on judgments of overall social benefit.

Kantianism: Obligation-Based Theory

A second type of theory denies much that utilitarian theories affirm. Often called *deontological* (i.e., a theory that some features of actions other than or in addition to consequences make actions right or wrong), this type of theory is now increasingly called *Kantian*, because the ethical thought of Immanuel Kant (1724–1804) has most deeply shaped its formulations.

Consider how a Kantian might approach the above-mentioned case of the five-year-old in need of a kidney. A Kantian would first insist that we should rest our moral judgments on reasons that also apply to others who are similarly situated. If the father has no generalizable moral obligation to his daughter, then no basis is available for morally criticizing him. The strict Kantian maintains that if the father chooses to donate out of affection, compassion, or concern for his dying daughter, his act would actually lack moral worth, because it would not be based on a generalizable obligation. Using one of the girl's younger siblings as a source of a kidney would be illegitimate because this recourse to children who are too young to consent to donation would involve using persons merely as means to others' ends. This principle would also exclude coercing the father to donate against his will.

Regarding the physician's options after the father requests deceiving the family, a strict Kantian views lying as an act that cannot without contradiction be universalized as a norm of conduct. The physician should not lie to the man's wife or to other members of the family, whether or not the lie would salvage the family (a consequentialist appeal). Even if the physician's statement was not, strictly speaking, a lie, he intentionally used this formulation to conceal relevant facts from the wife, an act Kantians typically view as morally unacceptable.

A Kantian will also consider whether the rule of confidentiality has independent moral weight, whether the tests the father underwent with the nephrologist established a relationship of confidentiality, and whether the rule of confidentiality protects information about the father's histocompatibility and his reasons for not donating. If confidentiality would prohibit the nephrologist from letting the family know that the father is histocompatible, then, even without considering possible effects on the family, the Kantian must face an apparent conflict of obligations: truthfulness in conflict with confidentiality. But before we can address such conflict, we need to understand Kantian theory.

Obligation from Categorical Rules

In an attempt to combat skeptical challenges to ethics, Kant argued that morality is grounded in reason, not in tradition, intuition, conscience, emotion, or attitudes such as sympathy. He saw human beings as creatures with rational powers to resist desire and with the freedom to do so.

One of Kant's most important claims is that the moral worth of an individual's action depends exclusively on the moral acceptability of the rule of obligation (or "maxim") on which the person acts. As Kant puts it, moral obligation depends on the rule that determines the individual's will, where the rule is understood as a morally valid reason that justifies the action.[18] For Kant, one must act not only *in accordance with* but *for the sake of* obligation. That is, to have moral worth, a person's motive for acting must come from a recognition that he or she intends what is morally required. For example, if an employer discloses a health hazard to an employee only because the employer fears a lawsuit, and not because of the importance of truth-telling, then the employer has performed the right action, but deserves no moral credit for the action. If agents do what is morally right simply because they are scared, because they derive pleasure from doing that kind of act, or because they are selfish, they lack the requisite good will that derives from acting for the sake of obligation.

To see how a Kantian would judge the moral worth of a proposed course of action, imagine a man who desperately needs money and knows that he will not be able to borrow it unless he promises repayment in a definite time, but who also knows that he will not be able to repay it within this period. He decides to make a promise that he knows he will break. Kant asks us to examine the man's reason, that is, his maxim: "When I think myself in want of money, I will borrow money and promise to pay it back, although I know that I cannot do so." This maxim, Kant says, cannot pass a test that he calls the *categorical imperative*. This imperative tells us what must be done irrespective of our desires. In its major formulation, Kant states the categorical imperative as follows: "I ought never to act except in such a way that I can also will that my maxim become a universal law." Kant says that this one principle justifies all particular imperatives of obligation (all "ought" statements that morally obligate).[19]

The categorical imperative is a canon of the acceptability of moral rules—that is, a criterion for judging the acceptability of the maxims that direct actions. This imperative adds nothing to a maxim's content. Rather, it determines which maxims are objective and valid. The categorical imperative functions by testing what Kant calls the "consistency of maxims": A maxim must be capable of being conceived and willed without contradiction. When we examine the maxim of the person who deceitfully promises, we discover, according to Kant, that this maxim is incapable of being conceived and willed universally without yielding a contradiction. It is inconsistent with what it presupposes. Lying works only if the person being lied to expects or presupposes that people are truthful, but in a world in which no one intended to keep promises, the maxim would make the purpose of promising impossible, because no one would believe the person who promises. Many examples from everyday life illustrate this thesis. For instance, maxims of lying are inconsistent with the practices of truth-telling they presuppose, and maxims permitting cheating on tests are inconsistent with the practices of honesty they presuppose.

Kant appears to have more than one categorical imperative, because his several formulations are very differently worded. His second formulation is at least as influential as the first: "One must act to treat every person as an end and never as a means only."[20] It has often been said that this principle categorically requires that we should never treat another as a means to our ends, but this interpretation misrepresents Kant's views. He argues only that we must not treat another *merely* or *exclusively* as a means to our ends. When human research subjects volunteer to test new drugs, they are treated as a means to others' ends, but they have a choice in the matter and retain control over their lives. Kant does not prohibit these uses of consenting persons. He insists only that they be treated with the respect and moral dignity to which every person is entitled.

Autonomy and Heteronomy

We saw in Chapter 3 that the word *autonomy* typically refers to what makes judgments and actions one's own. This conception of autonomy is emphatically not Kant's. Persons have "autonomy of the will" for Kant if and only if they knowingly act in accordance with the universally valid moral principles that pass the requirements of the categorical imperative. He contrasts this *moral* autonomy with "heteronomy," which refers to any controlling influence over the will other than motivation by moral principles.[21] If, for example, people act from passion, ambition, or self-interest, they act heteronomously, not from a rational will that chooses autonomously. Kant regards acting from desire, fear, impulse, personal projects, and habit as no less heteronomous than actions manipulated or coerced by others.

To say that an individual must "accept" a moral principle to be autonomous does not mean that the principle is subjective or that each individual must create (author or originate) his or her moral principles. Kant requires only that each individual *will the acceptance* of moral principles. If a person freely accepts objective moral principles, that person is a law-giver unto himself or herself. The importance of this account for Kant also extends beyond the *nature* of autonomy to its *value*. "The principle of autonomy," he contends, is "the sole principle of morals," and autonomy alone gives people respect, value, and proper motivation. A person's dignity—indeed, "sublimity"— comes from being morally autonomous.[22]

Contemporary Kantian Ethics

Several writers in contemporary ethical theory have accepted and developed a Kantian account, broadly construed.

1. A straightforward example is *The Theory of Morality* by Alan Donagan. He seeks the "philosophical core" of the morality expressed in the Hebrew–Christian tradition (which he interprets in secular rather than religious terms). Donagan's philosophical elaboration of this point of view relies heavily on Kant's theory of persons as ends in themselves, especially the imperative that one must treat humanity as an end and never as a means only. Donagan expresses the fun-

damental principle of the Hebrew–Christian tradition as a Kantian principle grounded in rationality: "It is impermissible not to respect every human being, oneself or any other, as a rational creature."[23] He believes that all other moral rules rely upon this fundamental principle.

2. A second Kantian theory derives from the work of John Rawls. Rawls has challenged utilitarian theories while attempting to develop Kantian themes of reason, autonomy, and equality. For example, he argues that vital moral considerations, such as individual rights and the just distribution of goods among individuals, depend less on social factors, such as individual happiness and majority interests, than on Kantian conceptions of individual worth, self-respect, and autonomy.[24] For Rawls, any philosophy in which the right to individual autonomy legitimately outweighs the dictates of rational moral principles is unacceptable. Even courageous and conscientious actions do not merit respect unless they accord with moral principles derived from reason.[25]

In his recent writings, Rawls has stressed that his work presents a political conception of justice, rather than a comprehensive moral theory. That is, his account is "a moral conception worked out for a specific subject, namely, the basic structure of a constitutional democratic regime." As such, it does not presuppose a comprehensive moral doctrine such as Kant's, and Rawls maintains that his theory is Kantian by "analogy not identity."[26] The upshot seems to be that Rawls expresses Kantian themes without commitment to a general Kantian moral theory.

3. Several philosophers, including Robert Nozick, Bernard Williams, and Thomas Nagel, have developed a doctrine of "deontological constraints" based on Kant's injunction never to use another person merely as a means.[27] These philosophers argue that Kant was correct to maintain that certain actions are impermissible regardless of the consequences. To see how these constraints should operate, consider the following experiment with human subjects. From April 1945 to July 1947, a program of human subjects research was initiated to try to learn how to protect personnel from plutonium exposure. Researchers intentionally injected 17 patients with plutonium at three university hospitals in the United States, including The University of California at San Francisco (UCSF). The purpose of this research was to determine the excretion rate of plutonium in humans. Investigators at the time did not regard these plutonium experiments as highly risky. Based on experiences with radium, they did not expect immediate side effects or illness, but they also knew virtually nothing about long-term risk.

Work began with some studies on rats and cancer conducted by Dr. Joseph Hamilton. In January 1945, Hamilton decided "to undertake, on a limited scale, a series of metabolic studies with [plutonium] using human subjects." The purpose "was to evaluate the possible hazards . . . to humans who might be exposed to them." Researchers did not expect the injections to have any therapeutic value for these three patients. It appears that the physicians did not obtain—and were not expected to obtain—consent in the first two cases. Even though the physicians obtained limited consent for experimentation from the third patient, it was not consent to *nontherapeutic* experimentation.[28]

In this case, the researchers thought that by experimenting on a few individuals they could help achieve several worthy social goals, such as protecting workers in the nuclear industry and developing an adequate system of military defense for Western nations during the Cold War. Even if achieving these goals would have good consequences for millions of people, deontologists maintain that the researchers treated their subjects unethically because they violated fundamental constraints on how we can permissibly treat persons. These "deontological constraints" limit our actions, even when we can bring about an overall good state of affairs.

Deontological constraints are essentially negative duties—that is, they specify what we cannot justifiably do to others, even in the pursuit of worthy goals; however, they do not specify any actions that we should perform for the sake of others. For example, while stealing a sibling's share of the family inheritance would violate deontological constraints, those constraints do not tell us how to divide wealth among siblings.

This conception of deontological constraints highlights an obvious difference between deontologists and utilitarians. The latter require us to determine the best possible objective state of affairs, irrespective of the position of particular agents who act in those states of affairs. Utilitarians demand an external, impartial view of the situation in order to weigh each person's interests equally. From this perspective, a person's own position, role, and sense of integrity have no independent force. They are only important in so far as they are factors in the calculus of utilities. For the utilitarian, it is unimportant who brings about the best possible state of affairs; all that matters is that good outcomes occur.[29]

By contrast, many deontologists maintain that such factors as one's role or sense of integrity have moral weight independent of consequences. Imagine that a terminally ill patient in extreme pain asks his physician to kill him. The man's family agrees with his decision, and the doctor realizes that everyone will be better off if the man dies. Nonetheless, a deontologist might believe that her role as a physician, as well as her own sense of moral integrity, prevent her from taking this man's life. Similarly, in the plutonium case, a physician might feel constrained from engaging in nontherapeutic human experimentation, regardless of the good consequences that would follow from the experimental work.

In these examples, deontological constraints are *agent-relative*, because they make reference to the values and judgments of particular persons, such as physicians and scientists. Deontologists argue that each individual agent's perspective is important in moral deliberation, and that who performs an action and how a good state of affairs is to be brought about are significant, irrespective of consequences. As moral agents, we should not directly cause certain harms to others, even if we cannot actually prevent those harms from occurring. For example, in the case of the doctor with a terminally ill patient, the doctor believes that she should not kill the patient, even though the patient will die soon anyway and the family agrees with the loved one's request.

A Critical Evaluation of Kantianism

Like utilitarianism, Kantian theory fails to provide a full and adequate theory of the moral life.

The problem of conflicting obligations. Kantianism has a severe problem with conflicting obligations. Suppose we have promised to take our children on a long-anticipated trip, but now find that if we do so, we cannot assist our sick mother in the hospital. A rule of promise-keeping and a rule of assistance or obligation of care generate this conflict. Conflict can also arise from a single moral rule rather than from two different rules—as, for example, when two promises come into conflict, although the promisor could not have anticipated the conflict when making the promises. To modify the previous example, consider a situation in which we have promised to take our children on a trip and promised to care for our mother when she is sick, and both promises come due at the same time.

Because moral rules are *categorical* for Kant, he seems to say that we are obligated to do the impossible and perform both actions. Although we cannot at the same time both take our children on a trip and help our mother in the hospital, Kant seems to require both. Any ethical theory that leads to this conclusion is incoherent, yet no clear way out exists for Kant or for any theory with truly categorical or absolutist rules. If even as many as two absolute rules exist, they will sometimes conflict. Either we must accept a system with only one absolute rule, or we must give up absolutes altogether (unless we can specify their meaning and scope in order to avoid conflict). Our own solution to the general problem of moral conflicts is found on pp. 15–23.

Overemphasizing law, underemphasizing relationships. Kant's arguments concentrate on lawful obligations, and recent Kantian theories, such as Rawls's, feature a contractual basis for obligations. But whether freedom, choice, equality, contract, law, and other staples of Kantianism deserve to occupy such a central position in a moral theory is questionable. (They are, we can nonetheless agree, central ingredients in legal and political theories.) These visions of the moral life fail to capture much in personal relationships that generate moral responsibilities, and in relationships among friends and family, we rarely think or act in terms of law, contract, or absolute rules.[30]

This perspective suggests that Kant's theory (like utilitarianism) is better suited for relationships among strangers than for relationships among friends or other intimates. Parents, for example, do not see responsibilities to their children in terms of contracts, but in terms of care, needs, sustenance, and loving attachment. Only if all forms of moral relationship—and our moral sentiments, motivations, and virtues—could be reduced to a law-governed exchange would Kantian theory become a cogent general moral theory.

Abstractness without content. G. W. F. Hegel once criticized Kant's theory for lacking the power to develop specific duties, such as those needed in professional ethics.[31] We agree that the notions of "rationality" and "humanity" offer too thin a basis for a determinate set of moral norms. Kant's relatively empty formalisms have little power to identify or assign specific obligations in almost any context of everyday morality, thereby raising questions about the theory's practicability. Its abstractness and impracticability give us another reason why method in ethics should start with considered judgments and then specify principles and test moral claims in light of overall coherence.

A Constructive Evaluation of Kantianism

Kant argued that when good reasons support a moral judgment, those reasons are good for all relevantly similar circumstances. Simple as it may seem, this claim is far-reaching. For example, if we are required to obtain valid consent for all subjects of biomedical research, we cannot make exceptions of certain persons merely because we could advance science by doing so. We cannot use institutionalized populations, for example, without consent any more than we can use people who are not in institutions without their consent. Kant and many Kantians have driven home the point that persons cannot act morally and privilege or exempt themselves or their favored group. If Kant had done nothing else than establish this point, he would have made a significant contribution to ethical theory.

Liberal Individualism: Rights-Based Theory

Thus far, we have concentrated on terms such as the following from moral discourse: *obligation, permissible action, virtue,* and *justification.* The language of *rights* is no less important. Statements of rights provide vital protections of life, liberty, expression, and property. They protect against oppression, unequal treatment, intolerance, arbitrary invasion of privacy, and the like. Some philosophers and framers of political declarations even regard rights as the basic language for expressing the moral point of view.

An ethical analysis of the case of the five-year-old needing a transplant would, from this perspective, focus on the rights of all the parties, in an effort to determine their meaning and scope, as well as their weight and strength. The father could be considered to have rights of autonomy, privacy, and confidentiality that protect his bodily integrity and sphere of decisionmaking from interference by others. In addition, he has a right to information, which he apparently received, about the risks, benefits, and alternatives of living kidney donation. The father's decision not to donate is within his rights, as long as it does not violate another's rights. No apparent grounds support a general right to assistance that could permit anyone, including his daughter, to demand a kidney. However, there are some special rights to assistance, and it might be argued that the daughter has a right to receive a kidney from her family, on the basis of either parental obligations or medical need. But even if such a right exists, which is doubtful, it would be sharply circumscribed. For example, it is implausible to suppose that such a right could be enforced against the girl's two siblings. Their right to noninterference, when the procedure is not for their direct benefit and carries risks, precludes their use as sources of a kidney.

Comprehensive analysis of this case in terms of rights would note that the father has exercised his rights of autonomy and privacy in allowing the physician to run some tests. He then seeks protection behind his right of confidentiality, which he believes allows him to control access to any information generated in his relationship with the physician. However, the scope and limits of these alleged rights and competing rights need careful attention. For example, does the mother herself have a right to the information generated in the relationship between the father and the nephrologist, particularly information bearing on the fate of the daughter?

An analysis using rights would also consider whether the physician has a right of conscientious refusal. For example, the physician might resist becoming an instrument of the father's desire to keep others from knowing why he is not donating a kidney. But even if the physician does have a right to protect his integrity, does this right outstrip or trump the rights of others? Can a physician justifiably say "I have a right of conscience" and use this trump to escape the clutches of a moral dilemma?

The Nature of Liberal Individualism

We analyze rights theory in this chapter as liberal individualism, the conception that, a democratic society must carve out a certain space within which the individual may pursue personal projects. Liberal individualism has, in recent years, challenged the reigning utilitarian and Kantian moral theories. H. L. A. Hart has described this challenge as a switch from an "old faith that some form of utilitarianism . . . *must* capture the essence of political morality" to a new faith in "a doctrine of basic human rights, protecting specific basic liberties and interests of individuals."[32]

This faith may be new, but liberal individualism is not a new development in moral and political theory. At least since Thomas Hobbes, liberal individualists have employed the language of rights to buttress moral and political arguments, and the Anglo–American legal tradition has heavily relied upon this language. The language of rights has served, on occasion, as a means to oppose the status quo, to assert claims that demand recognition and respect, and to promote social reforms that aim to secure legal protections for individuals. Historically, this language was instrumental in wresting certain freedoms from established orders of religion, society, and state, such as freedom of the press and freedom of religious expression.

The legitmate role of civil, political, and legal rights in protecting the individual from societal intrusions is now beyond serious dispute, but the idea that individual rights provide the fountainhead for moral and political theory has been strongly resisted—for example, by many utilitarians and Marxists. They note that individual interests are often at odds with communal and institutional interests. In discussions of health care delivery, for example, proponents of a broad extension of medical services often appeal to the "right to health care," whereas opponents sometimes appeal to the "rights of the medical profession." Many participants in these moral, political, and legal debates seem to presuppose that arguments cannot be made persuasive unless they can be stated in the language of rights, although other participants prefer to avoid this language because it seems confrontational and adversarial.

The Nature and Status of Rights

Rights are *justified claims* that individuals and groups can make upon other individuals or upon society; to have a right is to be in a position to determine, by one's choices, what others should do or need not do.[33] Claiming a right is a rule-governed activity. The rules may be legal rules, moral rules, institutional rules, or rules of games, but all rights exist or fail to exist because the relevant rules either allow or disallow the claim in question. As such, *legal* rights are claims that are justified by legal principles and rules, and *moral* rights are claims that are justified by moral principles and rules. A moral right, then, is a justified claim or entitlement, warranted by moral principles and rules.[34]

Absolute and Prima Facie Rights

Some rights may be absolute (e.g., the right to choose one's religion or to reject all religion) but, typically, rights are not absolute. Like principles of obligation, rights assert prima facie claims (in the sense of "prima facie" introduced in Chapter 1).

Some writers seem to insist that rights are absolute, at least in restricted contexts. Ronald Dworkin has argued the well-known thesis that some rights are so basic that ordinary justifications for interference with rights by the state, such as reducing inconvenience or promoting utility, are insufficient. The stakes must be far more significant to justify such invasions, he argues, because rights are "trumps" held by an individual against general plans and background justifications in a political state.[35] Democratic governments typically frame their policies to promote the general welfare and to conform to majority decisions. In response, rights function to guarantee that individuals cannot be sacrificed to these government or majority interests. Rights are above the state's utilitarian goals for Dworkin, much in the way deontologists maintain that we cannot trade off rights secured by justice through political bargaining or a utilitarian calculus of social interests.

However, as Dworkin recognizes, if the claims of public utility are highly significant, the individual may not justifiably play a trump card.[36] Rights are not so strong that they may never be overridden. Dworkin has argued that if the state needs to protect the rights of others (e.g., the state needs to prevent the spread of a catastrophic disease), then it may legitimately override individual rights. What we cannot do, Dworkin insists, is to act as if the right did not exist and so make decisions based entirely on net social utility. Mere benefit to the community is not of itself sufficient to override rights—that is the whole point of rights guarantees. Dworkin's qualifications make "trumps" rather tamer than they first appear to be, and many utilitarians would not protest his milder formulation. He seems to advance a sound theory about the *purpose* of having rights, rather than a theory of their stringency or absoluteness.

We believe that all rights, like all obligations, are prima facie—that is, presumptively valid—claims that sometimes must yield to other claims. Even the right to life is not absolute, irrespective of competing claims or social conditions, as evidenced by common moral judgments about killing in war and killing in self-defense. In light of this need to balance claims, we should distinguish a *violation* of a right from an *infringement* of a right.[37] Violation refers to an unjustified action against a right, whereas infringement refers to a justified action overriding a right.

Positive Rights and Negative Rights

A positive right is a right to receive a particular good or service from others, whereas a negative right is a right to be free from some action by others. A person's positive right entails another's obligation to do something for that person; a negative right entails another's obligation to refrain from doing something.[38] Examples of both sorts of rights appear in biomedical practice, research, and policy. If a right to health care exists, for example, it is a positive right to goods and services grounded in a claim of justice (see Chapter 6). The right to forgo a recommended surgical procedure, by contrast, is a negative right grounded in the principle of respect for autonomy. The liberal individualist tradition has generally found it easier to justify negative rights, but the recognition of welfare rights in modern societies has led to an extension of the scope of positive rights.

Confusion about public policies governing biomedicine often reflects a failure to distinguish positive and negative rights. One example involves the U.S. Supreme Court decisions on abortion. The Court first ruled that a woman's right to privacy gives her a right to pursue an abortion prior to fetal viability (and after fetal viability if her life or health is threatened). The constitutionally protected right of privacy is here construed exclusively as a negative right that limits state interference. Many people thought that the Court had concomitantly recognized a positive right in its early decisions, namely a right to receive aid and assistance. They were surprised when the Court later ruled that the federal and state governments do not have obligations to provide funds for nontherapeutic abortions.[39] They contended that the various abortion decisions are inconsistent, but they failed to see that the Court first recognized a negative right and later refused to recognize a positive right. The Court's reasoning is consistent. It affirms a negative right but denies a positive right.

The Correlativity of Rights and Obligations

How are rights connected to obligations? To answer this question, consider the meaning of "X has a right to do or have Y." X's right entails that some party has an obligation either not to interfere if X does Y or to provide X with Y. Suppose a physician agrees to take John Doe as a patient and commences treatment. The physician incurs an obligation to Doe, and Doe gains correlative rights. If a state has an obligation to provide goods, such as food or health care to needy citizens, then any citizen who meets the relevant criteria of need can claim an entitlement to food or health care.

This analysis suggests a firm but untidy *correlativity* between obligations and rights.[40] This correlativity is untidy because at least one use of the words *requirement, obligation,* and *duty* indicates that not all obligations imply corresponding rights. For example, although we sometimes refer to requirements or obligations of charity, no person can claim another person's charity as a matter of right. If such norms of charity express what we "ought to do," they do so not from obligation but from personal ideals that exceed obligation. We can best construe these commitments as self-imposed "oughts" that are not required by morality and that do not generate rights-claims for other persons.

We conclude that rights language is correlative to obligation language, but in an untidy way that requires careful attention to particular contexts and often entails further specification of both rights and their correlative obligations.

Waivers and Releases of Rights

If one person holds a right against another, the first person is entitled to, but not required to, press the claim against the second party. The first party can release the second of the obligation owed, because the claimant of a right has discretion over its exercise. With legal rights, for example, an agent has the option to sue over another's failure to discharge a legal obligation. Any rights holder may, under any circumstances, *waive* his or her right. In doing so, the party who waives the right releases the other party from his or her obligation. For example, if a person has a right to a yearly contract from a university, the university is obligated to supply the person with the appropriate signed agreement. However, if the person waives his or her right to the contract, the university is no longer obligated to provide it.

The Primacy of Rights

The correlativity thesis does not determine whether rights or obligations, if either, is the more fundamental or primary category. The proposal made by some philosophers that ethical theory should be "rights-based"[41] springs from a particular conception of the function and justification of morality. If the function of morality is to protect individuals' interests (rather than communal interests), and if rights (rather than obligations) are our primary instruments to this end, then moral action-guides are rights-based. Rights, on this account, precede obligations.

A theory we encountered in Chapter 6 illustrates this position: the libertarian theory of justice. One representative, Robert Nozick, maintains that "Individuals have rights, and there are things no person or group may do to them [without violating their rights]."[42] He takes the following rule to be basic in the moral life: All persons have a right to be left free to do as they choose. The obligation not to interfere with this right follows from the right itself. That it "follows" indicates the priority of a rule of right over a rule of obligation. That is, an obligation is derived from a right.

Alan Gewirth has proposed another rights-based argument that recognizes *positive* or *benefit* rights:

Rights are to obligations as benefits are to burdens. For rights are justified claims to certain benefits, the support of certain interests of the subject or right-holder. Obligations, on the other hand, are justified burdens on the part of the respondent or duty-bearer; they restrict his freedom by requiring that he conduct himself in ways that directly benefit not himself but rather the right-holder. But burdens are for the sake of benefits, and not vice versa. Hence obligations, which are burdens, are for the sake of rights, whose objects are benefits. Rights, then, are prior to obligations in the order of justifying purpose . . . in that respondents have correlative obligations *because* subjects have certain rights.[43]

These rights-based accounts do not reject the *correlativity* thesis. Rather, they accept a *priority* thesis that obligations follow from rights, not the converse. Rights form the justificatory basis of obligations, they maintain, because they best capture the purpose of morality, which is to secure liberties or other benefits for a rights-holder.

A Critical Evaluation of Liberal Individualism

Problems with rights-based theories. One problem with basing ethics on rights is that rights are only a piece of a more general account that identifies what makes a claim valid. Justification of the system of rules within which valid claiming occurs is not itself rights-based. Pure rights-based accounts also run the risk of truncating or impoverishing our understanding of morality, because rights cannot account for the moral significance of motives, supererogatory actions, virtues, and the like. Such a limited theory would fare poorly under the criteria of comprehensiveness and explanatory and justificatory power. Accordingly, we should not understand a rights-based account as a comprehensive or complete moral theory, but rather as a statement of certain minimal and enforceable rules that communities and individuals must observe in their treatment of all persons.

Normative questions about the exercise of rights. Often the question is not whether someone has a right, but whether rights-holders should or should not exercise their rights. If a person says, "I know you have the right to do X, but you should not do it," this moral claim goes beyond a statement of a right. One's obligation or character, not one's right, is in question. Even if we had a full and complete theory of rights, we would still need a theory of obligation and character, and it does not appear possible to develop a satisfactory account by attending only to rights and their limits.

The neglect of communal goods. Liberal individualists sometimes write as if social morality's major concern is to protect individual interests against government intrusion. This vision is too limited, because it excludes not only bona fide communal demands and group interests, but also communal goods and forms of life, such as public health, biomedical research, and the protection of animals. The better perspective is that social ideals and principles of obligation are as critical to social morality as rights, and that neither is dispensable.

The adversarial character of rights. Finally, the language of *claims* and *entitlements* is often unnecessarily adversarial. For example, the current interest in children's rights gives children many vital protections against abuse (for instance, when parents refuse to authorize life-saving therapies for children for inappropriate reasons), but the notion that children have claims against their parents provides an inadequate framework to express the moral character of the parent–child relationship. The attempt to understand this relationship and others, such as health care relationships, strictly in terms of rights, neglects and may even undermine the affection, sympathy, and trust at the core of the relationships. This is not to suggest either that rights are inherently adversarial or that they are dispensable, but rather to note that a rights-theory is a partial framework.

A Constructive Evaluation of Liberal Individualism

In recent ethical theory, some writers have sought to eliminate the language of rights. They suggest either that rights language can be replaced by another vocabulary (e.g., obligations and virtues) or that the assertion of valid individual claims against society has risky implications. We reject such views, and we accept both the correlativity thesis and the moral and social purposes served by traditional interpretations of basic human rights, in their positive as well as their negative forms.[44]

No part of the moral vocabulary has done more to protect the legitimate interests of citizens in political states than the language of rights. Predictably, injustice and inhumane treatment occur most frequently in states that fail to recognize human rights in their political rhetoric and documents. As much as any part of moral discourse, rights language crosses international boundaries and enters into treaties, international law, and statements by international agencies and associations. Rights thereby become acknowledged as international standards for the treatment of persons.

Being a rights-bearer in a society that enforces rights is both a source of personal protection and a source of dignity and self-respect. By contrast, to maintain that someone has an *obligation* to protect another's interest may leave the recipient in a passive position, dependent upon the other's good will in fulfilling the obligation. When persons possess enforceable rights correlative to obligations, they are enabled to be independent agents, pursuing their projects and making claims. What we often cherish most is not that someone is obligated to us, but that we have a right that secures for us the opportunity to pursue and claim as ours the benefit or liberty that we value.

Communitarianism: Community-Based Theory

Several approaches in contemporary philosophy and political theory have little sympathy with liberal individualism. In these theories, everything fundamental in ethics derives from communal values, the common good, social goals, traditional practices, and cooperative virtues. Communitarianism is such a theory. Conventions, traditions, loyalties, and the social nature of life and institutions figure more prominently in communitarianism than in the types of theory discussed to this point.

In the case of potential kidney transplantation discussed previously in this chapter, communitarians would not ask which rights are at stake, but which communal values and relationships are involved. They would focus on the family as a small community intermediate between the individual and the state. They would likely ask which acts, rules, and policies of organ donation, privacy, and confidentiality best reinforce and promote communal values, including family values.

Communitarian critics of the father's behavior, which reduces his daughter's chances of survival, would maintain that he is insufficiently committed to the goods of the family and that he asserts the values of liberal individualism in standing on his rights, without adequately attending to his responsibilities. The father contends that if the physician tells other members of the family the true reasons for his decision not to donate, it would wreck the family. The father's prediction about this negative impact may or may not be correct, but what his actions express about his own lack of commitment to the family's welfare is notable.

Communitarians might also view the physician as focused unduly on protecting rights, such as autonomy and privacy. From the communitarian perspective, the physician would be expected to consider whether his actions conform to traditions of medicine, with its communal goods, codes, and virtues. These traditions have often justified deception in treating patients, but the father asks the physician to deceive others, a relatively rare request and one with less clear historical precedent in medical practice (see our discussion in Chapter 7). By contrast, nondisclosure to others because of confidentiality does have clear historical precedent in medicine, although rules of confidentiality are not absolute and have often been overridden by a larger social interest.

The Repudiation of Liberalism

Unfortunately, no systematic account of communitarianism exists that rivals the systematic theories in Mill, Kant, and other liberal philosophers. Contemporary communitarianism is usually analyzed in terms of a few key themes that emerge from a few leading writers. The most prominent themes are the influence of society on individuals (by contrast to the alleged emphasis in theories like Kant's and Mill's on free individual choice) and the roots of values in communal history, traditions, and practices.

Contemporary communitarians repudiate central tenets in what is often called *liberalism*, a term that is defined through cardinal premises in the types of theory discussed in the three previous sections: utilitarian, Kantian, and liberal individualist theories. What makes them jointly "liberal" is their commitment to what Mill defended as *individuality*, what Kant called *autonomy*, and what liberal individualists protect as personal rights. Each type of theory protects the individual against the state, and—on the communitarian interpretation—each also asserts that the state should neither reward nor penalize different conceptions of the good life held by individuals. Postulates of individual autonomy, rights against the state, and community neutrality toward conflicting values, then, are the central liberal tenets that communitarians oppose.

Contemporary communitarians repudiate liberal *theory* and challenge *current societies* established on liberal premises, including many contemporary Western political states.[45] According to communitarians, these societies lack a commitment to the general welfare, to common purposes, and to education in citizenship, while expecting and even encouraging social and geographic mobility, distanced personal relations, welfare dependence, breakdowns in family life and marital fidelity, political fragmentation, and the like. The number of abandoned children and elderly parents, social and familial disintegration, the disappearance of meaningful democracy, and the lack of effective communal programs are, according to communitarians, the disastrous products of liberalism.

The meaning of *community* and its synonyms varies in these theories. Some communitarians refer almost exclusively to the political state as the community, whereas others refer to smaller communities and institutions with defined goals and role obligations. Some include the family as a basic communal unit, within which being a parent and being a child involve specific roles and responsibilities. Much of what a person ought to do in communitarian theories is determined by the social roles assigned to or acquired by this person as a member of the community. Understanding a particular system of moral rules, then, requires understanding the community's history, sense of cooperative life, and conception of social welfare.

With regard to theory, communitarian critics have regularly attacked Mill and Kant, but often they have aimed their criticisms at Rawls, particularly his liberal principle of justice that the rights of individuals cannot legitimately be sacrificed for the good of the community.[46] Communitarian criticisms of liberal theories seem to come to the following: Liberalism (1) fails to appreciate the constructive role of the cooperative virtues and the political state in promoting values and creating the conditions of the good life, (2) fails to acknowledge shared goals and obligations that come not from freely made contracts among individuals, but from communal ideals and responsibilities, and (3) fails to understand the human person as historically constituted by and embedded in communal life and social roles.[47]

Every major communitarian thinker has contested the thesis of the priority of individual rights over the common good. Charles Taylor's challenge is perhaps the most straightforward. He argues that all conceptions of the rights of individuals already contain within their fabric some conception of the individual and social good, at least in the form of the good of moral agency and the good of human associations, such as friendship. The liberal's claim of the priority of right is itself, from this perspective, premised on a conception of the human good (the good of autonomous moral agency, in particular). Furthermore, Taylor argues, the type of autonomy valued by liberals cannot be developed in the absence of family and other community structures. However, liberalism's emphasis on individual rights makes no provision for the development and maintenance of the necessary communities, and instead views individuals as isolated atoms existing independently of one another.[48]

Communitarians thus believe that liberals miss the essence of morality by unduly emphasizing abstract principles and abstract agents, while failing to see that both principles and agents are products of communal life.

Militant and Moderate Forms of Communitarianism

We can distinguish communitarianism into *militant* and *moderate* forms. Militants firmly support community control and reject liberal theories. Several influential contemporary moral, social, and political thinkers, including Alasdair MacIntyre, Charles Taylor, and Michael Sandel, have supported this approach. By contrast, moderates emphasize the importance of various forms of community—including the family and the political state—while attempting to accommodate strands in liberal theories. This kind of communitarianism includes figures as diverse as Aristotle, Hugo Grotius, David Hume, G. W. F. Hegel, John Mackie, and Michael Walzer. For them, social order and morality rest on historically developed norms, and moral rules derive their acceptability and correctness from these shared conventions. Although the term *communitarianism* was recently coined and typically applies to the militant form, we will use it for both forms. We will criticize militant theories, while relying on the moderate theories for our constructive evaluation.

Militant communitarianism sees liberalism as antagonistic to all tradition, and as opposed to rights and rights language. These communitarians aim to perpetuate and even impose on individuals conceptions of virtue and the good life that limit the rights conferred by liberal societies. Militant communitarians see persons as intrinsically *constituted* by communal values and as best suited to achieve personal goods through communal life.[49] In addition, MacIntyre argues that we have inherited many incoherent fragments of once-coherent schemes of thought and action, and only if we understand our peculiar historical and cultural situation can we recognize the problematic dimensions of moral evaluation and moral theory.[50]

The moderate communitarian takes a stance far less opposed to autonomy and individual rights. A typical example is J. L. Mackie's appeal to "intersubjective standards," meaning that community-wide agreements form the basis of acceptable moral rules and that these intersubjective agreements cannot be further validated or invalidated by appeals to rationality. Mackie understands morality entirely in terms of social practices that express what the community demands, allows, enforces, and condemns. Nonetheless, he insists that we need not view moral judgments as unchanging conventional rules beyond possibility of reform: "Of course there have been and are moral heretics and moral reformers. . . . But this can usually be understood as the extension, in ways which, though new and unconventional, seemed to them to be required for consistency of rules to which they already adhered as arising out of an existing way of life."[51]

The Primacy of Social Practices

MacIntyre and other communitarians have traced to Aristotle the thesis that local community practices and their corresponding virtues should have priority over ethical theory in normative decisionmaking. MacIntyre uses "practice" to designate a cooperative arrangement in pursuit of goods that are internal to a structured communal life. Social roles of parenting, teaching, governing, healing, and the like involve practices. "Goods internal to a practice" are achievable, according to MacIntyre, only by engaging in the practice and conforming to its constraints and standards of excellence. In the practice of medicine, for example, goods internal to the profession exist, and these determine what it means to be a good physician. The virtues of physicians flow from communal and institutional practices of care, practical wisdom, and education. Medicine, like other professions and political institutions, has a history that sustains a tradition requiring participants in the practice to cultivate certain virtues.[52]

The importance of traditional practices and the need for communal intervention to correct socially disruptive outcomes are standard themes in communitarian thought. For example, Sandel proposes that we disallow plant closings that devastate local communities and that we ban pornography when it deeply offends a community's way of life.[53]

As an example of communitarians' promotion of the common good in biomedical ethics, consider their debate with liberal individualists over policies of obtaining cadaveric organs for transplantation. Based on principles of liberal individualism, all states in the United States adopted the Uniform Anatomical Gift Act in the late 1960s and early 1970s. This act gives individuals the right to donate their organs after death and to express their decisions through a donor card or other documents of gift. If the individual has not made a decision prior to death, the law authorizes the family to decide whether to donate the decedent's organs. Opinion polls suggested that many individuals would sign donor cards and provide a sufficient supply of organs, thereby avoiding the need to search for living donors of kidneys.

In practice, however, few individuals sign donor cards, the cards are rarely available at the time of death, and procurement teams virtually always check with the family, even if the decedent left a valid donor card. As a result, a communitarian focus has emerged. The family has become the primary donor (that is, the decision-maker about donation) rather than the individual, and because the supply of organs has remained limited, various policies have been considered and some adopted that aim to promote the common good more vigorously. Even approaches that protect individual rights attempt to educate people about the need for organs, and some writers in ethics propose *requiring* people to make a decision about donation, for instance, when obtaining a driver's license. Recent laws and regulations require hospitals to ask families whether they know the wishes of the decedent and want to donate the decedent's organs.

Some communitarians now recommend still stronger laws and policies to make organ procurement a well-defined community project rather than a matter of individual or even family decisions. They defend *presumed consent* laws, which would parallel laws in several states for corneas (when bodies are under the auspices of the medical examiner's office) and laws in several countries for solid organs. These laws presume that individuals or families have decided to donate unless they have registered a dissent. A more straightforward rationale is the *routine salvaging* of organs unless objections are registered: Some communitarians defend such a policy of organ retrieval on grounds that members of a community should be willing to provide others objects of lifesaving value when they can do so at no cost to themselves.[54] A few commentators even recommend stricter policies of routine collection to reflect communal ownership of cadaveric body parts. The last approach conflicts so deeply with liberal individualistic values that it has, as yet, not received serious consideration.[55]

An emphasis on the community and the common good also appears in debates about the allocation of health care, as we observed in Chapter 6. According to Daniel Callahan's communitarian account, we should enact public policy from a shared consensus about the good society, not on the basis of individual rights. We should scrap liberal assumptions about government neutrality, and society should be free to implement a substantive concept of the good. Biomedical ethics should use communitarian values to implement or revise social laws and regulations governing the promotion of health, the use of genetic knowledge, the use of advances in medical technology, responsibilities to future generations, and the limits of health care for the elderly. In each case, Callahan would ask "What is most conducive to a good society?," not "Is it harmful or does it violate autonomy?"[56]

Although many communitarians critique and propose specific acts, practices, and policies, such as procuring organs or allocating health care, few systematic communitarian proposals have emerged for biomedical ethics. One exception is Ezekiel Emanuel's vision of medical ethics, which rests on the following claims: Public laws and public values have shaped the ends of medicine, as affirmed by the profession. These ends are understood through a framework of shared political convictions, conceptions of justice, and ideas of the good life. In place of the liberalism that has undergirded much of medical ethics, Emanuel proposes a communitarianism closely connected to political theory. This communitarianism is moderate by virtue of its acceptance of pluralistic conceptions of the good life and its recognition of some individual rights. Yet it remains communitarian because democratic initiatives are necessary to fashion a community's conceptions of the good life into policies and laws. Emanuel envisions thousands of community health plans in which citizen-members deliberate about conceptions of the good life and debate policies, such as those for termination of life-sustaining treatment for incompetent patients and for the allocation of medical resources.[57]

A Critical Evaluation of Communitarian Ethics

Several claims made by more militant communitarians rely on questionable accusations and arguments. We concentrate on these problems in our criticisms. Many themes in moderate communitarianism we believe to be unproblematic and even acceptable to advocates of liberal theories. We will focus on these unproblematic themes in our constructive comments.

An unfair account of liberal theories. Militant communitarians suggest that liberal theorists defend atomistic, isolated individuals and have a corrupting skepticism about communal goods. This characterization is inaccurate. Mill and Rawls, the figures most frequently attacked by communitarians, never depict either individuals or the communal good in these terms, and both philosophers develop a theory of the common good, as well as an account of social traditions and political community.[58] Mill thought he had captured how historical traditions converge to the principle of utility, which he construed as a principle of communal welfare. Even in *On Liberty* (Mill's treatise on individual liberty rights), Mill argued that a community should take steps to ensure adequate public discussion of what constitutes the good of the community. Liberty functions in his arguments to protect individuals against mistakes in planning communal pursuits of the good, and he defends individuality *because* it conduces to a constantly readjusted and improved community. Similarly, Rawls defends rights and liberties, in part, because an open society can correct and revise social ends better than a society controlled by tradition.[59]

A false dichotomy: community or autonomy. Communitarians present us with two false dichotomies: (1) either liberal accounts of rights and justice have priority or the communal good has priority,[60] and (2) either we protect radical autonomy in decision-making or we protect communal determination of social goals against the individual. A more accurate picture is that we inherit social roles and goals. We then critique, adjust, and attempt to improve our beliefs over time through free discussion and collective arrangements. Individuals and groups alike progressively interpret, revise, and sometimes even replace traditions with new conceptions that adjust and foster community values. This liberal outlook is, as Joel Feinberg notes, entirely compatible with communal interests: "It is impossible to think of human beings except as part of ongoing communities, defined by reciprocal bonds of obligation, common traditions, and institutions. . . . The ideal [in liberal accounts] of the autonomous person is that of an authentic individual whose self-determination is as complete as is consistent with the requirement that he is, of course, a member of a community."[61]

A failed challenge to rights. Communitarians sometimes argue against rights (especially natural rights) on grounds that they do not exist.[62] At other times, they argue against rights on grounds that rights function to give individuals too much power and that rights thereby stall communal organization and activities and dull our sense of social union. Both claims miss the valuable consequences that rights have for communities. We value rights because, when enforced, they provide protections against unscrupulous behavior, promote orderly change and cohesiveness in communities, and allow diverse communities to coexist peacefully within a single political state.[63] Rights are necessary both to enable individuals to live safely and to protect them from oppressive communities.

Even if we grant communitarian arguments that the best life is communal life, it would not follow that communities should determine the individual's goals or truncate individual rights. The major reason for the prominence of rights in moral and political theory is that they stand as a shield against communal intrusion.

A Constructive Evaluation of Communitarianism

By emphasizing historical traditions and institutional practices, communitarian theories have redirected ethical theory in recent years and have helped us rediscover the importance of community, even if we accept liberal values. Communitarians rightly emphasize the need to foster neighborhood associations, create communal ties, promote public health, and develop national goals. Also to be welcomed is the return in some communitarian theories to such landmarks in ethical theory as the writings of Aristotle, Hume, and Hegel. These more community-minded philosophers deserve status as great classical theorists, alongside Mill and Kant.

Ethics of Care: Relationship-Based Accounts

The *ethics of care* is another family of moral reflections that has no central moral principle. It shares some premises with communitarian ethics, including some objections to central features of liberalism and an emphasis on traits valued in intimate personal relationships, such as sympathy, compassion, fidelity, discernment, and love. *Caring* in these accounts refers to care for, emotional commitment to, and willingness to act on behalf of persons with whom one has a significant relationship. Noticeably downplayed are Kantian universal rules, impartial utilitarian calculations, and individual rights.

Proponents of an ethics of care would approach the case we have been examining by focusing on relationships involving care, responsibility, trust, fidelity, and sensitivity. The father who elects not to donate a kidney expresses some concern about his daughter's suffering, but his response is arguably grounded mainly in concern about himself. He does not think he can justify his behavior to his wife, who will, he believes, distrust his motives and "accuse him of allowing his daughter to die." Even if we give the father the benefit of the doubt about motives and trustworthiness, whether he responsibly expresses his care in donation or in nondonation will depend, in part, on the balance of risks and benefits and on his courage in confronting these risks.

The physician in this case faced several conflicts within relationships of care—to the dying daughter, her siblings, the reluctant father, the mother, and the family as a unit. Just as many moral theories face conflicts of principles and rights, the ethic of care faces conflicts among responsibilities in such situations. Traditional moral theory has concentrated on answers to questions about whether to lie or break confidentiality. The ethic of care, by contrast, emphasizes not only what the physician does—for example, whether he breaks or maintains confidentiality—but also how he performs those actions, which motives underlie them, and whether his actions promote or thwart positive relationships. The physician's trustworthiness and the quality of his care and sensitivity in the face of the father's request for deception are integral moral factors from the perspective of the ethics of care.

Two Speakers in a Different Voice

The ethic of care originated primarily in feminist writings. Its themes included how women display an ethic of care, by contrast to men, who predominantly exhibit an ethic of rights and obligations. We begin with two figures who have played prominent roles in this recent history, psychologist Carol Gilligan and philosopher Annette Baier.

Gilligan's psychological account. The hypothesis that "women speak in a different voice"—a voice that traditional ethical theory has drowned out—arose in Gilligan's book, *In a Different Voice.* She maintained that women's moral development is typically distinct from men's, a fact disregarded by influential psychological studies of moral development whose conceptions were based on studies of males only. She discovered "the voice of care" through empirical research involving interviews with girls and women. This voice, she said, stresses empathic association with others, not based on "the primacy and universality of individual rights, but rather on . . . a very strong sense of being responsible." In her studies, female subjects typically view morality in terms of responsibilities of care deriving from attachments to others, whereas male subjects typically see morality in terms of rights and justice. Men look to and are formed by freely accepted relationships and agreements; women look to and are formed by contextually given relationships, such as those of the family.[64]

Gilligan identified two modes of relationship, which constitute two modes of moral thinking: an ethic of care and an ethic of rights and justice. She did not claim that these two modes of thinking strictly correlate with gender or that all women or all men speak in the same moral voice.[65] Rather, she maintained that men *tend* to embrace an ethic of rights using quasilegal terminology and impartial principles, accompanied by dispassionate balancing and conflict resolution, whereas women *tend* to affirm an ethic of care that centers on responsiveness in an interconnected network of needs, care, and prevention of harm. The core notion involves caring for and taking care of others, and it is modelled on relationships, such as those between parent and child.[66]

Baier's philosophical account. Gilligan's interpretation of empirical data has parallels in philosophical ethics. In Annette Baier's account, the reasoning and methods of women who write in ethical theory differ noticeably from those found in traditional theories. She hears in contemporary female philosophers, despite their diversity, the same different voice that Gilligan heard in her studies, but one made "reflective and philosophical."[67] She deplores the near-exclusive emphasis in modern moral philosophy on universal rules and principles, and she sternly rejects Kantian contractarian models with their emphasis on justice, rights, law, and particularly autonomous choice by free and equal agents. The conditions of social cooperation, especially in families and in communal decision-making, are, Baier observes, typically unchosen and intimate, and they involve unequals in a relational network. She argues not that traditional ethical theories are false or outmoded, but that they capture only a piece of the larger moral world.[68]

Baier does not envision a grand system of ethics that holds together all the diverse strands, but rather smaller scale systems that pull together a few strands. In casting about for a connecting bridge to span an ethic of care with an ethic of obligation, she proposes "appropriate trust." She does not recommend that we discard categories of obligation, but that we make room for an ethic of love and trust, including an account of human bonding and friendship.[69]

Criticisms of Traditional Liberal Theories

Proponents of the care perspective offer a challenge to liberal theories. Two of their criticisms merit special attention.[70]

Challenging impartiality. According to the care perspective, liberalism has lost sight of the scope of morality by overemphasizing detached fairness. This orientation is suitable for some moral relationships, especially those in which persons interact as equals in a public context of impersonal justice and institutional constraints. But lost in this *detachment* is an *attachment* to what we care about most and is closest to us—for example, our loyalty to groups. In the absence of public and institutional constraints, partiality toward others is not only morally permissible but is the expected norm of interaction and is an ineliminable feature of the human condition. Without exhibiting partiality, we stand to sever important relationships and to alienate others. In seeking impartiality, liberalism risks making us blind and indifferent to the special needs of and relationships with others. Although impartiality is a moral virtue in some contexts, it is a moral vice in others. Traditional liberal theory overlooks this two-sidedness when it simply aligns good and mature moral judgment with moral distance.[71] The care perspective is especially meaningful for roles such as parent, friend, physician, and nurse, in which contextual response, attentiveness to subtle clues, and deepening special relationships are likely to be more important morally than impartial treatment.[72]

Challenging universal principles. A concern about abstract principles, the instruments of impartiality, also characterizes the ethics of care. As long as principles allow room for discretionary and contextual judgment, the ethics of care need not dispense with principles. However, like many proponents of virtue theory, defenders of the ethics of care find principles often irrelevant, unproductive, ineffectual, or constrictive in the moral life. A defender of principles could say that *principles* of care, compassion, and kindness tutor our responses in caring, compassionate, and kind ways. But this claim seems hollow. Our moral experience suggests that our responses rely on our emotions, our capacity for sympathy, our sense of friendship, and our knowledge of how caring people behave.

Consider, as an example, the following report by physician Timothy Quill and nurse Penelope Townsend of a discussion with a young woman who has just been told that she is HIV-infected:[73]

PATIENT: Oh God. Oh Lord have mercy. . . . Please don't do it again. Please don't tell me that. Oh my God. Oh my children. Oh Lord have mercy. Oh God, why did He do this to me? . . .

DR. QUILL: First thing we have to do is learn as much as we can about it, because right now you are okay.

PATIENT: I don't even have a future. Everything I know is that you gonna die anytime. What is there to do? What if I'm a walking time bomb? People will be scared to even touch me or say anything to me.

DR. QUILL: No, that's not so.

PATIENT: Yes they will, 'cause I feel that way . . .

DR. QUILL: There is a future for you . . .

PATIENT: Okay, alright. I'm so scared. I don't want to die. I don't want to die, Dr. Quill, not yet. I know I got to die, but I don't want to die.

DR. QUILL: We've got to think about a couple of things. . . .

Quill and Townsend have moral responsibilities to their patient, but it is difficult to capture all those responsibilities in principles and rules. We can produce rough generalizations about how caring physicians and nurses respond to patients, but these generalizations will not be subtle enough to provide helpful guidance for the next patient. Each situation calls for a set of responses outside any generalization, and behavior that in one context is caring may intrude on privacy or be offensive in another setting.

Relationship and Emotion

Two constructive themes are central to the ethics of care: mutual interdependence and emotional responsiveness.

Mutual interdependence in relationships. The ethics of care maintains that many human relationships (e.g., in health care and research) involve persons who are vulnerable, dependent, ill, and frail and that the desirable moral response is attached attentiveness to needs, not detached respect for rights. Feeling for and being immersed in the other person establish vital aspects of the moral relationship. Accordingly, this approach features responsibilities and forms of empathy that a rights-based account may ignore in the attempt to protect persons from invasion by others.[74]

A role for the emotions. Ethical theory since the late eighteenth century has exhibited a cognitivist proclivity—it has regarded theory and moral judgment as the affairs of reason, rather than of emotion or passion. Kant joined many other writers in the history of ethics, such as Plato, in depicting the emotions, feelings, passions, and inclinations as impediments to moral judgment. These philosophers call for a struggle against desire, impulse, and inclination in order to ensure a more rational course of deliberation and action. For these theories, actions done from desire, impulse, or inclination may be good, but not *morally* good, because they are not performed from an appropriate cognitive framework.

The ethics of care corrects this cognitivist bias by giving the emotions a moral role. Having a certain emotional attitude and expressing the appropriate emotion in action are morally relevant factors, just as having the appropriate motive for an action is morally relevant. The person seems morally deficient who acts from rule-governed obligations without appropriately aligned feelings, such as concern when a friend suffers. In addition to expressing their feelings in their responses, agents also need to attend to the feelings of persons toward whom they act. Insight into the needs of others and considerate attentiveness to their circumstances often come from the emotions more than reason.[75]

In the history of human experimentation, for example, those who first recognized that some subjects of research were being brutalized, subjected to misery, or placed at unjustifiable risk were persons who were able to feel compassion, disgust, and outrage through insight into the situation of these research subjects. They exhibited emotional discernment of and sensitivity to the feelings of subjects, where others lacked comparable responses. This emphasis on the emotional dimension of the moral life does not reduce moral response to emotional response. Caring also has a cognitive dimension, because it involves insight into and understanding of another's circumstances, needs, and feelings. As Hume pointed out, emotions motivate us and tell us much about a person's character, but human understanding directs us in choosing a path of action.

A Critical Evaluation of the Ethics of Care

The ethics of care emphasizes engaged, contextual, and even passionate moral thinking. As long as this approach acknowledges both passion and dispassion, it is subject to few, if any, crippling criticisms. Nonetheless, some problems need attention.

Underdeveloped theory. If one takes seriously the eight criteria for theory construction presented at the beginning of this chapter, then the ethics of care seems to fall short on criteria such as completeness, comprehensiveness, and explanatory and justificatory power. Of course, there may be a bias in these criteria: Because this list grows out of traditional accounts of theory that proponents of the ethics of care often oppose, it might be expected to support a critique of the ethics of care, which explicitly departs from traditional theory. But the heart of the problem is the lack of a developed and integrated body of reflections to supply the concepts and connections needed to satisfy these criteria. As Baier has pointed out, the ethics of care needs one or more central concepts and a set of bridging concepts to link it to the legitimate concerns of traditional theory. The ethic of care, then, is an underdeveloped theory, but not necessarily an incorrect one.[76]

Should we reject impartiality? In deemphasizing justice, impartiality, rights, and obligations, the ethics of care must confront situations in which bona fide requirements of impartiality conflict with acting partially from care. Acting partially clearly must sometimes yield to acting impartially (just as the converse relation may hold). On at least some occasions, we need an impartial judgment to arbitrate between conflicting moral judgments or feelings.[77] Many who endorse the ethics of care do not want to exclude all impartial judgments and considerations of justice and the public good. But a problem remains about the extent to which this approach can successfully incorporate these moral notions without losing much of its critical thrust and uniqueness.

A proper view of principles? One proponent of the ethics of care argues that in a defensible ethical theory, action should be sometimes principle-guided, but not necessarily always governed by or derived from principles.[78] This statement moves in the right direction of coherence. However, if an ethics of care can accommodate some principles, does this inclusion undercut its grounds for antipathy to principles? The question is one of coherence. Can a theory coherently trade on a rejection of some principles (Kantian principles, say), and, at the same time, accept a vital role for other principles (prima facie principles, say)?

We think principles will reappear in a more comprehensive theory and will enhance rather than weaken the ethics of care. We should not reject principles, but only avoid using them in such an abstract way that we neglect particular relations and personal moral judgments. If we agree that moral judgment involves more than applying abstract rules, we will be better prepared to accommodate a variety of legitimate moral points of view. Nevertheless, if we accept this perspective, together with the thesis that certain forms of sympathy and emotion are appropriate bases of motivation, we should be prepared for situations in which our actions are overly partial and need correction by impartial principles. We are likely to treat more favorably persons who are close to us in intimate relationships, although on some occasions those who are distant from us deserve more favorable treatment.

Feminist reservations. Some feminists have sharply criticized the ethics of care, despite its feminist origins, on the grounds that it attends to women's experiences as givers of care in traditional roles of self-sacrifice, but often neglects their oppression. Susan Sherwin argues that feminists should "be cautious about the place of caring in their approach to ethics; it is necessary to be wary of the implications of gender traits within a sexist culture. Because gender differences are central to the structures that support dominance relations, it is likely that women's proficiency at caring is somehow related to women's subordinate status."[79] Sherwin sees a need to examine the social context of care as well as to establish limits to the ethics of care. Both enterprises would involve appeals to justice and, perhaps, to rights.

Along the lines of this criticism, we can add that, without a broader framework, the ethics of care is too confined to the *private* sphere of intimate relationships and may serve to reinforce an uncritical adherence to traditional social patterns of assigning caretaker roles to women. Among health professionals, nurses have most often appropriated the ethic of care. A danger exists that the ethics of care, without further development, will be primarily located in nursing and primary care specialties in medicine to which many women are attracted, without having a major impact on health care as a whole.[80]

A Constructive Evaluation of the Care Ethic

The care ethic provides a needed corrective to two centuries of system-building in ethical theory and to the tendency to neglect themes such as sympathy, the moral emotions, and women's experiences. A morality centered on care and concern can potentially serve health care in a constructive and balanced way, because it is close to the processes of decision-making and feeling exhibited in clinical contexts. Sympathy, friendliness, compassion, and trust cannot easily be brought under rules of conduct or even under a principle of beneficence. Codes of physician and nursing ethics have recently stressed obligations (and occasionally rights), but the ethics of care can retrieve basic commitments of caring and caretaking and help liberate health professionals from narrow conceptions of their role responsibilities. Caring involves an open responsiveness to another's needs as the other sees those needs, and, therefore, runs counter to the assumption that a medical good will always best meet those needs.

The ethics of care seems particularly well-suited to disclosures, discussions, and decision-making in health care, which typically become a family affair, with support from a health care team. The ethics of care fits this context of relationships, whereas rights theory, for example, seems poorly equipped for it. Finally, correcting traditional theories' undue obsession with impartiality promises to have positive consequences because many aspects of character, forms of sensitivity, and modes of practical judgment exceed impartial principles.

Convergence Across Theories

Whenever several competing theories, systems, or general depictions of some phenomenon are available, we tend to seek out the best account and affirm it. However, affiliation with one type of ethical theory is precarious in both general ethics and biomedical ethics. If the two authors of this book were forced to rank the types of theory examined in this chapter, we would differ. We have reached different estimates after evaluating the available theories. But for both of us, the most satisfactory theory—if we could find only *one* to be most satisfactory—would be only slightly preferable, and no theory would fully satisfy all relevant criteria.

We would exaggerate differences among types of theory if we presented them as warring armies locked in combat. Many different theories lead to similar action-guides and to similar virtues. Several of these standpoints can defend roughly the same principles, obligations, rights, responsibilities, and virtues. For example, although utilitarianism often appears both starkly different from and hostile to other theories, utilitarian Richard Brandt's view is strikingly similar at the level of principle and obligation to W. D. Ross's deontological position, which sharply criticizes utilitarianism:

[The best code] would contain rules giving directions for recurrent situations which involve conflicts of human interests. Presumably, then, it would contain rules rather similar to W. D. Ross's list of prima facie obligations: rules about the keeping of promises and contracts, rules about debts of gratitude such as we may owe to our parents, and, of course, rules about not injuring other persons and about promoting the welfare of others where this does not work a comparable hardship on us.[81]

That Brandt appeals to utility and Ross to intuitive induction to justify similar sets of rules is a significant difference at the level of moral justification, and the two authors might interpret, specify, and balance their rules differently. Yet, their lists of primary obligations display only trivial differences. This convergence is not restricted to Brandt and Ross. Most of the theories this chapter addresses accept similar general principles (or values), including respect for autonomy, nonmaleficence, and the like, which we defended in previous chapters. Such agreement springs from an initial shared data base, namely, the norms of the common morality. Indeed, we can say without undue paradox that the proponents of these theories all accepted these principles before they devised their theory and that when they attend to practical problems they often rely as much on the principles they share with others as their own unique theory.

Convergence as well as consensus about principles among a group of persons is common in assessing *cases* and framing *policies*, even when deep theoretical differences divide the group. Agreement may similarly emerge about precedent cases. In the real world of practical judgments and public policies, we often need no more agreement than an agreement of principle—not an agreement regarding the foundation of the principle. At the same time, we should not confuse pragmatic advice about principled agreement with whether a theory adequately justifies the principles. Theoretical inquiry is appropriate even if practical agreement has been achieved.

Reasons exist, then, for holding that moral theory is an important enterprise, but that distinctions among types of theory are not as significant for *practical* ethics as some proclaim. It is a mistake to suppose that a series of continental divides separates moral theorists into distinct and hostile groups who reach different practical conclusions and fail to converge on principles. We should not overlook the fact that some theories are closer in substantive principles and rules to allegedly rival theories than they are to some theories of their own "type."

Conclusion

Contemporary biomedical ethics reflects theoretical conflicts of considerable complexity, and the diverse theories explored in this chapter help us see why. Competition exists among the various normative theories, and competing conceptions exist about how such theories relate to biomedical practice. Nonetheless, we stand to learn from all of these theories. Where one theory is weak in accounting for some part of the moral life, another is often strong. Although every general theory clashes at some point with our considered moral convictions, each also articulates convictions that we should be reluctant to relinquish. We can therefore focus on acceptable features in the different theories without having to choose one over the others.

Notes

1. Our views on pluralism are influenced by Thomas Nagel, "The Fragmentation of Value," in *Mortal Questions* (Cambridge: Cambridge University Press, 1979), pp. 128–37; and Baruch Brody's treatment in *Life and Death Decision Making* (New York: Oxford University Press, 1988), p. 9.

2. Our discussion has profited from Shelly Kagan, *The Limits of Morality* (Oxford: Clarendon Press, 1989), esp. pp. 11–15, and from criticisms by David DeGrazia.

3. For analysis of this utilitarian thesis, see Samuel Scheffler, *Consequentialism and its Critics* (Oxford: Clarendon Press, 1988).

4. Jeremy Bentham, *An Introduction to the Principles of Morals and Legislation*, ed. J. H. Burns and H. L. A. Hart (Oxford: Clarendon Press, 1970), pp. 11–14, 31, 34. John Stuart Mill, *Utilitarianism*, in vol. 10 of the *Collected Works of John Stuart Mill* (Toronto: University of Toronto Press, 1969), ch. 1, p. 207; ch. 2, pp. 210, 214; ch. 4, pp. 234–35.

5. A representative of the first list is G. E. Moore, *Principia Ethica* (Cambridge: Cambridge University Press, 1903), pp. 90ff; a representative of the latter list is James Griffin, *Well-Being: Its Meaning, Measurement and Moral Importance* (Oxford: Clarendon Press, 1986), p. 67.

6. This case is based on Melvin D. Levine, Lee Scott, and William J. Curran, "Ethics Rounds in a Children's Medical Center: Evaluation of a Hospital-Based Program for Continuing Education in Medical Ethics," *Pediatrics* 60 (August 1977): 205.

7. Among writers in bioethics, Joseph Fletcher and Peter Singer are good examples of act utilitarians, while R. M. Hare is a good example of rule utilitarianism. See, for example, Joseph Fletcher, *Humanhood: Essays in Biomedical Ethics* (Buffalo, NY: Prometheus Books, 1979); Peter Singer, *Practical Ethics*, 2nd ed. (Cambridge: Cambridge University Press, 1993); R. M. Hare, *Essays on Bioethics* (Oxford: Oxford University Press, 1993); and Hare, "A Utilitarian Approach to Ethics," in *A Companion to Bioethics*, ed. Helga Kuhse and Peter Singer (Oxford: Blackwell, 1998), pp. 80–85.

8. Worthington Hooker, *Physician and Patient* (New York: Baker and Scribner, 1849), pp. 357ff, 375–81.

9. J. J. C. Smart, *An Outline of a System of Utilitarian Ethics* (Melbourne: University Press, 1961); and "Extreme and Restricted Utilitarianism," in *Contemporary Utilitarianism*, ed. Michael Bayles (Garden City, NY: Doubleday and Co., 1968), esp. pp. 104–07, 113–15.

10. Richard B. Brandt, "Toward a Credible Form of Utilitarianism," in *Contemporary Utilitarianism*, pp. 143–86, and in Brandt's *Morality, Utilitarianism, and Rights* (Cambridge: Cambridge University Press, 1992).

11. This question is discussed in Madison Powers, "Repugnant Desires and the Two-Tier Conception of Utility," *Utilitas* 6 (1994): 171–76.

12. Alan Donagan, "Is There a Credible Form of Utilitarianism?" in *Contemporary Utilitarianism*, pp. 187–202.

13. A subtle argument to this conclusion is found in Kagan, *The Limits of Morality*, *passim*.

14. Williams, "A Critique of Utilitarianism," in J. J. C. Smart and Bernard Williams, *Utilitarianism: For and Against* (Cambridge: Cambridge University Press, 1973), pp. 116–17; and J. L. Mackie, *Ethics: Inventing Right and Wrong* (New York: Penguin Books, 1977), pp. 129, 133. For an extension, see Edward Harcourt, "Integrity, Practical Deliberation and Utilitarianism," *Philosophical Quarterly* 48 (1998): 189–98; for critical commentary, see Alastair Norcross, "Consequentialism and Commitment," *Pacific Philosophical Quarterly* 78 (1997): 380–403.

15. Milton Weinstein and William B. Stason, *Hypertension* (Cambridge, MA: Harvard University Press, 1977); and "Public Health Rounds at the Harvard School of Public Health: Allocating of Resources to Manage Hypertension," *New England Journal of Medicine* 296 (1977): 732–39; and "Allocation Resources: The Case of Hypertension," *Hastings Center Report* 7 (October 1977): 24–29.

16. Jane Morley, et al., "Hypertension Control and Access to Medical Care in the Inner City," *American Journal of Public Health* 88 (Nov. 1998): 1696–99; Steven Shea, et al., "Correlates of Nonadherence to Hypertension Treatment in an Inner-City Minority Population," *American Journal of Public Health* 82 (Dec. 1992): 1607–12.

17. Amartya Sen, *On Ethics and Economics* (Oxford: Basil Blackwell, 1987), p. 75.

18. Kant sought to show that unaided reason can be and should be a proper motive to action. What we should do morally is determined by what we would do "if reason completely determined the will." *The Critique of Practical Reason*, trans. Lewis White Beck (New York: Macmillan, 1985), pp. 18–19. Ak. 20. "Ak." designates the page-reference system of the 22-volume Preussische Akademie edition conventionally cited in Kant scholarship.

19. Kant, *Foundations of the Metaphysics of Morals*, trans. Lewis White Beck (Indianapolis, IN: Bobbs-Merrill Company, 1959), pp. 37–42; Ak. 421–24.

20. *Foundations*, p. 47; Ak. 429.

21. *Foundations*, pp. 51, 58–63; Ak. 432, 439–44.

22. *Foundations*, pp. 58; Ak. 439–40; and *Critique of Practical Reason*, p. 33; Ak. 33.

23. Alan Donagan, *The Theory of Morality* (Chicago: University of Chicago Press, 1977), pp. 63–66.

24. See *A Theory of Justice* (Cambridge, MA: Harvard University Press, 1971; revised edition, 1999), pp. 3–4, 27–31 (1999: 3–4, 24–28). For Rawls's more technical interests in and development of Kant, see his "Themes in Kant's Moral Philosophy," in *Kant's Transcendental Deductions*, ed. Eckart Förster (Stanford, CA: Stanford University Press, 1989), pp. 81–113.

25. Rawls, *A Theory of Justice*, pp. 252, 256, 515–20 (1999: 221–22, 226–27, 452–56). See also Rawls, "A Kantian Conception of Equality," *Cambridge Review* (February 1975): 97ff.

26. Rawls, "The Priority of Right and Ideas of the Good," *Philosophy & Public Affairs* 17 (1988): 252; and "Justice as Fairness: Political not Metaphysical," *Philosophy & Public Affairs* 14 (1985): 223–51, esp. 224–25.

27. See, for example, Thomas Nagel, "Personal Rights and Public Space," *Philosophy and Public Affairs* 24 (1995): 83–107, and his *The View from Nowhere* (New York: Oxford University Press, 1986); and Bernard Williams, *Ethics and the Limits of Philosophy* (Cambridge, MA: Harvard University Press, 1985), and his *Moral Luck: Philosophical Papers, 1973–1980* (Cambridge: Cambridge University Press, 1981).

28. See Advisory Committee on Human Radiation Experiments, *Final Report of the Advisory Committee on Human Radiation Experiments* (New York: Oxford University Press, 1996); Keay Davidson, "Questions Linger on 1940s UCSF Plutonium Shots," *The San Francisco Examiner* (February 23, 1995), p. A6; and University of California at San Francisco (UCSF), *Report of the UCSF Ad Hoc Fact Finding Committee on World War II Human Radiation Experiments* (February, 1995, unpublished but released to the public).

29. For an example of such a utilitarian approach to moral rules, see Richard B. Brandt, *Morality, Utilitarianism, and Rights*.

30. Annette Baier, "The Need for More than Justice," *Canadian Journal of Philosophy* 13 (1997), Supp. Vol. on *Science, Ethics, and Feminism*, ed. Marsha Hanen and Kai Nielsen: 41–56. Reprinted in Baier, *Moral Prejudices* (Cambridge, MA: Harvard University Press, 1994).

31. G. W. F. Hegel, *Philosophy of Right*, trans. T. M. Knox (Oxford: Clarendon Press, 1942), pp. 89–90, 106–07.

32. H. L. A. Hart, "Between Utility and Rights," in *Jurisprudence and Philosophy* (Ox-

ford: Clarendon Press, 1983), p. 198. For debates about liberalism, see Nancy L. Rosenblum, ed. *Liberalism and the Moral Life* (Cambridge, MA: Harvard University Press, 1989).

33. Compare H. L. A. Hart, "Bentham on Legal Rights," in *Oxford Essays in Jurisprudence*, 2nd series, ed. A. W. B. Simpson (Oxford: Oxford University Press, 1973), pp. 171–98.

34. See Joel Feinberg, *Social Philosophy* (Englewood Cliffs, NJ: Prentice-Hall, 1973), p. 67.

35. Ronald Dworkin, *Taking Rights Seriously* (Cambridge, MA: Harvard University Press, 1977), p. xi; and *Law's Empire* (Cambridge, MA: Harvard University Press, 1986), p. 223.

36. Ronald Dworkin, *Taking Rights Seriously* (Cambridge, MA: Harvard University Press, 1977), pp. xi, 92, 191, and "Is there a Right to Pornography?" *Oxford Journal of Legal Studies* 1 (1981): 177–212.

37. See Judith Jarvis Thomson, *The Realm of Rights* (Cambridge, MA: Harvard University Press, 1990), pp. 122ff.

38. See Feinberg, *Social Philosophy*, p. 59; and Eric Mack, ed., *Positive and Negative Duties* (New Orleans, LA: Tulane University Press, 1985).

39. The first decade of decisions began with *Roe v. Wade* 410 U.S. 113 (1973) and ran through *City of Akron v. Akron Center for Reproductive Health* (June 1983). Decisions of major importance pertaining to indigency and funding were *Maher v. Roe*, 432 U.S. 464 (1977) and *Harris v. McRae*, 448 U.S. 297 (1980). In *Planned Parenthood v. Casey* (June 28, 1992), the U.S. Supreme Court further upheld the pregnant woman's right to terminate her pregnancy within limits, while abolishing the trimester framework. It recognized the state's interest in fetal life from the beginning of the pregnancy and allowed states to institute requirements that do not impose an undue burden on the pregnant woman's decisions and actions.

40. See David Braybrooke, "The Firm but Untidy Correlativity of Rights and Obligations," *Canadian Journal of Philosophy* 1 (1972): 351–63; and Carl P. Wellman, *Real Rights* (New York: Oxford University Press, 1995).

41. Ronald Dworkin argues that political morality is rights-based in *Taking Rights Seriously*, pp. 169–77, esp. 171. John Mackie has applied this thesis to morality generally in "Can There Be a Right-Based Moral Theory?," *Midwest Studies in Philosophy* 3 (1978), esp. p. 350. For a view that the ancients had a theory of rights in place, but not a theory of the primacy of rights, see Myles Burnyeat, "Did the Ancient Greeks Have the Concept of Human Rights?" *Polis* 13 (1994): 1–11.

42. Robert Nozick, *Anarchy, State, and Utopia* (New York: Basic Books, 1974), pp. ix, 149–82. See also Jan Narveson, *The Libertarian Idea* (Philadelphia, PA: Temple University Press, 1988).

43. Alan Gewirth, "Why Rights Are Indispensable," *Mind* 95 (1986): 333. See Gewirth's later book, *The Community of Rights* (Chicago: University of Chicago Press, 1996); and a partial challenge to his theses that connects the theory to positive and negative rights in Jan Narveson, "Alan Gewirth's Foundationalism and the Well-Being State," *Journal of Value Inquiry* 31 (1997): 485–502.

44. For discussions of bioethical issues in the framework of human rights, see Lawrence O. Gaston and Zita Lazzarini, *Human Rights and Public Health in the AIDS Pandemic* (New York: Oxford University Press, 1997).

45. See Michael Sandel, "The Political Theory of the Procedural Republic," *Revue de métaphysique et de morale* 93 (1988): 57–68, esp. 64–67; Sandel, "Democrats and

Community," *The New Republic*, February 22, 1988: 20–23; Sandel, *Democracy's Discontent: America in Search of a Public Philosophy* (Cambridge, MA: Harvard University Press, 1996); Alasdair MacIntyre, *After Virtue*, pp. 235–37; Michael Walzer, "The Communitarian Critique of Liberalism," *Political Theory* 18 (1990): 6–23.

46. See Michael Sandel, *Liberalism and the Limits of Justice* (Cambridge: Cambridge University Press, 1982), pp. 15–17.

47. Sandel, "Introduction," in *Liberalism and Its Critics*, ed. Sandel (New York: New York University Press, 1984), p. 6; and "Morality and the Liberal Ideal," *The New Republic* (May 7, 1984), pp. 15–17; MacIntyre, *After Virtue*, ch. 1. For a balanced assessment of these theses, see Alisa L. Carse, "The Liberal Individual: A Metaphysical or Moral Embarrassment?" *Nous* 28 (1994): 184–209.

48. Charles Taylor, "Atomism," in *Powers, Possessions, and Freedom*, ed. Alkis Kontos (Toronto: University of Toronto Press, 1979): 39–62.

49. Sandel, *Liberalism and the Limits of Justice*, 15–23, 84–87, 92–94, 139–51; Alasdair MacIntyre, *Whose Justice? Which Rationality?* (Notre Dame, IN: University of Notre Dame Press, 1988), p. 10, and *After Virtue*, p. 206.

50. MacIntyre, *After Virtue*, p. 53.

51. Mackie, *Ethics*, pp. 30, 36–37; see also 106–10, 120–24. See also Michael Walzer's argument in *Interpretation and Social Criticism* (Cambridge, MA: Harvard University Press, 1987).

52. MacIntyre, *After Virtue*, pp. 17, 187, 190–94.

53. Sandel, "Morality and the Liberal Ideal," p. 17.

54. See James L. Nelson, "The Rights and Responsibilities of Potential Organ Donors: A Communitarian Approach," *Communitarian Position Paper* (Washington, DC: The Communitarian Network, 1992); and James Muyskens, "Procurement and Allocation Policies," *The Mount Sinai Journal of Medicine* 56 (1989): 202–06.

55. For the wide range of issues in organ procurement, see James F. Childress, *Practical Reasoning in Bioethics* (Bloomington and Indianapolis, IN: Indiana University Press, 1997), chs. 14–16.

56. Callahan, *What Kind of Life* (New York: Simon & Schuster, 1990), ch. 4, esp. pp. 105–13, and *Setting Limits* (New York: Simon & Schuster, 1987), esp. pp. 106–14.

57. Ezekiel J. Emanuel, *The Ends of Human Life: Medical Ethics in a Liberal Polity* (Cambridge, MA: Harvard University Press, 1991). See also Troyen Brennan, *Just Doctoring: Medical Ethics in the Liberal State* (Berkeley: University of California Press, 1991).

58. See arguments to this conclusion in Will Kymlicka, "Communitarianism, Liberalism, and Superliberalism," *Critical Review* 8 (1994): 263–84; "Liberalism and Communitarianism," *Canadian Journal of Philosophy* 18 (June 1988): 181–204; and "Liberal Individualism and Liberal Neutrality," *Ethics* 99 (July 1989): 883–905. Even John Locke and Thomas Hobbes—the communitarians' arch-enemies (see MacIntyre, *After Virtue*, pp. 233–34)—have a considerable emphasis on promoting the commonweal. Locke, for example, gives an elegant statement in *Two Treatises of Civil Government*, *Works* (London: C. and J. Rivington, 1824), 12th ed., bk. 2, note 8, p. 357.

59. See Amy Gutmann, "Communitarian Critics of Liberalism," *Philosophy and Public Affairs* 14 (Summer 1985): 308–22; and Andrew Jason Cohen, "A Defense of Strong Voluntarism," *American Philosophical Quarterly* 35 (1998): 251–65.

60. Sandel interprets Rawls as creating this dilemma by his account of the alleged priority of the right over the good. See *Liberalism and the Limits of Justice*, pp. 1–10, 17–24, 168–72, and "Morality and the Liberal Ideal," pp. 16–17.

61. Joel Feinberg, *Harm to Self*, Vol. 3, in *The Moral Limits of the Criminal Law* (New York: Oxford University Press, 1986), p. 47.

62. See MacIntyre, *After Virtue*, pp. 67–68.

63. See William R. Lund, "Politics, Virtue, and the Right To Do Wrong: Assessing the Communitarian Critique of Rights," *Journal of Social Philosophy* 28 (1997): 101–22; Allen Buchanan, "Assessing the Communitarian Critique of Liberalism," *Ethics* 99 (July 1989): 852–82, esp. 862–65; and William A. Galston, *Liberal Purposes* (Cambridge: Cambridge University Press, 1991).

64. Carol Gilligan, *In a Different Voice* (Cambridge, MA: Harvard University Press, 1982), esp. p. 21. See also her "Mapping the Moral Domain: New Images of Self in Relationship," *Cross Currents* 39 (Spring 1989): 50–63.

65. Gilligan and many others deny that the two distinct voices correlate strictly with gender. See Gilligan and Susan Pollak, "The Vulnerable and Invulnerable Physician," in *Mapping the Moral Domain*, ed. C. Gilligan, J. Ward, and J. Taylor (Cambridge, MA: Harvard University Press, 1988), pp. 245–62.

66. See Gilligan and G. Wiggins, "The Origins of Morality in Early Childhood Relationships," in *The Emergence of Morality in Young Children*, ed. J. Kagan and S. Lamm (Chicago: University of Chicago Press, 1988). See also Margaret Olivia Little, "Care: From Theory to Orientation and Back," *Journal of Medicine and Philosophy* 23 (1998): 190–209.

67. Annette Baier, "What Do Women Want in a Moral Theory?" *Nous* 19 (March 1985): 53.

68. Ibid, pp. 53–56.

69. Cf. Baier, *Postures of the Mind* (Minneapolis, MN: University of Minnesota Press, 1985), pp. 210–19.

70. Our formulation of these criticisms of liberalism is influenced by Alisa L. Carse, "The 'Voice of Care': Implications for Bioethical Education," *The Journal of Medicine and Philosophy* 16 (1991): 5–28, esp. 8–17.

71. Baier, "Trust and Antitrust," *Ethics* 96 (1986): 248.

72. See the treatment of these issues in Alisa L. Carse, "Impartial Principle and Moral Context: Securing a Place for the Particular in Ethical Theory," *Journal of Medicine and Philosophy* 23 (1998): 153–69.

73. Timothy Quill and Penelope Townsend, "Bad News: Delivery, Dialogue, and Dilemmas," *Archives of Internal Medicine* 151 (March 1991): 463–64.

74. See Nel Noddings, *Caring: A Feminine Approach to Ethics and Moral Education* (Berkeley: University of California Press, 1984).

75. See Nancy Sherman, *The Fabric of Character* (Oxford: Oxford University Press, 1989), pp. 13–55; and Martha Nussbaum, *Love's Knowledge* (Oxford: Oxford University Press, 1990).

76. See the useful defense of care ethics against this and other criticisms in Alisa L. Carse and Hilde Lindemann Nelson, "Rehabilitating Care," *Kennedy Institute of Ethics Journal* 6 (1996): 19–35. See also Monique Deveaux, "Shifting Paradigms: Theorizing Care and Justice in Political Theory," *Hypatia* 10 (1995): 115–19.

77. See the Kantian arguments in Barbara Herman, "Integrity and Impartiality," *Monist* 66 (April 1983): 233–50, and Marcia Baron, "The Alleged Repugnance of Acting from Duty," *Journal of Philosophy* 81 (April 1984): 197–220.

78. Carse, "The 'Voice of Care,'" p. 17.

79. Susan Sherwin, *No Longer Patient: Feminist Ethics and Health Care* (Philadelphia, PA: Temple University Press, 1992), pp. 49–50. See also Laura Purdy, "A Call To

Heal Ethics," in *Feminist Perspectives in Medical Ethics,* ed. Helen Bequaert Holmes and Purdy (Bloomington, IN: Indiana University Press, 1992), p. 10.

80. See Hilde L. Nelson, "Against Caring," Nel Noddings, "In Defense of Caring," and Toni M. Vezeau, "Caring: From Philosophical Concerns to Practice," in *The Journal of Clinical Ethics* 3 (Spring 1992): 8–20; and Helga Kuhse, *Caring: Nurses, Women and Ethics* (Oxford: Blackwell Publishers, 1997). See the following for a good entry point for these debates: Special Issue: *Journal of Medicine and Philosophy* 23 (1998); Rosemarie Tong, *Feminist Approaches to Bioethics: Theoretical Reflections and Practical Applications* (Boulder, CO: Westview Press, 1997); Rita C. Manning, "A Care Approach," in *A Companion to Bioethics,* ed. Helga Kuhse and Peter Singer (Malden, MA: Blackwell, 1998): 98–105; Eve Browning Cole and Susan Coultrap-McQuin, eds., *Explorations in Feminist Ethics: Theory and Practice* (Bloomington, IN: Indiana University Press, 1992); Mary Jeanne Larrabee, ed., *An Ethic of Care: Feminist and Interdisciplinary Perspectives* (New York: Routledge, 1993); and Virginia Held, ed., *Justice and Care: Essential Readings in Feminist Ethics* (Boulder, CO: Westview Press, 1995).

81. Brandt, "Toward a Credible Form of Utilitarianism," p. 166.

9

Method and Moral Justification

Wide agreement exists that we can teach and practice biomedical ethics, but little agreement exists about the methods for achieving these goals. Related disagreement exists about how to justify moral conclusions. In this chapter, we step back from the first-order problems of normative ethics that have occupied us in this book. Here we reflect on second-order problems of whether there is method in bioethics, and, if so, which methods are preferable.

Our conclusions about method are intimately connected to our views on moral justification. The first three major sections of this chapter explicate three models of justification and, in the process, examine the views of several critics of our methods and principles. Later in the chapter, we connect our account of method to the common-morality theory introduced in Chapter 1 and also to the account of moral character developed in Chapter 2.

Justification in Ethics

Morally good people typically have little difficulty in making moral judgments about whether to tell the truth, to injure another person, or to abandon someone in danger. Moral beacons that we learn early in life suffice to guide us in these decisions. However, when we experience moral perplexity or moral conflict, we often need moral justification and reasoning. What, then, is justification in ethics, and by what method of reasoning do we achieve it?

Justification has several meanings in English, some specific to disciplines. In law, for example, justification is a showing in court that one has a sufficient reason for one's claim or for what one has been called to answer. In ethical discourse, the objective is to establish one's case by presenting sufficient grounds for it. A mere listing of reasons will not suffice, because those reasons may not support the conclusion. Not all reasons are good reasons, and not all good reasons are sufficient for justification. We therefore need to distinguish a reason's *relevance* to a moral judgment from its final *adequacy* for that judgment; we also need to distinguish an *attempted* justification from a *successful* justification.

For example, chemical companies in the United States at one time took the presence of toxic chemicals in a work environment to be a legally and morally sound reason to exclude women of childbearing age from a hazardous workplace, but the U.S. Supreme Court overturned these policies on grounds that they are discriminatory.[1] The dangers to health and life presented by hazardous chemicals constitute a *good* reason for excluding employees from a workplace, but this reason may not be a *sufficient* reason for a ban that impacts women alone. Even a worthy attempt at justification may not succeed, because a successful justification requires a sufficient reason.

Several models of justification operate in ethical theory and contemporary biomedical ethics. We will evaluate three particularly influential models, which also provide methods of ethics. The first model approaches justification and method from a top-down perspective that emphasizes general norms and ethical theory. The second approaches justification and method from a bottom-up perspective that emphasizes moral tradition, experience, and particular circumstances. The third refuses to assign priority to either a top-down or a bottom-up strategy. We defend a version of the third.

Top-Down Models: Theory and Application

A top-down model holds that we reach justified moral judgments through a structure of normative precepts that cover the judgment. This model is inspired by disciplines such as mathematics, in which a claim follows logically (deductively) from a credible set of premises. The idea is that justification occurs if and only if general principles and rules, together with the relevant facts of a situation, support an inference to the correct or justified judgment(s).

This model is simple and conforms to the way virtually all persons learn to think morally: Its method involves applying a general rule (principle, ideal, right, etc.) to a clear case falling under the rule. The deductive form is therefore sometimes considered an "application" of general precepts—a conception that moti-

vated use of the term *applied ethics*. The following is the deductive form involved
in "applying" a rule (here using what is *obligatory*, rather than what is *permitted* or *prohibited*, although the deductive model is the same for all three):

1. Every act of description A is obligatory.
2. Act b is of description a.

Therefore,

3. Act b is obligatory.

A simple example is:

1x. Every act in a patient's overall best interest is obligatory for the patient's doctor.
2x. Act of resuscitation b is in this patient's overall best interest.

Therefore,

3x. Act of resuscitation b is obligatory for this patient's doctor.

Covering precepts, such as (1) and (1x), occur at various levels of generality.
We may justify a particular judgment, belief, or hypothesis by bringing it under
one or more moral rules; or justify the rules by bringing them under general principles; or defend both rules and principles by a full ethical theory. Consider the
example of a nurse who refuses to assist in an abortion procedure. The nurse
might attempt to justify the act of refusal by the rule that it is wrong to kill an
innocent human being intentionally. If pressed further, the nurse may justify this
moral rule by reference to a principle of the sanctity of human life. Finally, the
particular judgment, rule, and principle might all find support in an ethical theory that is only implicit and inchoate in the nurse's original judgment. In a pure
deductivist model (as instanced, for example, by utilitarianism), the primary problem of practical ethics is choosing a general ethical theory.

This model functions smoothly in the simple case of a judgment brought directly and unambiguously under a rule or a principle. Consider the following justification: "You must tell Mr. Sanford that he has cancer and will probably die
soon, because a clinician must observe rules of truthfulness in order to properly
respect the autonomy of patients." The top-down model suggests that the judgment, "You should not lie to Mr. Sanford" descends in its moral content directly
from the covering principle, "You should respect autonomy," from which we derive the covering rule, "You shouldn't lie to patients."

Problems in the model. This model is overrated if presented as the one correct
account of moral thinking and method in ethics. It suggests an ordering in which
theories and principles enjoy priority in ethics over traditional practices, institutional rules, and case judgments. While much in the moral life does conform

roughly to this linear-dependence conception, much does not. Particular moral judgments in hard cases almost always require that we specify and balance norms, not merely that we bring a particular instance under a covering rule or principle. The abstract rules and principles in moral theories are extensively indeterminate; that is, the content of these rules and principles is too abstract to determine the acts that we should perform. In the process of specifying and balancing norms and in making particular judgments, we often must take into account factual beliefs about the world, cultural expectations, judgments of likely outcome, and precedents previously encountered to help fill out and give weight to rules, principles, and theories.

The moral life often requires even more than *specified* general norms. The facts of a situation can be such that no general norm (principle or rule) clearly applies. Or the facts of cases may be complex, and the different moral norms that can be brought to bear on the facts may yield inconclusive, even contradictory, results. For example, destroying a nonviable human fetus does not clearly violate rules against killing or murder, nor does the rule that a person has a right to protect bodily integrity and property clearly apply to this moral issue. Even if we have our facts straight, the choice of facts and the choice of rules that we deem relevant will generate a judgment that is incompatible with another choice of facts and rules. Selecting the right set of facts and bringing the right set of rules to bear on these facts are not reducible either to a deductive form of judgment or to the resources of a general ethical theory.

The top-down model also creates a potentially infinite regress of justification— a never-ending demand for final justification—because each level of appeal to a covering precept requires some further general level to justify it. Theoretically, we could handle this problem by presenting a principle that is self-justifying or one that it is irrational not to hold, but proof that some principles occupy this status and that they justify all other principles or rules is an arduous demand that current ethical theory cannot meet. Yet, if all standards are unjustified until brought under a justified covering precept, it would appear, on the assumptions of this approach, that there are no justified principles or judgments.

Finally, the appeal to theory in the covering-precept model suggests that only one correct normative theory exists, yet many distinct theories exist, each with attractive defenses (as we saw in Chapter 8). There is no authoritative or even dominant theory. To the surprise of many philosophers in the last 20 years, often little is lost in practical moral decision-making by dispensing with general moral theories. The rules and principles shared by various theories seem to serve practical judgment more adequately, at least as starting points, than the theories themselves.

Impartial-rule theory. An important version of top-down theory (though not a pure deductivism) has been developed over the last four decades by Bernard Gert and his coauthors H. Danner Clouser and Charles Culver. When challenges arose to our framework of principles in the late-1980s, these authors emerged as our most unsparing critics. Clouser and Gert wrote several articles and part of a book to express concerns about prima facie principles. They coined the label "principlism" to refer to all accounts of ethics comprised of a plurality of potentially conflicting prima facie principles. They directed their criticism primarily at our framework of four principles and offered, as a substitute, a framework centered on rules. This impartial-rule theory, as we will call it, allegedly provides an alternative methodology in biomedical ethics.[2]

Clouser and Gert bring several accusations against our proposed use of principles.[3] First, they charge that principles function like names, checklists, or headings for values worth remembering, but lack deep moral substance and capacity to guide action. That is, principles point to moral themes that merit consideration by grouping those themes under broad headings, but do little more. A second and related criticism is that, because moral agents confronted with bioethical problems receive no directive guidance from principles, they are left free to deal with the problems in their own way. They may give a principle whatever weight they wish, or even no weight at all. From this perspective, our account is insubstantial and permissive, in part because it lacks a controlling theory. A third criticism is that the prima facie principles (and other action guides in our framework) often conflict, and our account is too indeterminate to provide a decision procedure to adjudicate the conflicts.

Clouser and Gert are particularly fond of pointing to these deficiencies in the principles of justice discussed in Chapter 6 of this book. There is, they say, no specific guide to action that derives from these principles. All principles of justice mentioned in this chapter merely instruct persons to attend to matters of justice and think about justice; they give no specific normative guidance. Since such vagueness and generality underdetermine solutions to problems of justice, agents are free to decide what is just and unjust, as they see fit.

Gert and Clouser also criticize principlism for making *both* nonmaleficence *and* beneficence principles of obligation. They maintain that there are no moral rules of beneficence (though they encourage *moral ideals* of beneficence). The only obligations in the moral life, apart from duties encountered in professional roles and other specific stations of duty, are captured by moral rules that prohibit causing harm or evil. For Gert and colleagues, the general goal of morality is to minimize evil or harm, not to promote good (a basic thesis that they find intuitively attractive, but do little to justify). Rational persons can act impartially at all times in regard to all persons with the aim of not causing evil, they say, but rational persons cannot impartially promote the good for all persons at all times.[4]

The limitations of impartial-rule theory. We do not deny that the problems Gert, Clouser, and Culver present deserve sustained reflection. We reject, however, certain assumptions that they make, especially their requirement that there be "a single, clear, coherent, and comprehensive decision procedure for arriving at answers."[5] We are skeptical of this enterprise, even as a model for ethical theory, for reasons presented in Chapters 1 and 8.

Moreover, we believe that the same criticisms they direct at our account affect their impartial-rule theory. In particular, their criticism that our principles lack specific, directive moral substance (being unspecified principles) applies to their rules in a near-identical way one level down in the order of abstraction. Any norm—rule or principle—will have this problem if it is underspecified for the task at hand. A basic norm is intrinsically general, designed to cover a vast range of circumstances.[6] If general rules are not specified in biomedical ethics, they are almost always too general and will fail to provide adequate normative guidance. Clouser and Gert's rules (e.g., "Don't cheat," "Don't deceive," and "Do your duty") are comparable to our principles in just this way: They lack specificity in their original general form. Being one tier less abstract than principles, their rules constitute a first level of specified principles, which explains why their rules do, indeed, have a more directive and specific content than our abstract principles. However, our full account of principles and rules already includes a set of rules almost identical to the rules embraced by Gert and colleagues.[7]

Regarding their criticism that our principles are checklists or headings without deep moral substance, we agree that principles order, classify, and group moral norms that need additional content and specificity. Until we analyze and interpret the principles (as we do in every first section of Chapters 3–6) and then specify and connect them to other norms (as we do in later sections of each of these chapters), it is unreasonable to expect much more than a classification scheme that organizes the normative content and gives very general moral guidance.[8]

Regarding the criticism that principles compete in ways that our account cannot handle, we acknowledge that our moral framework does not resolve a priori conflicts among principles and rules. No framework of guidelines could reasonably anticipate the full range of conflicts; and the impartial-rule system does no more to settle the problem than our system does. However, it does not follow that our principles are inconsistent or that we encounter incompatible moral commitments in embracing them. A virtue of our theory is that it requires specification (see Chapter 1), and a problem in Clouser and Gert's account is that it supposes that its "more concrete" rules escape the need for specification. Only a theory that could put enough content in its norms to escape conflicts and dilemmas in all contexts could live up to the Clouser–Gert demand, but no theory approximates this ideal.[9]

Experience and sound judgment are indispensable allies in resolving these problems. No one has attained or will ever attain a fully specified system of norms for health care ethics. Thomas Nagel has forcefully argued that an unconnected heap of obligations and values is an ineradicable feature of morality, and W. D.

Ross rightly argued that his Kantian and utilitarian critics forced an "architec-tonic" of "hastily reached simplicity" on ethics.[10] Whereas critics of Ross's ac-count (and ours) rely on an ideal of systematic unity, we regard disunity, conflict, and moral ambiguity as pervasive features of the moral life. Untidiness, com-plexity, and conflict may be perplexing, but a theory of morality cannot be faulted for realistically incorporating these dimensions of morality.

Regarding the criticism that our principle–analysis fails to provide a general ethical theory,[11] we see the criticism as correct but irrelevant. We do not attempt a general ethical theory and do not claim that our principles mimic, are analo-gous to, or substitute for the foundational principles in leading classical theories, such as utilitarianism (with its principle of utility) and Kantianism (with its cat-egorical imperative). We expressed a constrained skepticism about this founda-tionalism in Chapter 8 and doubt that such a unified foundation for ethics is possible without distortion of the moral life.

In response to the criticism that the principle of beneficence expresses an ideal, never a moral obligation, we believe that this thesis is false. Their claim implies that one is never morally required (except by role and professional duties) to pre-vent or remove harm or evil, but only to avoid causing harm or evil. They rec-ognize no requirement to *do* anything, only to avoid causing harmful events. We believe that their thesis seriously misreads the commitments of the common morality.

Moreover, the claim that beneficence is never morally required is not even sup-ported within Gert and Clouser's own account of moral obligations. Gert relies in his book, *Morality: A New Justification of the Moral Rules*, on the premise that one is morally obligated to act beneficently under various conditions. He in-terprets his general rule, "Do your duty," to incorporate what we call obligations of beneficence. Gert explains his system and its commitments as follows:

Although duties, in general, go with offices, jobs, roles, etc., there are some duties that seem more general. . . . A person has a duty . . . because of some special circumstances, for example, his job or his relationships. . . . In any civilized society, if a child collapses in your arms, you have a duty to seek help. You cannot simply lay him out on the ground and walk away. In most civilized societies, one has a duty to help when (1) one is in phys-ical proximity to someone in need of help to avoid a serious evil, usually death or seri-ous injury, (2) one is in a unique or close to unique position to provide that help and (3) it would be relatively cost-free for one to provide that help.[12]

Although Gert insists that these requirements are all supported by the moral rule, "Do your duty," they are effectively *identical* to the obligations that follow from what we call—following traditions in ethical theory in the eighteenth, nineteenth, and twentieth centuries—beneficence. It therefore cannot be the case that Gert's system lacks obligations of beneficence in our sense of beneficence. From this perspective, Gert and Clouser's criticism of principles of beneficence is throughly misplaced.[13]

To generalize, much in principlism that Clouser and Gert appear to reject is presupposed by Gert's final rule, "Do your duty" (or "Don't avoid doing your duty"). Our theories are therefore more compatible than these critics allow (which is not to say entirely compatible). It is hard to see how their impartial-rule theory provides a real alternative to our substantive claims about the nature and scope of obligations. It is also unlikely that their theory can function any better than ours can, without also relying heavily on specification.

A reason for preferring our theory to theirs is that some substantive requirements of the common morality can be better expressed in the language of principles than in the language of rules. Consider respect for autonomy, which Gert and colleagues find as problematic as justice and beneficence. Their disregard of this principle renders their assessments of some cases convoluted and puzzling. Here is a typical problem-case: Following a serious accident, a patient, while still conscious, refuses a blood transfusion on religious grounds; he then falls unconscious and his physicians believe that he will die unless he receives a transfusion. Gert and Culver argue that the provision of a blood transfusion under these circumstances is paternalistic and wrong because, after the patient regains consciousness, the physicians would violate either the moral rule against deception or the moral rule against causing pain: If they did not tell the patient about the transfusion, they would violate the rule against deception; if they did tell him, they would cause pain.[14]

Gert and Culver's inattention to the principle of respect for autonomy forces them to this misleading analysis. They lack the resources to argue that the transfusion, in this case, is paternalistic and prima facie wrong because it violates the patient's expressed wishes and choices (in order to provide him with a medical benefit). Paradoxically, their analysis implies that if the patient dies without regaining consciousness, the physicians did not act wrongly because they violated no moral rules. One of Gert's basic moral rules is "Do not deprive of freedom." In order to address the problems that arise from this case, and similar cases, Gert and colleagues have come *in recent years* to interpret this moral rule to include "freedom from being acted upon as well as depriving of opportunity to act."[15] This expanded interpretation is reasonable, but their rule, so interpreted, approximates the principle of respect for autonomy. If they had a clearer statement of this principle, they could handle a still broader range of cases.

Bottom-Up Models: Cases and Inductive Generalization

Many writers in biomedical ethics concentrate not on principles or theories, but on practical decision-making. They believe that moral justification proceeds inductively (bottom up) by contrast to deductively (top down). Inductivists, as we will call them, argue that we reason inductively from particular instances to general statements or positions. Inductivists hold that we use existing social agreements and practices, insight-producing novel cases, and comparative case analysis as the initial starting points from which to make decisions in particular cases and to generalize to norms. Inductivists emphasize an evolving moral life that reflects exemplary lives and narratives, experience with hard cases, and analogy from prior practice. From this perspective, "inductivism" and "bottom-up models" are broad categories that contain several methodologies critical of top-down theories. Pragmatism[16] and particularism,[17] as well as some forms of feminism and virtue theory, would qualify as accounts of this kind.

Inductivists propose that certain kinds of cases and particular judgments provide warrants to accept moral conclusions independently of general norms. Inductivists see rules and principles as derivative in the order of knowledge, not primary. That is, the meaning, function, and weight of a principle derive from previous moral struggles and reflection in particular circumstances. For example, physicians once regarded withdrawing various medical technologies from patients as acts of impermissible killing. But progressively, after dealing with many agonizing cases, they and society came to frame many of these acts as forms of permissible allowing to die and even as morally required acts of acknowledging refusals of treatment. All moral rules arise and are refined over time; they never become more than provisionally secure points in a cultural matrix of guidelines. A society's moral views find their warrant through an embedded moral tradition and a set of procedures that often permit and even foster new insights and judgments. This account does not support a static or conservative conception of morality, as long as the tradition presents methods and procedures for reflecting on and developing that tradition.

Consider an example from the explosion of interest since 1976 in surrogate decision-making. A series of cases beginning with the Quinlan case challenged medical ethics and the courts to develop virtually an entire new framework of substantive rules for responsible surrogate decision-making about life-sustaining treatments, as well as authority rules regarding who should make those decisions. This framework was created by working through cases analogically, and testing new hypotheses against preexisting norms. In both ethics and law, a string of cases with some similar (and some dissimilar) features set the terms of the ethics of surrogate decision-making. Even if a principle or rule was not entirely novel in a proposed framework, its content was shaped by problems needing resolution in the cases at hand. Gradually, a loose consensus emerged in the courts and in ethics about a framework for such decision-making.

Casuistry: case-based reasoning. Casuistry, an influential version of bottom-up thinking, revives a model that enjoyed an impressive influence in medieval and early modern philosophy and refashions it for modern biomedical ethics.[18] *Casuistry* refers to the use of case-comparison and analogy to reach moral conclusions.[19] Albert Jonsen and Stephen Toulmin, who spearheaded this approach to method in contemporary biomedical ethics, have in the process criticized our framework of principles.[20]

Casuists are skeptical of rules, rights, and general theories divorced from cases, history, precedents, and circumstances. Appropriate moral judgments occur, they say, through an intimate acquaintance with particular situations and the historical record of similar cases. Casuists dispute, in particular, the goal of a tidy, unified theory containing general and universal principles.[21] Although a foundational and absolute principle is not inconceivable, casuists maintain that moral beliefs and reasoning, in fact, do not assume or stand in need of such a principle.

Casuists do not always exclude rules and principles from moral thinking, but they insist that moral judgments can be and often are made when no appeal to principles is possible. For example, we make moral judgments when principles, rules, or rights conflict and no further recourse to a higher principle, rule, or right is available. When principles are interpreted inflexibly irrespective of the nuances of the case, some casuists see a "tyranny of principles."[22] As a result, attempts to resolve moral problems suffer from a gridlock of conflicting principles, and moral debate becomes intemperate and interminable. This impasse can often be avoided, Jonsen and Toulmin argue, by focusing on points of shared agreement about cases rather than on principles. The following is their prime example, drawn from their experiences during four years of work with the National Commission for the Protection of Human Subjects of Biomedical and Behavioral Research:

> The one thing [individual commissioners] could not agree on was *why* they agreed. . . . Instead of securely established universal principles . . . giving them intellectual grounding for particular judgments about specific kinds of cases, it was the other way around.
>
> The *locus of certitude* in the commissioners' discussions . . . lay in a shared perception of what was specifically at stake in particular kinds of human situations. . . . That could never have been derived from the supposed theoretical certainty of the principles to which individual commissioners appealed in their personal accounts.[23]

Jonsen and Toulmin believe that casuistical reasoning rather than universal principles forged agreement. The commission functioned successfully by appeal to paradigms and families of cases, despite the diverse principles and theoretical perspectives held by individual commissioners. Although commissioners did often cite moral principles to justify their collective conclusions, Jonsen and Toulmin argue that these principles were less certain and less central than particular judgments about cases.[24]

A simple example illustrates their claim that moral certitude resides in case judgments and appeals to tradition rather than in principles or theory: We know (in most cases) that it is morally wrong to run significant risks with children in biomedical research. We are sure of the statement, "We should not give this healthy baby the flu in order to test a new decongestant," but we may be unsure which principle controls this judgment or whether some viable theory sanctions the judgment. The casuist believes that we are almost always more certain about particular moral conclusions than we are about *why* they are correct. In this sense, practical knowledge takes priority over theoretical knowledge. Moreover, if a principle or a theory were to instruct us to give the flu to children in order to test drugs (as some versions of utilitarianism might), this outcome would provide us with a good reason for rejecting the principle or theory. Moral certitude, then, is found at the bottom—in the case and traditions of practical judgment—not at the top in a principle or theoretical judgment.

Casuists must decide where a new case fits, relative to paradigmatically right and wrong actions. They must place difficult cases in the context of similar and acceptable cases, as well as similar and unacceptable cases. Thus, precedent cases and analogical reasoning are paramount in this method. For example, if a case involves a problem of medical confidentiality, casuists consider analogous cases in which breaches of confidentiality were justified or unjustified in order to see whether such a breach is justified in the present case. The leading cases—often called "paradigm cases"—become the most enduring and authoritative sources of appeal in the underlying consensus. For example, the current literature of biomedical ethics constantly invokes cases, such as the Quinlan case, the Tuskegee syphilis experiments, the Cowart case, and the Quill case not only to illustrate claims, but as sources of authority for new judgments. Decisions reached about moral rights and wrongs in these seminal cases serve as a form of authority for new cases, as they profoundly affect prevailing standards of fairness, negligence, paternalism, and the like.[25]

A similar method appears in case law. When the decision of a majority of judges becomes authoritative in a case, their judgments are positioned to become authoritative for other courts hearing cases with *similar* facts. This is the doctrine of precedent. Casuists see moral authority similarly: Ethics develops from a social consensus formed around cases. This consensus is then extended to new cases by analogy to the past cases, around which the consensus was formed. As similar cases and similar conclusions evolve, a society becomes increasingly confident in its moral conclusions and acknowledges secure generalizations in its evolving tradition of ethical reflection.

The limits of casuistry. Casuists sometimes overstate the power of their account and understate the value of competing accounts, but a more balanced assessment of the role of cases in moral reasoning should remedy these defects.

First, casuists sometimes write as if paradigm cases speak for themselves or inform moral judgment by their facts alone. Clearly, they do not. For the casuist to move constructively from case to case, some recognized rule of moral relevance must connect the cases. The rule is not part of the case, but rather a way of interpreting and linking cases. All analogical reasoning requires a connecting norm to indicate that one object or event is like or unlike another in relevant respects. The creation or discovery of these norms cannot be achieved by analogy itself. Jonsen seems to treat this problem by distinguishing descriptive elements in a case from moral maxims that inform judgment about the case: "These maxims provide the 'morals' of the story. For most cases of interest, there are several morals, because several maxims seem to conflict. The work of casuistry is to determine *which maxim* should *rule the case* and to what extent."[26] We accept this thesis, which conforms perfectly to our views about prima facie principles and rules. So understood, casuistry presupposes principles, rules, or maxims as essential moral elements *in the case*.

The casuists' "paradigm cases" actually combine *facts* that can be generalized to other cases (e.g., "The patient refused the recommended treatment") and *settled values* (e.g., "Competent patients have a right to refuse treatment"). These settled values are analytically distinct from the facts of particular cases. In casuistical appeals, values and facts are bound together and the central values are preserved from one case to the next. The more general the central values or connecting norms, the closer they come to the status of prima facie principles.

Just as other philosophers have a problem with conflicting principles (ostensibly a reason to favor casuistry), so casuists have a problem with conflicting analogies, judgments, and case interpretations. Casuists stress that cases point beyond themselves and evolve into generalizations, but they also may evolve in the wrong way if they were improperly resolved from the outset. Casuists have no clear methodological resource to prevent a biased development of cases or a neglect of relevant features of cases.

These problems lead to questions about the justificatory power of casuistry. How does *justification* occur? The casuists' answer seems to rest on social convention and analogy. However, different analogies and novel cases might generate competing "right" answers on any given occasion. Without some stable framework of norms, we lack both control on judgment and ways to prevent prejudiced or poorly formulated social conventions.

This criticism is a variant of a much discussed problem about casuistry: Because casuistry works only bottom up, it lacks critical distance from cultural blindness, rash analogy, and mere popular opinion.[27] How is the casuist to identify unjust practices, predisposing bias, and prejudicial use of analogy in order to avoid one-sided judgments? In casuistry, identification of the morally relevant features of a case depends on those who make judgments about cases, and these individuals could operate from very partial perspectives. In this respect, the ethics of casuistry contrasts sharply with a stable system of impartial principles and human rights. Even if we are confident that morally mature cultures have built-in resources for critical distancing and self-evaluation, these resources do not clearly emerge from the methods of casuistry.

The root of this problem is that casuistry is a *method without content*. It is a tool of thought that displays the fundamental importance of case-comparison and analogy in moral thinking, but it lacks initial moral premises. It also lacks any substantive ground of "certitude," as Jonsen and Toulmin put it. It is true enough that we reason by analogy every day, and we are often confident in our conclusions. For example, if we feel better after using a certain medicine, then we feel comfortable in recommending it to other persons, in the expectation that they too will feel more comfortable. A logical form is present in all analogy: If some person or thing has one property associated with a second property, and another person or thing also has the first property, we may feel justified in inferring that the second person or thing also has the second property. However, such analogies often fail: Our friends may not feel better after they take our favored medicine. Analogies never warrant a claim of truth, and we often do not know something by analogy that we think we know. The method of casuistry leaves us in precisely this position: No matter how many properties one case and another share, our inference to yet another property in the second case may mislead or produce false statements.

These are not reasons for rejecting the casuistical method any more than for rejecting the use of analogy. Both are helpful as long as we have a solid knowledge base that allows us to use them. However, to obtain that knowledge, the casuistical method needs to be supplemented by principles of moral relevance that incorporate prior judgments of right and wrong conduct.[28] We will return to this problem of a proper knowledge base when we come to the subject of "considered judgments" later in this chapter (see pp. 398-401).

Finally, Jonsen and Toulmin appear to us to confuse the lack of a practical need for *theory* (a view with which we have considerable sympathy) with the lack of a practical need for *principles*. They also seem to confuse certitude about principles with certitude about theory. We believe the general public and the mainstream of moral philosophy have found a "locus of certitude" in universal moral principles. We agree that in practical deliberation we often have more certitude about particular cases and conclusions than we do about moral theories, but principles that form the cement of the common morality do not lack certitude. In one of his later methodological statements, Jonsen describes connections between principles and casuistry:

Principles, such as respect, beneficence, veracity, and so forth, are invoked necessarily and spontaneously in any serious moral discourse. . . . Moral terms and arguments are imbedded in every case, usually in the form of maxims or enthymemes. The more general principles are never far from these maxims and enthymemes and are often explicitly invoked. Thus, casuistry is not an alternative to principles, in the sense that one might be able to perform good casuistry without principles. In another sense, casuistry is an alternative to principles: they are alternative scholarly activities.[29]

We agree that the two are complementary, but it is unclear that *alternative* scholarly activities are at work. Prima facie principles of the sort we accept are not subject to the casuists' critique and are not excluded by their methodology. Moreover, the movement from principles to specified rules is similar to Jonsen's account of casuistical method, which involves tailoring maxims to fit a case through progressive interactions with other relevant cases. Casuists and principlists should be able to agree that when they reflect on cases and policies, they rarely, if ever, have in hand either principles that were formulated without reference to experience with cases or paradigm cases that have not become paradigmatic because of a prior commitment to general norms.

Finally, casuists disagree among themselves about the value and limitations of theory in practical ethics. While some casuists sharply criticize theory, others encourage theory construction. Baruch Brody, for example, insists that ethical theory is both possible and desirable. Case-based judgment that rests on plausible intuition "is only the *first* stage in the process of coming to have moral knowledge. The *next* stage is that of theory formation. . . . The goal is to find a theory that systematizes these intuitions, explains them, and provides help in dealing with cases about which we have no intuitions. In the course of this systematization, it may be necessary to reject some of the initial intuitions on the grounds that they cannot be systematized into the theory."[30] We find this theoretical casuistry more appealing than a casuistry that denounces or avoids theoretical reflection.[31]

In general, the problems exhibited by casuistry also emerge in other bottom-up models. Despite its many plausible features, pure inductivism faces a familiar problem. We frequently criticize morally inadequate judgments or traditions by appeal to general standards, such as human rights. A bottom-up theory appears to lack reasons to justify the use of general standards that stand outside the framework of the very traditions and judgments that need to be criticized. By contrast, we have argued from Chapter 1 to the present that the common morality incorporates precepts that bind all persons in all places. When cultural groups compromise, ignore, or abuse universal moral standards, their practices do not become immune from moral criticism merely because they regard their views as deriving from their own moral tradition.

It is no accident that all major codes of international bioethics promulgated in the last half-century have insisted on fundamental principles and have linked them to human rights. These categories alone give us a universalist basis that allows us to judge immoral conduct across cultures.

An Integrated Model: Coherence Theory

"The top" (principles, theories) and "the bottom" (cases, individual judgments) are not solely sufficient for biomedical ethics. Neither general principles nor paradigm cases have sufficient power to generate conclusions with the needed reliability. Principles need to be made specific for cases, and case analysis needs illumination from general principles. Whether an action-guiding norm depends on particular experiences or on a general principle is a matter of what is known and inferred in specific contexts (so-called inferential support as a matter of epistemic context). In short, no essential order of inference or dependence fixes how we come to have moral knowledge.

Instead of a top-down or bottom-up model, we support a version of another model, variously referred to as "reflective equilibrium" and "coherence theory." John Rawls used the term *reflective equilibrium* to refer to his influential statement of this method.[32] He views justification as a reflective testing of our moral beliefs, moral principles, theoretical postulates, and other relevant moral beliefs in order to make them as coherent as possible. Method in ethics properly begins with our "considered judgments," the moral convictions in which we have the highest confidence and believe to have the lowest level of bias. The term *considered judgments* refers to "judgments in which our moral capacities are most likely to be displayed without distortion." Examples are judgments about the wrongness of racial discrimination, religious intolerance, and political repression. These considered judgments occur at all levels of generality in moral thinking, "from those about particular situations and institutions through broad standards and first principles to formal and abstract conditions on moral conceptions."[33] Whenever some feature in a moral theory that we hold conflicts with one or more of our considered judgments, we must modify one or the other in order to achieve equilibrium.

Even the considered judgments that we accept "provisionally as fixed points" are, Rawls argues, "liable to revision." The goal of reflective equilibrium is to match, prune, and adjust considered judgments in order to render them coherent with the premises of our most general moral commitments. We start with paradigm judgments of moral rightness and wrongness, and then construct a more general and more specific account that is consistent with these paradigm judgments, rendering them as coherent as possible. We then test the resultant action-guides to see if they yield incoherent results. If so, we readjust these guides or give them up and then renew the process.

We can never assume a completely stable equilibrium. The pruning and adjusting occur continually in view of the perpetual goal of reflective equilibrium. To refer again to the rule about putting the patient's interests first, we seek in biomedical ethics to make this rule as coherent as possible with other considered judgments about clinical teaching responsibilities, responsibilities to subjects in the conduct of research, responsibilities to patients' families, legitimate forms of financial investment in medical facilities, responsibilities to corporate sponsors of clinical trials, and so forth.

It is demanding to bring our diverse moral commitments into coherence and then to test the results against all other moral commitments. Even the rule about putting the patient's interests first is not categorical for all possible cases; it is an acceptable starting premise as a considered judgment, but no more. We are left with a range of options about how we should and should not specify this rule and balance it against other norms. As long as contingent conflicts occur under recognized and legitimate principles and rules, some incoherence will remain.

To take an example in the ethics of organ transplantation, imagine that we are attracted to each of two moral considerations: (1) distribute organs by expected number of years of survival (in order to maximize the beneficial outcome of the procedure), and (2) distribute organs by time on the waiting list (in order to give every candidate an equal opportunity). As they stand, these two distributive principles are not coherent, because using either will undercut or even eliminate the other. We can retain both (1) and (2) in a defensible theory of fair distribution, but to do so we will have to introduce limits on these principles, as well as accounts of how to specify our commitments and balance these commitments against others. These limits and accounts will, in turn, have to be made coherent with other principles and rules, such as norms regarding discrimination against the elderly and the role of ability to pay in the allocation of expensive medical procedures. (See our discussion of justice in Chapter 6.)

All organized sets of moral belief are somewhat indeterminate and unable to eliminate contingent conflicts among principles and rules. So-called wide reflective equilibrium occurs when we evaluate the strengths and weaknesses of all plausible moral judgments, principles, and relevant background theories. Here we incorporate as wide a variety of kinds and levels of legitimate beliefs as possible, including hard test cases in experience. We include beliefs about particular cases, about rules and principles, about virtue and character, about consequentialist and nonconsequentialist forms of justification, about the moral standing of fetuses and animals, about the role of moral sentiments, and so forth.[34]

We emphasize again the ideal, although not Utopian, character of this procedure: No matter how wide the pool of beliefs, we have no reason to anticipate that the process of pruning, adjusting, and rendering coherent will either come to an end or be perfected. A moral framework is more a process than a finished product; and moral problems, such as developing the most suitable system for organ procurement and distribution, should be considered projects in need of continual adjustment by reflective equilibrium. Virtually any set of theoretical generalizations achieved by this method will fall short of full coherence with considered judgments. We should assume that we face a never-ending search for incoherence, for counterexamples to our beliefs, and for novel situations that challenge our moral framework.[35]

From this perspective, moral thinking is analogous to hypotheses in science that we test, modify, or reject through experience and experimental thinking. Justification is no more deductivist (giving general norms preeminent status) than inductivist (giving experience and analogy preeminent status). Many different considerations provide reciprocal support in the attempt to fit moral beliefs into a coherent whole. This is how we test, revise, generalize, specify, and balance moral beliefs.

Although justification is a matter of coherence in this model, bare coherence never provides a sufficient basis for justification, because the body of substantive judgments and principles that cohere could themselves be morally unsatisfactory. An example of this problem appears in the "Pirates' Creed of Ethics or Custom of the Brothers of the Coast."[36] Formed under a democratic confraternity of marauders circa 1640, this creed for pirates is a coherent, carefully delineated set of rules governing mutual assistance in emergencies, penalties for prohibited acts, the distribution of spoils, modes of communication, compensation for injury, and "courts of honour" that resolve disputes. This body of substantive rules and principles, although coherent, is a moral outrage. Its appeal to "spoils," its awarding of slaves as compensation for injury, and the like involve immoral activities. But what justifies us in saying this coherent code does not constitute an acceptable code of ethics?

This question points to the importance of starting with considered judgments that are settled moral convictions and then casting the net more broadly in specifying, generalizing, testing, and revising those convictions. Coherentism does not involve the relentless reduction of a chosen set of beliefs to coherence. We start in ethics, as elsewhere, with a particular set of beliefs—the set of considered judgments that are acceptable initially without argumentative support. We cannot justify every moral judgment in terms of another moral judgment without generating an infinite regress or vicious circle of justification in which no judgment is justified. The avenue of escape is to accept some judgments as justified without recourse to other judgments.

These considered judgments typically have a history rich in moral experience that undergirds our confidence that they are credible and trustworthy. Considered judgments therefore cannot be mere matters of individual intuition. Any moral certitude associated with these norms should derive from beliefs that are acquired, tested, and modified over time. It is on the basis of these beliefs that the Pirates' Creed, while coherent and acceptable among pirates, fails the test of initial moral acceptability.

Although we start with initially credible premises, the persons, codes, institutions, or cultures from which the premises descend may not themselves be in every case highly reliable or comprehensive. For example, the Hippocratic tradition—the starting point in medical ethics for centuries—has turned out to be a limited and generally unreliable basis for medical ethics. A coherence theory can overcome this problem by calling on a wider body of experience to collect points of convergence.

To use an analogy to eye witnesses in a courtroom, if a sufficient number of entirely independent witnesses converge to agreement in recounting the facts of a story, the story gains credibility beyond the credibility of the individuals who tell it. We can eliminate the witnesses' stories that do not converge and cannot be made consistent with the main lines of convergence. The greater the coherence in a broadly based account that descends from initially credible premises, the more likely we are to believe it. Similarly in moral theory, as we increase the number of accounts, establish convergence, and increase coherence, we become increasingly confident that the beliefs are justified and should be accepted. When we find wider and wider confirmation of hypotheses, the best explanation of this confirmation is that these hypotheses are the right ones.

In conclusion, we note a few unresolved problems about the method of coherence that we will not be able to address here.[37] First, vagueness surrounds the precise scope of the method: We might be reflecting on communal policies, constructing a moral philosophy, or improving an individual's set of moral beliefs. The focus might be on judgments, on policies, on cases, or on finding moral truth. Second, it is not entirely clear how we should and should not achieve coherence, or how to know when we have done so. Third, a theory of moral justification requires that the reasons offered can be (or perhaps must be) publicly stated. Public justification is especially important when dealing with rules for constraints on public policy, a common task in biomedical ethics. This publicity condition is not well-developed in the account we have provided above or in coherence theory more generally.[38] Finally, available work using the method of coherence lacks the power to eliminate various conflicts among principles and rules. This insufficiency is not surprising, because all moral theories experience this problem, and coherence theory has no magical powers to settle these conflicts.

Common-Morality Theory[39]

We have argued that justification requires considered judgments, but we have yet to establish the nature and source of these judgments. To do so, we reach back to Chapter 1, where we first appealed to the common morality. This shared morality is the source of the initial moral content needed in our account of justification and method. No more basic moral data exist than principles requiring that we respect persons, take account of their well-being, treat them fairly, and the like. Theoretical reflection augments this initial content, making the various strands coherent, and specifying and balancing the emergent norms. In this section, we develop the idea that the common morality supplies appropriate considered judgments and further develop our methods and their connection to coherence theory.

Two Examples of Common-Morality Theory

We begin by outlining two moral philosophies that, like our own, build from foundations in the common morality and appeal to principles as their structural basis. These two twentieth-century theories epitomize appeals to the common morality. We have learned a great deal from both, although we do not believe that either captures quite the right set of basic principles for general moral theory or for biomedical ethics.

Frankena's theory. An elegant and simple example of a common-morality account that preceded and influenced ours is William Frankena's version of David Hume's postulate that the two major "principles of morals" are *beneficence* and *justice.* Frankena accepts what Bishop Joseph Butler called "the moral institution of life," together with what Frankena calls "the moral point of view," meaning a controlled attitude of sympathy that reaches moral decisions by appeal to principled good reasons. For Frankena, the principle of beneficence resembles, but is not identical to, the utilitarian demand that we maximize good over evil, whereas the principle of justice (primarily an egalitarian principle) guides "our distribution of good and evil" independently of judgments about maximizing and balancing good outcomes. He maintains that these two general principles capture the substance of the moral point of view.[40]

Ross's theory. A second example is W. D. Ross, who has had a particularly imposing influence on twentieth-century ethical theory, and more influence on the present authors than any twentieth-century writer. Ross's starting point is the premise that the moral convictions of thoughtful persons are "the data of ethics just as sense-perceptions are the data of a natural science. Just as some of the latter have to be rejected as illusory, so have some of the former."[41] The moral beliefs of the "plain" person are, for Ross, the beginning, not the end. Ross also holds that *acts* are right and wrong, whereas *motivation* and *character* are good and bad. This distinction allows him to say that a right act can be done from a bad motive and that a good motive may eventuate in a wrong act.

Ross defends several basic and irreducible moral principles that express prima facie obligations. For example, promises create obligations of fidelity, wrongful actions and debts create obligations of reparation, and the generous services or gifts of others create obligations of gratitude. In addition to fidelity, reparation, and gratitude, Ross lists obligations of self-improvement, justice, beneficence, and nonmaleficence. This list of obligations is not grounded in an overarching principle.[42]

In a methodological statement, Ross maintains that principles are "recognized by intuitive induction as being implied in the judgments already passed on particular acts."[43] He also says that we know principles in the same way the plain person knows the main lines of moral obligation. Here we have *knowledge*, not *opinion*. However, when two or more obligations conflict and balancing judgments are necessary, Ross says we must examine the situation carefully until we form a "considered opinion (it is never more)" that one obligation is weightier in the circumstances than another.[44]

Principal Features of Common-Morality Theory

We turn now to the commitments of our own version of common-morality ethics. In doing so, we make no attempt to present or to justify a *general* ethical theory. Our concern is with the account of common morality assumed or developed in previous chapters and its connection to questions of method and justification in biomedical ethics.[45]

There is, we maintained in Chapter 1, a single, universal common morality. However, there is more than one *theory* of the common-morality, as the theories of Frankena and Ross indicate. Despite their differences, these theories share several features: First, all common-morality theories rely on ordinary, shared moral beliefs for their starting content; they make no appeal to pure reason, rationality, natural law, a special moral sense, or the like. Second, all common-morality theories hold that any ethical theory that cannot be made consistent with these pretheoretical commonsense moral judgments falls under suspicion. Third, all common-morality theories are pluralistic: Two or more nonabsolute (prima facie) principles form the general level of normative statement.[46] The four principles developed in Chapters 3–6 form such a set of principles.

Our common-morality theory does not hold that all *customary* moralities qualify as part of the *common* morality; and use of the common morality in moral reasoning need not lead to conclusions that are customarily accepted. An important function of the general norms in the common morality is to provide a basis for the evaluation and criticism of groups or communities whose customary moral viewpoints are in some respect deficient. Critical reflection may ultimately vindicate moral judgments that at the outset were not widely shared. In short, the common morality is a pretheoretic moral point of view that transcends local customs and attitudes. Conclusions that criticize those customs and attitudes are warranted when they maintain fidelity to the common morality.

Our book unites the common morality with the coherence model of justification delineated earlier. This strategy allows us to rely on the authority of the principles in the common morality, while incorporating tools to refine and correct unclarities and to allow for additional specification of the principles. As ethical reasoning progresses, the insights gathered along the way form a body of more specific moral guidelines (specifications of the principles). This way of understanding how to specify general principles is consistent with the claim that sound moral reasoning can occur at any level of generality and can motivate revisions of ethical belief either "upward" or "downward."

Of course, serious questions arise about how to justify particular specifications when *competing* specifications emerge. As we maintained in Chapter 1, different resolutions by specification are often possible, and nothing in our method can prevent them from occurring or can declare only one justifiable in many cases. Our general position is that a particular specification, or any revision in moral belief, is justified if it maximizes the coherence of the overall set of beliefs that are accepted upon reflection. While this thesis is very abstract and cannot here be defended or refined further than it has been, we believe it can be tested in, and is supported by, everyday moral thinking.

Why the Common Morality Is Central

We can now consider why the common morality is better suited to play a foundational role in bioethics than the ethical theories examined in Chapter 8.

If we could be confident that some abstract moral theory was a better source for codes and policies than the common morality, we could work constructively on practical and policy questions by progressively specifying the norms in that theory. At present, we have no such theory, and even proponents of the same type of general theory typically disagree about its commitments, how to apply it, and how to address specific issues. The general norms and schemes of justification found in philosophical ethical theories are invariably more contestable than the norms in the common morality. We cannot reasonably expect that a contested moral theory will be better for practical decision-making and policy development than the morality that serves as our common heritage. Far more social consensus exists about principles and rules drawn from the common morality (e.g., our four principles) than about theories. This is not surprising, given the central social role of the common morality and the fact that its principles appear in some form in all major theories.

Nor do we need a theory in order to introduce moral reform. Innovation in ethics almost always occurs by extending and interpreting norms that are within rather than beyond the common morality. For example, if our policies on AIDS are so uncompassionate and unfair that we need to alter our conception of how therapeutic drugs are brought to the market, purchased, and distributed (as, in effect, has now occurred), this reevaluation will invoke available conceptions of compassion, fair funding, and just distribution, rather than totally new principles of justice. Any "new" norms will creatively extend old norms. Very rarely is a moral theory the sole source of innovation, and rarely does a theory lead us to give up a norm developed from the common morality. This approach to construction invites evolutionary change while insisting that the common morality provides both the starting point and the constraining framework.

Many moral philosophers convey the impression that if only we could find a correct theory we could resolve our problems by bringing that theory to bear on them. They imply that the hard work in ethics is to find and defend such a theory; the rest is comparatively uncomplicated. In truth, however, there is no direct, uncontroverted passage from theory to practice or resolution, even among persons who hold the same theory. Concepts are too general, principles too indefinite, and the facts of cases too difficult to bring under principles. Even if we had a theory to supply our initial norms, we have no direct way to move with confidence from the theory to decisions in particular cases. Applying a moral theory would still require specification.

Many writers in biomedical ethics also seem to think that we would rightly have more confidence in our principles and considered judgments if only we could justify them on the basis of a comprehensive ethical theory. This outlook has matters upside-down: We would have more confidence in an ethical theory if it could be shown coherent in a comprehensive way with the principles and considered judgments comprising the common morality. If an ethical theory were to reject any of the four clusters of principles defended in this book, for example, we would have a sound reason for healthy scepticism about the theory, not for scepticism about the principle(s). Our presentation of the principles—together with arguments to show the coherence of these principles with other aspects of the moral life, such as the moral emotions, virtues, and rights—constitute the normative account in the present volume. In this "theory," there is no single unifying principle or concept—a traditional goal of ethical theory that seems now to be fast fading.

In conclusion, we return to the question, "What is a moral theory a theory of?" The appropriate answer is that it is a theory of morality. A moral theory attempts to capture the moral point of view. Morality is the anchor of theory; theory is not the anchor of morality.

The Prima Facie Nature of Principles

Like Ross, we construe principles as prima facie (see the introduction to this topic in Chapter 1). Some theories recognize principles and rules, but treat them as expendable rules of thumb. Other theories contain absolute principles. Still other theories give a hierarchical (or lexical) ordering to moral norms. All three interpretations fail to capture the nature of moral norms. Rules of thumb permit too much discretion, as if principles or rules had no binding moral force. Absolute principles and rules disallow all discretion for moral agents and also encounter unresolvable moral conflicts. A hierarchy of rules and principles suffers from devastating counterexamples.

The latitude to balance prima facie principles in cases of conflict leaves room for compromise, mediation, and negotiation; and the need to specify them allows for moral growth and progress. The charge that principles are rigid and tyrannical, therefore, cannot be sustained. In stubborn cases of conflict, there may even be no single right action, because two or more morally acceptable actions are un-avoidably in conflict and have equal weight in the circumstances. In these cases, we can give good but not decisive reasons for more than one action. For instance, although murder is absolutely prohibited because of the normative content in the word *murder*, killing is not absolutely prohibited. Killing persons is *prima facie* wrong, but killing to prevent a person's further extreme pain or suffering is not wrong in every circumstance, as we argued in Chapter 4.

When a prima facie obligation is outweighed or overridden, it does not sim-ply disappear or evaporate: It leaves moral residues or what Nozick called "moral traces."[47] Even when moral agents act correctly in overriding a prima facie oblig-ation, regret is the morally appropriate attitude. The act of overriding a prima fa-cie obligation may generate *residual obligations* (e.g., of compensation), but we can best address this question in a specific context rather than in the abstract. Our point is about *perception* and *attitude*: A moral residue remains whether or not residual obligations remain, and attitudes of regret, contrition, sorrow, and the like are often appropriate and even expected in a person of good moral char-acter.

Problems for Common-Morality Theory

We acknowledge that our appeal to the common morality leaves unsettled prob-lems that we would have to address in a more complete account of this theory. Three problems are particularly important.

Specification and judgment. Do principles, when specified, enable us to reach practical judgments, or are they still too indeterminate to eventuate in judgments? Our theory requires that we specify carefully in order to escape abstractness, but we also must not overspecify a principle or rule, which then may become too rigid and insensitive to circumstances. Many specified principles and rules will encounter this problem of too little or too much for some contexts, and this is one reason why balancing and judgment are as necessary as specification for moral thinking. But without tighter controls on permissible balancing than com-mon-morality theories usually propose, critics will charge that too much room remains for judgments that are unprincipled and yet sanctioned or permitted by the theory. Can the conditions on balancing presented in Chapter 1 reduce intu-ition to an acceptable level? Can the constraints of coherence be tightened to re-spond to these concerns?

Throughout this book, we have tried to illustrate how a cautious form of spec-ification (combined with balancing) can make progress in bioethics, and we be-lieve that proper safeguards can be put in place that will adequately manage the problems that specification and balancing confront. A sense of the need for safe-guards (e.g., procedures in reviews by ethics committees) will generally arise from practical experience, and what works in one context may not suffice for another.

Coherence in the common morality? We have linked a coherence theory of justification to a common-morality theory, but can the common morality be made coherent? If one argues, as we do, that a heap of obligations and values unconnected by a first principle comprises the common morality, is there any hope of coherence, short of so radically reconstructing the norms that they only vaguely resemble the common morality? Is our goal of coherence more an article of faith than a demonstrable achievement?

Consider, for example, the use of animals as research subjects. Individuals and societies disagree regarding the "considered judgments" that might form our starting place for reflecting on this issue, and we too doubt that the common morality can be tapped to find shared considered judgments. On the one hand, we might search for a wider body of beliefs that can be brought into reflective equilibrium. On the other hand, we might simply specify our personal considered judgments. Either way, no clear starting point and body of beliefs exist to be rendered coherent, mainly because of a lack of agreement about the status of animals and our obligations, if any, to them. Many other controversies similarly invite disagreement over appropriate initial beliefs.

We should not expect to resolve all these disagreements in the direction of a single set of coherent norms. The goal of unified coherence is a worthy ideal, but not one that can always be realized.

Theory construction. These problems of coherence lead to connected problems about theory. The language of a "common-morality *theory*" suggests that we can philosophically construct one or more theories from it. Is there good reason to believe that a theory (not merely an unconnected group of coherent principles and rules) is possible? Perhaps mid-level principles, polished analyses of the moral virtues, and coherent statements of transnational human rights are all that we should attempt, rather than a theory that conforms to the criteria delineated at the beginning of Chapter 8. Perhaps "moral theory" has been so diluted in meaning in the case of "common-morality theories" that we should abandon the goal of a theory altogether, in favor of a more modest goal, such as "moral reflection and construction."

A related problem is that attempts to bring the common morality into greater coherence through specification risk decreasing rather than increasing moral agreement in society. That is, a theory can introduce claims that generate disagreements not found in the initial considered judgments; or, as we have often seen in the history of ethics, the theory may turn out to be less clear and reliable for practical decision-making than the common morality as it stands.

In part, these problems turn on legitimate expectations for a "theory." Clouser and Gert expect a strong measure of unity and systematic connection among rules, a clear pattern of justification, and a practical decision procedure that flows from a theory, whereas other philosophers are skeptical of one or more of these conditions, and even of the language of "theory."[48] The latter perspective is more congenial to the views we have taken throughout this book. A common-morality theory will certainly not satisfy the full set of criteria we delineated at the beginning of Chapter 8.

Conclusion

The image of working "down" by applying theories or principles to cases has attracted many who work in biomedical ethics, but we have resisted this model. Often, we have more reason to trust our responses to specific cases and the characteristic responses of moral persons than a theory, principle, or rule. We also have reason to trust principles in the common morality more than theories. In our model, no level or type of moral reasoning—comprehensive theories, principles, rules, or case judgments—has priority or serves as the groundwork of the other levels. Moral justification proceeds from an expansive coherentist framework of norms that originate at all "levels." These norms can emerge from institutions, individuals, and cultures, and no norm is immune to revision.

In everyday moral reasoning, we effortlessly blend appeals to principles, rules, rights, virtues, passions, analogies, paradigms, narratives, and parables.[49] We should be able to do the same in biomedical ethics. To assign priority to any one of these moral categories as the key ingredient in the moral life is a dubious project of certain writers in ethics who wish to refashion in their own image what is most central in the moral life. The more general (principles, rules, theories, etc.) and the more particular (case judgments, feelings, perceptions, practices, parables, etc.) are integrally linked in our moral thinking, and neither should have pride of place.

Notes

1. U.S. Supreme Court, *United Automobile Workers v. Johnson Controls, Inc.*, Slip opinion (Argued October 10, 1990—Decided March 20, 1991).
2. K. Danner Clouser and Bernard Gert, "A Critique of Principlism," *The Journal of Medicine and Philosophy* 15 (April 1990): 219–36. Each article they published was spearheaded by Clouser's concerns about principles and by a desire to defend Gert's book, *Morality: A New Justification of the Moral Rules* (New York: Oxford University Press, 1988). Later, Gert and Clouser published, with Charles M. Culver, *Bioethics: A Return to Fundamentals* (New York: Oxford University Press, 1997). This book contains a sustained criticism of our views. However, Gert, Culver, and Clouser accept both the language of the common morality and a conception of it very similar to ours; see *Bioethics: A Return to Fundamentals*, ch. 1; Clouser, "Common

Morality as an Alternative to Principlism," *Kennedy Institute of Ethics Journal* 5 (1995): 219–36; and Gert, Culver, and Clouser, "Common Morality Versus Specified Principlism: Reply to Richardson," *Journal of Medicine and Philosophy* 25 (2000): 308–22.

3. Clouser and Gert, "A Critique of Principlism"; "Morality vs. Principlism," in *Principles of Health Care Ethics*, ed. Raanan Gillon and Ann Lloyd (London: John Wiley & Sons, 1994), pp. 251–66; and Gert, Culver, and Clouser, *Bioethics: A Return to Fundamentals*, ch. 3, esp. pp. 74ff.

4. Gert, Culver, and Clouser, *Bioethics: A Return to Fundamentals*, pp. 7–8, 62, 75–76, 82–88.

5. "A Critique of Principlism," p. 233. Cf. their demand for "a complete system that provides guidance" and "an explicit account of the entire moral system," in Gert and Clouser, "Concerning Principlism and Its Defenders: Reply to Beauchamp and Veatch," in *Building Bioethics: Conversations with Clouser and Friends on Medical Ethics*, ed. Loretta Kopelman (Boston: Kluwer Academic, 1999), pp. 191–93; and their "Common Morality versus Specified Principlism: Reply to Richardson."

6. As we narrow the territory governed by a norm (principle, rule, paradigm case, etc.), the conditions become more specific—for example, making a shift from "all persons" to "all competent patients." As these shifts to the specific occur, it becomes increasingly less likely that the norm will qualify as a principle. For instance, the principle of respect for autonomy applies to all autonomous persons and autonomous actions, whereas a norm of respecting informed refusals by competent patients is, due to its narrowed scope, more plausibly a rule than a principle.

7. Moreover, Gert and associates, like us, appeal to a relatively small number of norms drawn from the common morality. See Gert, Culver, and Clouser, *Bioethics: A Return to Fundamentals*, pp. 16–17, 33–35.

8. Gert's moral rules can be treated as falling under broader principles. Gert has told us in private conversation that once principles are interpreted as normative headings under which rules fall, they become unobjectionable, but also expendable. His view is that "if specified principlism develops properly, it will become our account." See Gert, Culver, and Clouser, *Bioethics: A Return to Fundamentals*, p. 90. See also a clarification and partial retraction of their earlier criticism in Gert and Clouser, "Concerning Principlism and Its Defenders: Reply to Beauchamp and Veatch," pp. 190–91.

9. For a proposed method to handle this problem, see Gert, Culver, and Clouser, *Bioethics: A Return to Fundamentals*, pp. 26–31, 36–41, 55–58; and "Morality vs. Principlism," pp. 261–63. They propose that a moral rule may be violated only if "an impartial person [would] advocate that violating it be publicly allowed." However, this "solution" is subject to many competing judgments, and there is no method in their theory for determining how one harm is greater than or outweighs another. See other problems mentioned in B. Andrew Lustig, "The Method of 'Principlism': A Critique of the Critique," *Journal of Medicine and Philosophy* 17 (1992): 487–510; and Tom L. Beauchamp, "Principlism and Its Alleged Competitors," *Journal of the Kennedy Institute of Ethics* 5 (September 1995): 181–98, esp. 186–90.

10. Thomas Nagel, *Mortal Questions* (Cambridge: Cambridge University Press, 1979), pp. 128–37; and W. D. Ross, *The Right and the Good* (Oxford: Clarendon Press, 1930; reprinted Indianapolis, IN: Hackett, 1988). Ross anticipated some parts of Nagel's criticism and acknowledged that his catalogue of obligations is unsystematic and probably incomplete.

11. Ronald Green has directed a variant of this criticism at our position in "Method in

Bioethics: A Troubled Assessment," *The Journal of Medicine and Philosophy* 15 (1990): 188–89. See also the comments on this subject in Robert M. Veatch, "Contract and the Critique of Principlism," pp. 122ff.

12. Gert, *Morality: A New Justification of the Moral Rules*, pp. 154–55.

13. Cf. Gert, Culver, and Clouser, *Bioethics: A Return to Fundamentals*, pp. 62–68, and the later formulation in Gert and Clouser, "Concerning Principlism and Its Defenders: Reply to Beauchamp and Veatch," pp. 190–91. Often, when Clouser and Gert critique our views, it appears that they want to categorize all norms of beneficence as moral ideals, but it would be inconsistent to take this line given the latent commitments to *duties of beneficence* in Gert's book.

14. See Bernard Gert and Charles Culver, "The Justification of Paternalism," *Ethics* 89 (1979): 199–210; for a critique, see James F. Childress, *Who Should Decide? Paternalism in Health Care* (New York: Oxford University Press, 1982), pp. 237–41.

15. See Gert, Culver, and Clouser, *Bioethics: A Return to Fundamentals*, p. 34.

16. See the comments, formulations, and frameworks in Glenn McGee, ed., *Pragmatic Bioethics* (Nashville, TN: Vanderbilt University Press, 1999); Benjamin H. Levi, "Four Approaches to Doing Ethics," *Journal of Medicine and Philosophy* 21 (1996): 7–39; Susan M. Wolf, "Shifting Paradigms in Bioethics and Health Law: The Rise of a New Pragmatism," *American Journal of Law and Medicine* 20 (1994): 395–415; and Henry Richardson, "Beyond Good and Right: Toward a Constructive Ethical Pragmatism," *Philosophy and Public Affairs* 24 (1995): 108–41. In *The Perfect Baby* (Lanham, MD: Rowman & Littlefield, 1997), Glenn McGee offers "the first book-length attempt to use classical American pragmatism to solve a problem in bioethics (p. viii). On "clinical pragmatism" in the context of clinical ethics, see Franklin G. Miller, Joseph J. Fins, and Matthew D. Bacchetta, "Clinical Pragmatism: John Dewey and Clinical Ethics," *The Journal of Contemporary Health Law and Policy* 13 (1996): 27–51; and Fins, Miller, and Bacchetta, "Clinical Pragmatism: A Method of Moral Problem Solving," *Kennedy Institute of Ethics Journal* 7 (1997): 129–45. For commentary and criticisms, see Rosemarie Tong, "The Promises and Perils of Pragmatism: Commentary on Fins, Bacchetta, and Miller," *Kennedy Institute of Ethics Journal* 7 (1997): 145–52; and Lynn A. Jansen, "Assessing Clinical Pragmatism," *Kennedy Institute of Ethics Journal* 8 (1998): 23–36. Fins, Bacchetta, and Miller respond in "Clinical Pragmatism: Bridging Theory and Practice," *Kennedy Institute of Ethics Journal* 8 (1998): 37–42.

17. A number of positions are particularistic in nature. For interpretations, defenses, and critiques of narrative approaches to bioethics, see Hilde Lindemann Nelson, ed., *Stories and Their Limits: Narrative Approaches to Bioethics* (New York: Routledge, 1997). For other strategies, see Daniel Callahan, "Universalism & Particularism: Fighting to a Draw," *Hastings Center Report* 30 (2000): 37–44; and Earl Winkler, "Moral Philosophy and Bioethics: Contextualism vs. the Paradigm Theory," in *Philosophical Perspectives on Bioethics*, ed. L. W. Sumner and Joseph Boyle (Toronto: University of Toronto Press, 1996), pp. 50–78.

18. See Albert R. Jonsen and Stephen Toulmin, *The Abuse of Casuistry: A History of Moral Reasoning* (Berkeley: University of California Press, 1988); Carson Strong, "Specified Principlism: What Is It, and Does It Really Resolve Cases Better than Casuistry?" *Journal of Medicine and Philosophy* 25 (2000): 323–41 (with a Reply by Tom L. Beauchamp) and his "Justification in Ethics," in *Moral theory and Moral Judgments in Medical Ethics*, ed. Baruch Brody (Boston: Kluwer Academic, 1988), pp. 193–211; John D. Arras, "Getting Down to Cases: The Revival of Casuistry in

Bioethics," *Journal of Medicine and Philosophy* 16 (1991): 29–51; Baruch Brody, *Life and Death Decision Making* (New York: Oxford University Press, 1988); and James F. Keenan and Thomas Shannon, *The Context of Casuistry* (Washington, DC: Georgetown University Press, 1995).

19. Casuists have had relatively little to say about the nature or definition of a "case," or about the meaning of the term "casuistry," but see the helpful analyses in Albert R. Jonsen, "Casuistry as Methodology in Clinical Ethics," *Theoretical Medicine* 12 (1991): 297–98; and Albert R. Jonsen, Mark Siegler, and William J. Winslade, *Clinical Ethics*, 4th ed. (New York: McGraw-Hill, 1998), pp. 1–12.

20. Albert R. Jonsen, "Casuistry: An Alternative or Complement to Principles?" *Journal of the Kennedy Institute of Ethics* 5 (1995), esp. pp. 246–47; "Strong on Specification," *Journal of Medicine and Philosophy* 25 (2000): 348–60; and "Morally Appreciated Circumstances: A Theoretical Problem for Casuistry," in *Philosophical Perspectives on Bioethics*, ed. Sumner and Boyle, pp. 37–49. See also John Arras, "Principles and Particularity: The Roles of Cases in Bioethics," *Indiana Law Journal* 69 (1994): 983–1014.

21. Here are two candidates as defenders of the ideal of a unified theory. (1) Jeremy Bentham: "From utility then we may denominate a principle, that may serve to preside over and govern . . . several institutions or combinations of institutions that compose the matter of this science." From *A Fragment on Government*, ed. Burns and Hart (Oxford: Clarendon Press, 1977), p. 416. (2) Henry Sidgwick: "Utilitarianism may be presented as [a] scientifically complete and systematically reflective form of th[e] regulation of conduct." *Methods of Ethics* (Indianapolis, IN: Hackett Publishing Co., 1981), bk. 4, ch. 3, § 1, p. 425.

22. Stephen Toulmin, "The Tyranny of Principles," *Hastings Center Report* 11 (December 1981): 31–39.

23. Jonsen and Toulmin, *Abuse of Casuistry*, pp. 16–19.

24. Ibid. See also Toulmin, "The National Commission on Human Experimentation: Procedures and Outcomes," in *Scientific Controversies: Case Studies in the Resolution and Closure of Disputes in Science and Technology*, ed. H. T. Engelhardt, Jr., and A. Caplan (New York: Cambridge University Press, 1987), pp. 599–613; and Jonsen, "American Moralism and the Origin of Bioethics in the United States," *Journal of Medicine and Philosophy* 16 (1991): 113–30.

25. See John D. Arras, "Getting Down to Cases: The Revival of Casuistry in Bioethics," 31–33; Jonsen and Toulmin, *Abuse of Casuistry*, pp. 16–19, 66–67; and Jonsen, "Casuistry and Clinical Ethics," *Theoretical Medicine* 7 (1986): 67, 71.

26. Jonsen, "Casuistry as Methodology in Clinical Ethics," p. 298.

27. See Cass Sunstein, "On Analogical Reasoning," *Harvard Law Review* 106 (1993): 741–91, esp. 767–78; Loretta M. Kopelman, "Case Method and Casuistry: The Problem of Bias," *Theoretical Medicine* 15 (1994): 21–37; John D. Arras, "Getting Down to Cases"; Kevin Wildes, *Moral Acquaintances: Methodology in Bioethics* (Notre Dame, IN: University of Notre Dame, 2000), chs. 3–4; Tom Tomlinson, "Casuistry in Medical Ethics: Rehabilitated, or Repeat Offender?" *Theoretical Medicine* 15 (1994): 5–20, esp. 13–14; and Mark G. Kuczewski, "Casuistry and Its Communitarian Critics," *Kennedy Institute of Ethics Journal* 4 (1994): 99–116, esp. 106–12. For an attempt to combine casuistry with communitarianism, both rooted in the Aristotelian tradition, see M. Kuczewski, *Fragmentation and Consensus: Communitarian and Casuistic Bioethics* (Washington, DC: Georgetown University Press, 1997).

28. See the argument in John Arras, "A Case Approach," in *A Companion to Bioethics*,

ed. Helga Kuhse and Peter Singer (Oxford: Blackwell Publishers, 1998), pp. 106–13, esp. 112–13.

29. Jonsen, "Casuistry: An Alternative or Complement to Principles?" pp. 246–47.

30. Brody, *Life and Death Decision Making*, p. 13

31. Jonsen and Toulmin sometimes seem to criticize all theory and at other times only abuse and overstatement in theory. We interpret them as hostile primarily to theory, that is, deductivist or composed of allegedly universal, eternal, and unchallengeable principles. Pragmatic and nondogmatic theories, such as those of Aristotle and William James, seem to them to be laudable. See *Abuse of Casuistry*, pp. 23–27, 279–303.

32. John Rawls, *A Theory of Justice* (Cambridge, MA: Harvard University Press, 1971; revised edition, 1999), esp. pp. 20ff, 46–50, 579–80 (1999: 17ff, 40–45, 508–09). See also Rawls's comments on reflective equilibrium in his later book, *Political Liberalism* (New York: Columbia University Press, 1996), esp. pp. 8, 381, 384, and 399.

33. John Rawls, "The Independence of Moral Theory," *Proceedings and Addresses of the American Philosophical Association* 48 (1974–75): 8.

34. See Norman Daniels, "Wide Reflective Equilibrium and Theory Acceptance in Ethics," *Journal of Philosophy* 76 (May, 1979): 257ff; "Wide Reflective Equilibrium in Practice," in *Philosophical Perspectives on Bioethics*, ed. Sumner and Boyle, pp. 96–114; and *Justice and Justification: Reflective Equilibrium in Theory and Practice* (New York: Cambridge University Press, 1996). Henry Richardson has pointed out to us that Rawls does not make it a logically necessary condition of considered judgments that they be *shared* with others; nor does he make it a logically necessary condition of wide reflective equilibrium that judgments be shared. However, to make his enterprise of social justice work, the considered judgments Rawls selects would have to be widely shared. The importance of shared agreement seems highlighted in Rawls's emphasis on his theory of justice as a liberal political theory.

35. Compare Rawls, *A Theory of Justice*, pp. 195–201 (1999: 171–76).

36. Circa 1640. Published 1974 by Historical Documents Co.

37. For these and other problems, see Michael R. DePaul, *Balance and Refinement: Beyond Coherence Models of Moral Inquiry* (London: Routledge, 1993); M. Holmgren, "The Wide and Narrow of Reflective Equilibrium," *Canadian Journal of Philosophy* 19 (1989): 43–60; and Kai Nielsen, "Relativism and Wide Reflective Equilibrium," *Monist* 76 (1993): 316–32.

38. However, see Rawls's account of public justification fused to reflective equilibrium in *Political Liberalism*, pp. 381–87.

39. Revisions in our theory in this and the previous edition have benefited from David DeGrazia's criticisms. See his "Moving Forward in Bioethical Theory: Theories, Cases, and Specified Principlism," *Journal of Medicine and Philosophy* 17 (October 1992): 511–39. We have also benefited from criticisms and constructive suggestions received from Ruth Faden, Norman Daniels, Bernard Gert, Danner Clouser, Sissela Bok, Albert Jonsen, Earl Winkler, and Frank Chessa.

40. William K. Frankena, *Ethics*, 2nd ed. (Englewood Cliffs, NJ: Prentice-Hall, 1973), pp. 4–9, 43–56, 113; and *Thinking about Morality* (Ann Arbor: University of Michigan Press, 1980), pp. 26, 34. Frankena cites Butler on p. 6 of the former. See also Annette Baier, "Frankena and Hume on Points of View," *Monist* 64 (1981): 342–58.

41. Ross, *The Right and the Good*, p. 41.

42. Ibid, pp. 21–22.

43. W. D. Ross, *The Foundations of Ethics* (Oxford: Clarendon Press, 1939), pp. 169–70.

44. Ross, *The Right and the Good*, p. 19.

45. For a sensible account of our "common values," see Sissela Bok, *Common Values* (Columbia, MO: University of Missouri Press, 1995).

46. H. A. Prichard presented powerful arguments in the common-morality tradition to show that all single or absolute-principle theories disintegrate in the face of the diversity in the considered judgments of pretheoretic commonsense morality. See his *Moral Obligation: Essays and Lectures*, ed. W. D. Ross (Oxford: Clarendon Press, 1949).

47. Robert Nozick, "Moral Complications and Moral Structures," *Natural Law Forum* 13 (1968): 1–50. See also Thomas E, Hill, Jr., "Moral Dilemmas, Gaps, and Residues: A Kantian Perspective," in *Moral Dilemmas and Moral Theory*, ed. H. E. Mason (New York: Oxford University Press, 1996).

48. See Annette Baier, *Postures of the Mind* (Minneapolis: University of Minnesota Press, 1985), pp. 139–41, 206–17, 223–26, 232–37.

49. For reservations about this thesis, see David H. Smith, "A Response to Beauchamp," and Karen Hanson, "Are Principles Ever Properly Ignored? A Reply to Beauchamp on Bioethical Paradigms," both in *Indiana Law Journal* 69 (1994): 973–74, 975–81.

Appendix

Cases in Biomedical Ethics

Case 1: The Tarasoff Case

Facts in the Case

On October 27, 1969, Prosenjit Poddar killed Tatiana Tarasoff. Plaintiffs, Tatiana's parents, allege that two months earlier Poddar confided his intention to kill Tatiana to Dr. Lawrence Moore, a psychologist employed by the Cowell Memorial Hospital at the University of California at Berkeley. They allege that on Moore's request, the campus police briefly detained Poddar, but released him when he appeared rational. They further claim that Dr. Harvey Powelson, Moore's superior, then directed that no further action be taken to detain Poddar. No one warned plaintiffs of Tatiana's peril.

   Plaintiffs, Tatiana's mother and father, . . . [allege] that on August 20, 1969, Poddar was a voluntary outpatient receiving therapy at Cowell Memorial Hospital. Poddar informed Moore, his therapist, that he was going to kill an unnamed girl, readily identifiable as Tatiana, when she returned home from spending the summer in Brazil. Moore, with the concurrence of Dr. Gold, who had initially

This case is edited from *Tarasoff v. Regents of the University of California*, 17 Cal.3d 425 (1976); 131 California Reporter 14 (July 1, 1976). The language is that of the court. The facts and majority opinion are written by Justice Tobriner. The dissenting opinion is written by Justice Clark.

examined Poddar, and Dr. Yandell, assistant to the director of the department of psychiatry, decided that Poddar should be committed for observation in a mental hospital. Moore orally notified Officers Atkinson and Teel of the campus police that he would request commitment. He then sent a letter to Police Chief William Beall requesting the assistance of the police department in securing Poddar's confinement.

Officers Atkinson, Brownrigg, and Halleran took Poddar into custody, but, satisfied that Poddar was rational, released him on his promise to stay away from Tatiana. Powelson, director of the department of psychiatry at Cowell Memorial Hospital, then asked the police to return Moore's letter, directed that all copies of the letter and notes that Moore had taken as therapist be destroyed, and "ordered no action to place Prosenjit Poddar in a 72-hour treatment and evaluation facility."

Plaintiff's second cause of action, entitled "Failure to Warn of a Dangerous Patient," . . . adds the assertion that defendants negligently permitted Poddar to be released from police custody without "notifying the parents of Tatiana Tarasoff that their daughter was in grave danger from Prosenjit Poddar." Poddar persuaded Tatiana's brother to share an apartment with him near Tatiana's residence; shortly after her return from Brazil, Poddar went to her residence and killed her.

Majority Opinion   TOBRINER, Justice

We shall explain that defendant therapists cannot escape liability merely because Tatiana herself was not their patient. When a therapist determines, or pursuant to the standards of his profession should determine, that his patient presents a serious danger of violence to another, he incurs an obligation to use reasonable care to protect the intended victim against such danger. The discharge of this duty may require the therapist to take one or more of various steps, depending upon the nature of the case. Thus it may call for him to warn the intended victim or others likely to apprise the victim of the danger, to notify the police, or to take whatever other steps are reasonably necessary under the circumstances. . . .

In each instance the adequacy of the therapist's conduct must be measured against the traditional negligence standard of the rendition of reasonable care under the circumstances. . . . In sum, the therapist owes a legal duty not only to his patient, but also to his patient's would-be victim and is subject in both respects to scrutiny by judge and jury. . . . Some of the alternatives open to the therapist, such as warning the victim, will not result in the drastic consequences of depriving the patient of his liberty. Weighing the uncertain and conjectural character of the alleged damage done the patient by such a warning against the peril to the victim's life, we conclude that professional inaccuracy in predicting violence cannot negate the therapist's duty to protect the threatened victim. . . .

We recognize the public interest in supporting effective treatment of mental illness and in protecting the rights of patients to privacy . . . and the consequent public importance of safeguarding the confidential character of psychotherapeutic communication. Against this interest, however, we must weigh the public interest in safety from violent assault.

The revelation of a communication under the above circumstances is not a breach of trust or a violation of professional ethics; as stated in the Principles of Medical Ethics of the American Medical Association (1957), section 9: "A physician may not reveal the confidence entrusted to him in the course of medical attendance . . . unless he is required to do so by law or unless it becomes necessary in order to protect the welfare of the individual or of the community." We conclude that the public policy favoring protection of the confidential character of patient–psychotherapist communications must yield to the extent to which disclosure is essential to avert danger to others. The protective privilege ends where the public peril begins.

Dissenting Opinion   CLARK, Justice (dissenting)

Until today's majority opinion, both legal and medical authorities have agreed that confidentiality is essential to effectively treat the mentally ill, and that imposing a duty on doctors to disclose patient threats to potential victims would greatly impair treatment. . . .

Policy generally determines duty. Principal policy considerations include foreseeability of harm, certainty of the plaintiff's injury, proximity of the defendant's conduct to the plaintiff's injury, moral blame attributable to defendant's conduct, prevention of future harm, burden on the defendant, and consequences to the community.

Overwhelming policy considerations weigh against imposing a duty on psychotherapists to warn a potential victim against harm. While offering virtually no benefit to society, such a duty will frustrate psychiatric treatment, invade fundamental patient rights and increase violence.

The importance of psychiatric treatment and its need for confidentiality have been recognized by this court. "It is clearly recognized that the very practice of psychiatry vitally depends upon the reputation in the community that the psychiatrist will not tell. . . . "

Assurance of confidentiality is important for three reasons.

DETERRENCE FROM TREATMENT. First, without substantial assurance of confidentiality, those requiring treatment will be deterred from seeking assistance. It remains an unfortunate fact in our society that people seeking psychiatric guidance tend to become stigmatized. Apprehension of such stigma—apparently increased by the propensity of people considering treatment to see themselves in the worst possible light—creates a well-recognized reluctance to seek aid. This reluctance is alleviated by the psychiatrist's assurance of confidentiality.

FULL DISCLOSURE. Second, the guarantee of confidentiality is essential in eliciting the full disclosure necessary for effective treatment. The psychiatric patient approaches treatment with conscious and unconscious inhibitions against revealing his innermost thoughts. . . .

SUCCESSFUL TREATMENT. Third, even if the patient fully discloses his thoughts, assurance that the confidential relationship will not be breached is necessary to maintain his trust in his psychiatrist—the very means by which treatment is effected. . . .

Given the importance of confidentiality to the practice of psychiatry, it becomes clear the duty to warn imposed by the majority will cripple the use and effectiveness of psychiatry. Many people, potentially violent—yet susceptible to treatment—will be deterred from seeking it; those seeking it will be inhibited from making revelations necessary to effective treatment; and, forcing the psychiatrist to violate the patient's trust will destroy the interpersonal relationship by which treatment is effected.

VIOLENCE AND CIVIL COMMITMENT. By imposing a duty to warn, the majority contributes to the danger to society of violence by the mentally ill and greatly increases the risk of civil commitment—the total deprivation of liberty—of those who should not be confined. The impairment of treatment and risk of improper commitment resulting from the new duty to warn will not be limited to a few patients but will extend to a large number of the mentally ill. Although under existing psychiatric procedures only a relatively few receiving treatment will ever present a risk of violence, the number making threats is huge, and it is the latter group—not just the former—whose treatment will be impaired and whose risk of commitment will be increased.

Case 2: Nondisclosure of Prostate Cancer

A 69-year-old male, estranged from his children and with no other living relatives, underwent a routine physical examination in preparation for a brief and much anticipated trip to Australia. The physician suspected a serious problem and ordered more extensive testing, including further blood analysis (detailing an acid phosphatase), a bone scan, and a prostate biopsy. The results were quite conclusive: The man had an inoperable, incurable carcinoma—a small prostate nodule commonly referred to as cancer of the prostate. The carcinoma was not yet advanced and was relatively slow growing. Later, after the disease had progressed, it would be possible to provide good palliative treatment. Blood tests and X rays showed the patient's renal function to be normal. (The physician con-

This case was prepared especially for this volume. David Bloom, M.D., was a contributing consultant.

sulted with the urologist who had performed the prostate biopsy in order to confirm the diagnosis.)

The physician had treated this patient for many years and knew that he was fragile in several respects. The man was quite neurotic and had an established history of psychiatric disease—although he functioned well in society and was clearly capable of rational thought and decision making. He had recently suffered a severe depressive reaction, during which he had behaved irrationally and attempted suicide. This episode immediately followed the death of his wife, who had died after a difficult and protracted battle with cancer. It was clear that he had not been equipped to deal with his wife's death, and he had been hospitalized for a short period before the suicide attempt. Just as he was getting back on his feet, the opportunity to go to Australia materialized, and it was the first excitement he had experienced in several years.

This patient also had a history of suffering prolonged and serious depression whenever informed of serious health problems. He worried excessively and often could not exercise rational control over his deliberations and decisions. His physician thought that disclosure of the carcinoma under his present fragile state would almost certainly cause further irrational behavior and render the patient incapable of thinking clearly about his medical situation.

When the testing had been completed and the results were known, the patient returned to his physician. He asked nervously, "Am I OK?" Without waiting for a response, he asked, "I don't have cancer, do I?" Believing his patient would not suffer from or even be aware of his problem while in Australia, the physician answered, "You're as good as you were ten years ago." He was worried about telling such a bald lie but firmly believed that it was justified.

Case 3: A Son's Request for Nondisclosure

Mr. Johnson, a man in his late sixties, is brought to his physician by his son who is concerned about his father's apparent problems in interpreting and dealing with what used to be normal day-to-day activities. He worries that his father may have Alzheimer's disease, but he asks the physician not to tell his father if Alzheimer's disease is confirmed as the diagnosis. After the appropriate tests, the physician believes that she has a firm diagnosis of Alzheimer's disease and discusses with a nurse and a social worker the son's "impassioned plea" not to tell his father the diagnosis. The nurse notes that a strong consensus has developed over the last 25 years about disclosing the diagnosis of cancer to patients and wonders whether the same reasons apply to patients with Alzheimer's disease.

This case has been formulated on the basis of and incorporates language from Margaret A. Drickamer and Mark S. Lachs, "Should Patient with Alzheimer's Disease Be Told Their Diagnosis?" *New England Journal of Medicine* 326 (April 2, 1992): 947–51.

The physician responds that "many of the arguments that support telling the patient with cancer assume the relative accuracy of diagnosis, an array of therapeutic options, a predictable natural history, and a fully competent patient." She is not sure that these arguments apply to patients with Alzheimer's disease because the diagnosis is made on the basis of clinical criteria and diagnostic algorithms (documented through autopsies to be as high as 92 percent), the prognosis is "unusually imprecise," life expectancy varies greatly, therapeutic options are limited, and patients with Alzheimer's disease "inevitably have an erosion of decisionmaking capacity and competency" and may also have limited coping mechanisms.

The social worker adds that although there is empirical evidence that most patients now want to know if they have cancer, there is less evidence about the preferences of patients with Alzheimer's disease. Nevertheless, the nurse responds, "It is important to maximize individual autonomy whenever possible. We can be truthful with our patients about what we think is happening and our degree of certainty, whatever it is. Mr. Johnson may be able to make an advance directive about treatment and nontreatment. At the very least, he may be able to express his feeling and fear." "But wait," the physician responds, "Mr. Johnson will lose his ability to change his mind once he loses his ability to make decisions." "That's true," the nurse agrees, "but still the best indication we could have of what he would want under those circumstances would be his advance directive." The physician, nurse, and social worker agree to discuss the case tomorrow before deciding what to do.

Case 4: A Family of Potential Kidney Donors

A 40-year-old widow with chronic glomerulonephritis has been on maintenance hemodialysis for ten years. Over the past two years she has been progressively deteriorating from multiple complications, including severe renal osteodystrophy, inability to obtain adequate blood access, and malnutrition from intermittent depression. Peritoneal dialysis cannot be accomplished because of multiple abdominal surgical procedures with adhesions. Her physician has recommended transplantation because he feels she will not survive more than four to six months on dialysis.

The patient has four children (ages 11 to 14 years) and wants a transplant to allow her to live and provide for the future well-being of her children.

The patient's 44-year-old brother is a farmer with eight children. He refused to donate or be tissue typed. The patient has a 42-year-old sister who was will-

A case history at St. Francis Hospital, Honolulu, written by Arnold W. Siemsen, M.D., Institute of Renal Diseases.

ing to donate but was not tissue typed because she has been an insulin-requiring diabetic for ten years.

The patient also has a 35-year-old mentally retarded brother who has been institutionalized since age eight. This brother is an A match with four antigens being identified. He is so severely retarded that he cannot comprehend or understand any of the risks of nephrectomy. He is able to take care of his own personal needs and ambulate with guidance. He neither recognizes his own family members nor interacts with medical staff. The patient would regularly drive 300 miles to see her brother four times per year until 12 years ago, when her own personal and family needs reduced the frequency to one to two times per year. She has not seen her brother for three years, because of her own medical illnesses. At the present time she feels she has an obligation to her brother, but there is no particular closeness.

Her 14-year-old daughter would like to donate a kidney, even though she is a two-antigen mismatch. The daughter has demonstrated a perceptive, thorough, and reasonably unemotional grasp of her mother's situation and needs, and of the seriousness of her own potential donation. ABO blood types for the retarded brother and the daughter are compatible.

The patient's older brother and sister feel the donor should be the younger, mentally retarded brother. The diabetic sister is the legal guardian of the retarded brother. Both parents are dead. The patient has been on the cadaveric transplant waiting list for two years.

The following statements are reasonable projections based on known data:

	2-yr. kidney survival (%)	2-yr. patient survival (%)
Retarded brother to patient	70	85
Minor child to patient	60	75
Cadaveric to patient	40	65

Case 5: The Spring Case

In November 1977, 78-year-old Earle Spring suffered a mild scratch on the instep of his foot. A fiercely independent outdoorsman, he left the cut unattended until his foot finally became gangrenous. Hospitalization was followed by pneumonia and then a diagnosis of kidney failure. After undergoing three five-hour dialysis sessions a week, Spring soon improved enough to return home. Meanwhile, his mental deterioration, which had been diagnosed before his injury as "chronic organic brain syndrome," became markedly pronounced.

This case was prepared by John J. Paris, S.J. It derives from his "Death, Dying, and the Courts: The Travesty and Tragedy of the Earle Spring Case," *Linacre Quarterly* 49 (February 1982): 26–41.

After more than a year of treatment, the nephrologist informed Spring's son, Robert, that his father was not benefiting from dialysis. He suggested it may have been a mistake to have initiated it on a man his age and that it might be best if the treatments were ended. The son and the wife agreed with the physician and requested that the treatments be stopped. However, because of the Massachusetts Supreme Judicial Court's 1977 *Saikewicz* ruling, decisions of such significance in that state had to be made by courts rather than by families and physicians.

On January 25, 1979, Robert Spring, who had been appointed temporary guardian, petitioned the Franklin County Probate Court for an order to terminate the hemodialysis treatments. They began a full adversary hearing in which the guardian *ad litem*, an attorney appointed by the court to represent the best interests of the patient, had the responsibility for presenting "all reasonable arguments in favor of administering treatment to prolong the life of the individual involved."

Mark I. Berson, Spring's guardian *ad litem*, insisted (contrary to *Saikewicz*) that the court not render a "substituted judgment" (a statement of what Spring himself would have wanted) without some evidence from Spring's lucid moments on that subject. On May 15, 1979, Judge Keedy entered a judgment permitting the temporary guardian, Robert Spring, "to refrain from authorizing further life-prolonging medical treatment" for his father. Attorney Berson was not satisfied that there was sufficient evidence that Spring would have wanted to terminate the treatments, and he appealed. Judge Keedy vacated his original order and on July 2 entered a new one to the effect that Spring's wife and son, together with the attending physician, were to make the decision. Again Berson appealed.

The court of appeals upheld the probate court's action. It rejected Berson's position on the need for an express statement of intent to withhold treatment. In its words, "Such a contention would largely stifle the very rights of privacy and personal dignity which the *Saikewicz* case sought to secure for incompetent persons." Berson appealed.

On January 10, the supreme judicial court heard the case. It concluded that the trial judge's finding that Earle Spring "would, if competent, choose not to receive the life-prolonging treatment" was correct. But, unlike the trial judge and the court of appeals, the supreme judicial court found that the facts "bring the case within the rule of *Saikewicz*." It therefore held "it was an error to delegate the decision to the attending physician and the ward's wife and son." Once again, Spring's guardian was directed by the probate court to "refrain from authorizing any further life-prolonging treatment" for his father.

Meanwhile, it was becoming clear that the staff of the Holyoke Geriatric Center were, in their own words, "appalled over the decision to stop the dialysis treatment." Two nurses on the 3 p.m. to 11 p.m. shift asked Spring if he wanted to die. Reportedly, he replied, "No." Although a psychiatrist had previously evaluated Spring as "incompetent," the nurses taking his statement as proof of Spring's desires brought their story to a local newspaper, which used it as headline news. Berson responded immediately. On the basis of an affidavit filed by a right-to-life group, he petitioned Judge Keedy to reinstate the dialysis treatments until new evidence of Spring's competence could be gathered. The right-to-life activists hired a lawyer to petition the probate court to admit them as parties to the case. In the sixth judicial determination on Spring's case, Judge Keedy denied the petition to reinstate dialysis treatment. Berson appealed once more.

This appeal was granted by the supreme judicial court, which then appointed five psychiatrists and geriatric specialists to determine Spring's mental status. During that time, Spring had been admitted to the hospital suffering from an infection and pneumonia. He responded to medical treatment and returned to the nursing home on March 25, but in an extremely weakened condition. The following Sunday, the day before the competency hearing was scheduled, Earle Spring died. The next day, the five court-appointed physicians filed their report: Spring "was suffering from such profound mental impairment that he had no idea where he was or what was going on. The dementia was not related to the kidney failure, was untreatable, and irreversible." Had he not died the day before, the responsibility for deciding to stop the dialysis treatments would have rested where it had 14 months previously—with the court.

Case 6: The Wanglie Case

Mrs. Helga Wanglie, an 85-year-old resident of a nursing home, was taken to Hennepin County Medical Center on January 1, 1990, to receive emergency treatment for her dyspnea that resulted from chronic bronchiectasis. Emergency intubation was provided, and Mrs. Wanglie was placed on a respirator. During the period that followed, she was not able to communicate clearly, but she did occasionally acknowledge discomfort and she recognized her family members who visited. The staff was unable to wean her from the respirator, and in May she was transferred to a chronic care hospital. A week later, during another effort to wean her from the respirator, her heart stopped. She was resuscitated and then taken to another hospital for intensive care. When she did not regain consciousness, a physician indicated to the family that it would be appropriate to consider withdrawing the life-support systems. The family responded by transferring her to the Hennepin County Medical Center on May 31. Tests over the next two weeks convinced the medical staff that she was in a persistent vegetative state

Sources: Steven H. Miles, "Informed Demand for Non-Beneficial Medical Treatment," *New England Journal of Medicine* 325 (August 15, 1991): 512–15, with additional information from Ronald E. Cranford, "Helga Wanglie's Ventilator," *Hastings Center Report* 21 (July/August 1991): 23–24; "Brain-Damaged Woman at Center of Lawsuit Over Life-Support Dies," *New York Times* (July 6, 1991), p. 8; and Edward Walsh, "Recasting 'Right to Die'," *Washington Post* (May 29, 1991), pp. A1, A6.

(PVS) as a result of severe anoxic encephalopathy. Her care included maintenance on the respirator, with repeated courses of antibiotics, frequent airway suctioning, tube feedings, an air flotation bed, and biochemical monitoring.

During June and July, 1990, physicians indicated to the family that the life-sustaining treatment was not benefiting the patient and recommended that it be withdrawn. However, Mrs. Wanglie's husband, daughter, and son insisted on continued treatment. As reported by Dr. Steven Miles, the family stated that "physicians should not play God, that the patient would not be better off dead, that removing her life support showed moral decay in our civilization, and that a miracle could occur." According to her husband, Mrs. Wanglie had never indicated her preferences about life-sustaining treatment. Nevertheless, with reluctance, the family did accept a do-not-resuscitate (DNR) order because of the improbability that Mrs. Wanglie would survive a cardiac arrest. The family declined the counseling recommended by an ethics committee consultant and asked in late July that the question of removal of the respirator not be raised again.

In August the nurses involved in Mrs. Wanglie's care expressed their consensus view that continued life support was inappropriate. In October, 1990, a new attending physician in consultation with specialists confirmed that the patient's cerebral and pulmonary conditions were permanent and concluded that she was "at the end of her life and that the respirator was 'non-beneficial,' in that it could not heal her lungs, palliate her suffering, or enable this unconscious and permanently respirator-depended woman to experience the benefit of the life afforded by respirator support." He did not characterize the respirator as "futile," because it could prolong her life.

In November, the physician, with the concurrence of Steven Miles, the ethics consultant for the hospital since August, informed the family that he was unwilling to continue the respirator. When the husband rejected this option and also refused to transfer the patient to another facility or to seek a court order to require this exceptional treatment, the hospital indicated that it would seek a court determination about its obligation to continue treatment. A follow-up conference two weeks later indicated that neither party had budged. The family had hired an attorney, and the husband indicated that the patient had consistently indicated her desire for respirator support under such conditions.

The Hennepin County Board of Commissioners, who serve as the medical center's board of directors, by a 4-to-3 vote authorized the hospital to go to court to try to resolve the dispute. Despite their efforts during the first several months of 1991, the family could not locate another facility that would accept Mrs. Wanglie. Even those with space declined because of her poor prognosis for rehabilitation.

The hospital first asked the court to appoint an independent conservator to determine whether the respirator was benefiting the patient. Then the hospital intended to seek a second hearing to determine whether it was obligated to continue the respirator if the conservator held that it was non-beneficial. The trial court held a hearing in late May and on July 1, 1991, appointed Mr. Wanglie as the conservator, as he had requested, on the grounds that he could best represent his wife's interests. The court did not address the speculative question about whether a request to stop treatment would have been granted, because no request had been made, and the hospital indicated that it would continue the respirator because of the uncertainty about its legal obligation to provide it.

However, the patient died three days later (on July 4) of multisystem organ failure as a result of septicemia. The family did not want an autopsy and affirmed that the patient's care had been excellent, but, as the daughter put it, "we just had a disagreement on ethics." In the words of Mr. Wanglie, "We felt that when she was ready to go that the good Lord would call her, and I would say that's what happened."

The hospital and the county had no financial interest in withdrawing treatment to allow Mrs. Wanglie to die, because Medicare paid most of the $200,00 bill for the first hospitalization, and a private insurer paid the $500,000 bill for the second hospitalization.

Case 7: The Saikewicz Case

By 1976, 67-year-old Joseph Saikewicz had lived in state institutions for more than 40 years. His IQ was ten, and his mental age was approximately two years and eight months. He could communicate only by gestures and grunts, and he responded only to gestures or physical contacts. He appeared to be unaware of dangers and became disoriented when removed from familiar surroundings.

His health was generally good until April 1976, when he was diagnosed as having acute myeloblastic monocytic leukemia, which is invariably fatal. In approximately 30% to 50% of cases of this type of leukemia, chemotherapy can bring about temporary remission, which usually lasts between two and 13 months. The results are poorer for patients older than 60. In addition, chemotherapy often has serious side effects, including anemia and infections.

At the petition of the Belchertown State School, where Saikewicz was located, the probate court appointed a guardian *ad litem* with authority to make the necessary decisions concerning the patient's care and treatment. The guardian *ad litem* noted that Saikewicz's illness was incurable, that chemotherapy had significant adverse side effects and discomfort, and that Saikewicz could not understand the treatment or the resulting pain. For all these reasons, he concluded "that not treating Mr. Saikewicz would be in his best interests." The Supreme Judicial Court of Massachusetts upheld this decision on July 9, 1976 (although its

This case is drawn from *Superintendent of Belchertown v. Saikewicz*, Mass. 370 N.E. 2d 417 (1977).

opinion was not issued until November 28, 1977). Mr. Saikewicz died on September 4, 1976.

Case 8: The Brophy Case

Paul E. Brophy, Sr., a firefighter and emergency medical technician in Easton, Massachusetts, suffered a ruptured brain artery on March 22, 1983. Surgery was performed in April, but it was unsuccessful, and Brophy never regained consciousness. He was transferred to the New England Sinai Hospital in a persistent vegetative state. When he developed pneumonia in August, both his physicians and Patricia Brophy, his wife and legal guardian, concurred in an order not to resuscitate him if he suffered a cardiac arrest. In December 1983, Mrs. Brophy gave the physicians permission for a surgical procedure to insert a feeding tube into his stomach. He received seven and a half hours of nursing care each day, consisting of bathing, shaving, turning, and so on. Brophy's medical bills, approximately $10,000 per month, were paid entirely by Blue Cross/Blue Shield.

Brophy had often told family members that he did not want to be kept alive if he ever became comatose. In a discussion of the Karen Ann Quinlan case, he had indicated to his wife that "I don't ever want to be on a life-support system. No way do I want to live like that; that's just not living." Several years earlier, the town of Easton had given Brophy and his partner a commendation for bravery after they had pulled a man from a burning truck. When he learned that the victim had suffered a great deal before dying several months after being saved, Brophy threw his commendation into the wastebasket, exclaiming to his wife, "I should have been five minutes later. It would have been all over for him." He told his brother, Leo, "If I'm ever like that, just shoot me, pull the plug." And prior to his own neurosurgery, he told one of his daughters, "If I can't sit up to kiss one of my beautiful daughters, I may as well be six feet under."

Mrs. Brophy, a devout Catholic and a nurse who worked part-time with the mentally retarded, decided to question the continuation of artificial feeding when her husband's condition remained unchanged through the next year. There was no hope that he would regain consciousness, and, though he had never expressed a specific judgment about artificial feeding, she recalled his previously expressed wishes about "pulling the plug." She consulted with clergy, ethicists, and a lawyer before requesting withdrawal of artificial nutrition with the understanding that

This case summary has been drawn from *Brophy v. New England Sinai Hospital, Inc.*, 497 N.E. 2d 626 (Mass. 1986), and Robert Steinbrook and Bernard Lo, "Artificial Feeding—Solid Ground, Not Slippery Slope," *New England Journal of Medicine* 286 (February 4, 1988): 286–90.

her husband would die in one to two weeks. Her decision received the unanimous support of their five children and other family members, including Brophy's seven brothers and sisters and his elderly mother, who was in her nineties. However, the physicians and the hospital administration refused to act on this request.

In February 1985, Mrs. Brophy asked a probate court for a declaratory judgment ordering the hospital to act affirmatively on her request. The New England Sinai Hospital responded that the physician-in-chief of the hospital could not "in good conscience, consistent with the ethical codes of the medical profession, participate in the discontinuation of all nutrition and hydration." And it requested that Brophy be transferred to another facility if the court ordered discontinuation of artificial nutrition and hydration.

The court-appointed guardian *ad litem* (a person appointed by the court to protect the interests of a ward in a legal proceeding) found that "removal of the G [gastrostomy] tube is not comparable to cessation of dialysis or removal of a respirator because removal of the aforesaid artificial mechanisms permits the illness or injury to run its natural course. Nutrition, however, is not a need required by Mr. Brophy as a result of his illness, but rather, it is a need common to all human beings." Furthermore, the guardian *ad litem* continued, "Brophy is a chronically ill patient, but is not terminally ill. He is entitled to the same fundamentals of comfort, i.e., food, shelter and bedding, as is any other chronically ill patient, and it is the duty of the medical facility to provide him with the aforesaid care." The probate judge ruled that the feeding tube must be continued, even though he found that Brophy would have preferred to be dead than to have his life prolonged in a persistent vegetative state and that if competent he would reject artificial nutrition. Mrs. Brophy appealed this verdict.

In September 1986, in a split decision (4 to 3), the Supreme Judicial Court of Massachusetts held that Brophy's feeding tube could be removed. Three U.S. Supreme Court justices declined to review the decision. The Massachusetts court did not require the hospital to compromise its principles by terminating feeding, but it did require the hospital's cooperation in transferring Brophy to Emerson Hospital in Concord, which was willing to honor Mrs. Brophy's request.

In October 1986, Brophy was transferred to Emerson Hospital under the care of a neurologist who had earlier testified that Brophy was in a persistent vegetative state. Many of the hospital staff volunteered to help care for Brophy by providing supportive care, including anticonvulsants and antacids, while he died. Brophy, age 49, died of pneumonia on October 23, 1986, eight days after the feeding tube was removed. He was surrounded by his wife, who had remained with him around the clock, their children, and a grandchild. According to the attending physician, Brophy's death was an "amazing, peaceful, quiet time."

Case 9: Willowbrook

The Willowbrook State School is an institution for mentally retarded children on Staten Island, New York. The number of its residents increased from 200 in 1949 to more than 6000 in 1963. Hepatitis was first noticed among the children in 1949, and in 1954 Dr. Saul Krugman and his associates, including Dr. Joan Giles and Dr. Jack Hammond, began to study the disease in the institution. Of the 5200 residents at Willowbrook during one part of their study, 3800 were severely retarded, with IQs of less than 20. In addition, at least three thousand of the children were not toilet-trained. Because infectious hepatitis is transmitted via the fecal–oral route, and because susceptible children were constantly admitted to the institution, contagious hepatitis was persistent and endemic.

As Dr. Krugman (1971) describes the situation, "viral hepatitis is so prevalent that newly admitted susceptible children become infected within 6 to 12 months after entry in the institution. These children are a source of infection for the personnel who care for them and for their families if they visit with them. We were convinced that the solution of the hepatitis problem in this institution was dependent on the acquisition of new knowledge leading to the development of an effective immunizing agent. The achievements with small pox, diphtheria, poliomyelitis, and more recently measles represent dramatic illustrations of this approach."

Krugman continues, "It is well known that viral hepatitis in children is milder and more benign than the same disease in adults. Experience has revealed that hepatitis in institutionalized, mentally retarded children is also mild, in contrast to measles which is a more severe disease when it occurs in institutional epidemics involving the mentally retarded. Our proposal to expose a small number of newly admitted children [ultimately 750 to 800 children were involved altogether] to the Willowbrook strains of hepatitis virus was justified in our opinion for the following reasons: (1) they were bound to be exposed to the same strains under the natural conditions existing in the institution; (2) they would be admitted to a special, well-equipped, and well-staffed unit where they would be isolated from exposure to other infectious diseases which were prevalent in the institution—namely, shigellosis, parasitic infections, and respiratory infections—thus, their exposure in the hepatitis unit would be associated with less risk than the type of institutional exposure where multiple infections could occur; (3) they

Sources: Saul Krugman and Joan P. Giles, "Viral Hepatitis: New Light on an Old Disease," *Journal of the American Medical Association* 212 (May 10, 1970): 1019–29; Henry Beecher, *Research and the Individual* (Boston: Little, Brown, 1970); letters to the editor of *Lancet*: by Stephen Goldby (April 10, 1971), Saul Krugman (May 8, 1971), Edward N. Willey (May 22, 1971), Benjamin Pasamanick (May 22, 1971), Joan Giles (May 29, 1971), M. H. Pappworth (June 5, 1971), Geoffrey Edsall (July 10, 1971); F. J. Ingelfinger, "Ethics of Experiments on Children," *New England Journal of Medicine* 288 (April 12, 1973): 791–92; Saul Krugman, "The Willowbrook Hepatitis Studies Revisited: Ethical Aspects," *Reviews of Infectious Diseases* 8 (January-February 1986): 157–62.

were likely to have a subclinical infection followed by immunity to the particular hepatitis virus; and (4) only children with parents who gave informed consent would be included."

Critics have leveled several charges against the Willowbrook hepatitis studies. First, some contend that it is "indefensible to give potentially dangerous infected material to children, particularly those who were mentally retarded, with or without parental consent, when no benefit to the child could conceivably result" (Goldby). Hence, these critics reject the claim by Krugman and Giles that "the artificial induction of hepatitis implies a 'therapeutic' effect because of the immunity which is conferred." The ground for rejecting this claim is that most of the children would have become infected anyway and that this therapeutic effect is not different from what the natural environment would have bestowed. Thus, one major question is whether this experiment offered some therapeutic benefit to the subjects themselves or only to others. The aim of the study was to determine the period of infectivity of infectious hepatitis. Even if the experiment produced good results, as it did (see Krugman, 1986), critics contend that an experiment is justified not by its results but "is ethical or not at its inception" (Beecher). In this case, "immunization was not the purpose of these Willowbrook experiments but merely a by-product that incidentally proved beneficial to the victims" (Pappworth).

Second, critics contend that there were alternative ways to control hepatitis in the institution. According to the head of the State Department of Mental Hygiene in New York, for much of the period of the experiment a gamma-globulin inoculation program had already reduced the incidence of viral hepatitis in Willowbrook by eighty to eighty-five percent (Beecher). And the pediatrician's duty is to improve the situation, not to take advantage of it for experimental purposes (Goldby).

Third, questions have been raised about whether the parents' consent for their children to participate in the research was informed and voluntary. Originally, information was conveyed to individual parents by letter or personal interview, but later information was disclosed through a detailed discussion of the project with groups of six to eight parents who were invited to enroll their children in the research. Krugman and Giles contend that the "group method" enabled them "to obtain more thorough informed consent." In either setting, "it was not clear whether any or all parents were told that hepatitis sometimes progresses to fatal liver destruction or that there is a possibility that cirrhosis developing later in life may have had its origin in earlier hepatitis" (Beecher). Serious questions emerged about the voluntariness of parental consent when parents of prospective residents of Willowbrook were told in late 1964 that overcrowding prevented further admissions but were subsequently informed, often within a week or so, that there were some vacancies in the hepatitis unit and that if the parents wanted to volunteer their children for the research project the children could be admitted to Willowbrook.

Defenders of Willowbrook reject most of these criticisms and ask "is it not proper and ethical to carry out experiments in children, which would apparently incur no greater risk than the children were likely to run by nature, in which the children generally receive better medical care when artificially infected than if they had been naturally infected, and in which the parents as well as the physician feel that a significant contribution to the future well-being of similar children is likely to result from the studies?" (Edsall).

Case 10: The Case of Baby M

Mrs. Mary Beth Whitehead, a 29-year-old housewife from Brick Township, New Jersey, signed a contract on February 6, 1985, to bear a child for William and Elizabeth Stern. As part of the 16-page contract, arranged by the Infertility Center of New York, Mrs. Whitehead agreed "that in the best interests of the child, she will not form or attempt to form a parent–child relationship with any child . . . she may conceive . . . and shall freely surrender custody to William Stern, Natural Father, immediately upon birth of the child; and terminate all parental right to said child pursuant to this agreement." Mrs. Whitehead was to receive $10,000 for "compensation for services and expenses" from the Infertility Center as part of the total of approximately $25,000 Mr. Stern agreed to pay the center. Of the remainder, $5000 went to Mrs. Whitehead's medical, legal and insurance costs during pregnancy, and $7500 to $10,000 went to the center as its fee.

When the child, conceived through artificial insemination with Mr. Stern's sperm, was born on March 27, 1986, Mrs. Whitehead and her husband, who already had two children, were reluctant to part with the child. They turned her over to the Sterns on March 30, but Mrs. Whitehead would not accept the $10,000, and within a few days she went to the Stern residence and begged to be allowed to take the child for a week. The Sterns agreed. But by early May, it was clear that Mrs. Whitehead would not willingly return the child, and the Sterns filed a successful petition for temporary custody with the family court. Mrs. Whitehead managed to hand the baby out a bedroom window to her husband when six policemen arrived to take the baby. The husband left with the baby, and Mrs. Whitehead was able to join them later without detection. The Whiteheads were able to elude law enforcement officials in Florida for three months. When the infant, known in the court records as "Baby M," was finally located, she was turned over to the Sterns, and Family Judge Harvey R. Sorkow's temporary custody order was extended, along with limited visitation rights to Mrs. Whitehead.

A court-ordered paternity test established that Mrs. Whitehead's husband, Richard Whitehead, who had had a vasectomy, could not have fathered the child.

Source: *In the Matter of Baby M*, 109 N.J. 396, 537 A. 2d. 1227 (1988).

After a 32-day trial, Judge Sorkow declared the surrogacy contract valid and enforceable, terminated Mrs. Whitehead's parental rights, and awarded sole custody of Baby M to Mr. Stern. Judge Sorkow required specific performance of the surrogate contract on the grounds that it was in Baby M's best interests. He also immediately granted Mrs. Stern an order of adoption.

Upon appeal, the New Jersey Supreme Court (February 3, 1988) held that a surrogacy contract that provides money to the surrogate mother and requires her irrevocable agreement to surrender her child at birth is invalid and unenforceable. The surrogacy contract in the case of Baby M violates New Jersey statutes that prohibit the use of money in connection with adoptions, that limit termination of parental rights to situations in which there has been a valid showing of parental unfitness or abandonment of the child, and that allow a mother to revoke her consent to surrender her child in private placement adoption. In addition, the surrogacy contract conflicts with New Jersey's public policy that custody be determined on the basis of the child's best interests (the surrogacy contract makes a determination of custody prior to the child's birth), that children be brought up by their natural parents (the surrogacy contract guarantees the separation of the child from its natural mother), that the rights of the natural father and the natural mother are equal (the surrogacy contract elevates the natural father's right by destroying the natural mother's right), that a natural mother receive counseling before agreeing to surrender her child (the surrogacy contract in this case did not have such a provision), and that adoptions not be influenced by the payment of money (the surrogacy contract was based on such a payment).

Regarding the point that Mrs. Whitehead "agreed to the surrogacy arrangement, supposedly fully understanding the consequences," the court responded: "Putting aside the issue of how compelling her need for money may have been, and how significant her understanding of the consequences, we suggest that her consent is irrelevant. There are, in a civilized society, some things that money cannot buy. In America, we decided long ago that merely because conduct purchased by money was 'voluntary' did not mean that it was good or beyond regulation and prohibition." In addition, the court expressed concern about the unknown long-term effects of surrogacy contracts on various parties: "Potential victims include the surrogate mother and her family, the natural father and his wife, and most importantly, the child." However, the court did not find any legal prohibition of surrogacy "when the surrogate mother volunteers, without any payment, to act as a surrogate and is given the right to change her mind and to assert her parental rights."

The New Jersey Supreme Court affirmed the lower court's grant of custody to the natural father, but reversed the lower court's termination of the natural mother's parental rights and required the lower court to determine the terms of the natural mother's visitation with Baby M.

Index